The Dissociative Child

The Dissociative Child:

Diagnosis,
Treatment,
and Management

Edited by Joyanna L. Silberg, Ph.D.
Foreword by Richard P. Kluft, M.D.

The Sidran Press
Lutherville, Maryland

Printed in the United States of America

Library of Congress Cataloging-in-Publication Data

   The dissociative child : diagnosis, treatment & management / edited by Joyanna L.
Silberg : foreword by Richard P. Kluft.
       p.   cm.
   Includes bibliographical references.
   ISBN 1-886968-03-9 (alk. paper). — ISBN 1-886968-01-2 (pbk. : alk. paper)
   1. Dissociative disorders in children.   I. Silberg, Joyanna L.
RJ506.D55D57   1996
618.92'89—dc20   96-33496

Cover art: "The Navaho" was painted by a child who dissociated, when she was eleven years
old. The face of her Navaho child may reflect a wish to be able to move undetected through
a dangerous world. The artist, now 26 and a "true survivor," says she is studying counseling
in order to help others overcome the effects of early and severe abuse.

For all cases presented in this book, names and relevant historical details have been altered
to preserve patient confidentiality. Informed consent was obtained for the use of any patient
artwork or writing.

This book is dedicated to the memory of my mother, Edythe Samson, whose compassion, intelligence, and creativity helped guide my career path.

Contents

Foreword

Richard P. Kluft, M. D.

The Dissociative Child: Diagnosis, Treatment, and Management addresses subjects of the greatest importance for the dissociative disorders field and for the economics of the delivery of mental health care. The identification and treatment of dissociative disorders in children demonstrates that DID (Dissociative Identity Disorder) and related forms of DDNOS (Dissociative Disorder Not Otherwise Specified) are naturalistically-occurring psychopathologies and that the adult forms of this disorder do not suddenly develop de novo in response to contemporary stimuli (Kluft, 1985a & b). Furthermore, antecedent traumata can be documented in 95% of these younger patients, whose circumstances usually are investigated vigorously by appropriate professionals and agencies (Hornstein & Putnam, 1992; Coons, 1994). This is an important foundation finding, because it is much more difficult to document the naturalistic nature and traumatic background of adults with DID/MPD, whose psychopathology typically evolves with a certain degree of autonomy from early adolescence through adult life (Kluft, 1985a, 1991; Kluft & Schultz, 1993), and can take on a life of its own, often deeply imbued with fantasy materials and ego-syntonic reconfigurations and subject to post-event influences.

Also, by adult life DID/MPD usually is a fairly entrenched psychopathology with considerable comorbidity that requires years of intensive therapy to reach a successful resolution and sometimes defies treatment efforts. It is more economical in terms of both fiscal cost and humanitarian concerns to spare the dissociative patient years of morbidity and misery by identifying and treating the dissociative psychopathology during childhood. By adolescence it is already much more difficult to treat the condition, and developmental pressures within the adolescent are likely to oppose the treatment process (Dell & Eisenhower, 1990; Kluft & Schultz, 1993). As early as 1984 I observed:

> It is difficult to overstate the preventive potential of the early diagnosis and treatment of multiple personality in childhood. The phenomena that proved so responsive to simple interventions in this age group become more fixed and more elaborated when allowed to mature into the adult condition. Over the intervening years personalities develop their own lives and histories. They often become more invested in separateness and less amenable to modest measures. Adult patients with multiple personality disorder average 6.8 years between initial mental health assessment and accurate diagnosis, and then often require years of therapy. Including time prior to correct diagnosis, psychiatric careers of over a decade are not uncommon. All this while, these individuals' condition is likely to diminish their productivity, cause morbidity, pain, and incapacity in themselves, create severe difficulty for others and society..., and cost untold thousands in medical bills and disability.
>
> Kluft, 1984, p. 133

Therefore, any advance in our understanding of dissociative children is a cause for celebration by both the most compassionate clinician and the most cost-conscious administrator alike. Dr. Silberg and her colleagues have made many substantial contributions in this book, many of which will be of immediate use to any clinician working with traumatized children.

I have long believed that improvements in the identification and treatment of children with dissociative disorders should be the foremost priority of the dissociative disorders field. Within weeks of identifying my first patient with dissociative identity disorder/multiple personality disorder (DID/MPD), I became preoccupied with a question that dictated the direction of many of my projects in clinical research for over a decade: Where does this condition come from? A few moments before my first DID/MPD patient switched in front of me I had thought I understood her. She was a severe borderline, capable of massive regression. Steeped in the psychoanalytic literature on borderline states, I believed I was capable of comprehending the etiology of my patient's distress in terms of childhood difficulties and biological factors. Furthermore, I could explain her to colleagues in a language we shared and in terms that allowed us to communicate easily with one another.

Suddenly, within seconds, and with no preparation, I had been transported into a whole new world. This vista, lurching unwelcome into my reluctant awareness, introduced me to an unexpected terrain in which at first I recognized neither familiar pathways nor informative landmarks. I was lost and confused. Worse still, I could not explain my clinical concerns to colleagues without their either becoming confused or expressing disbelief. Most distressing to me was that the clinical manifestations of my patient's DID/MPD appeared to have virtually erupted. They seemed to come from some psychiatric left field or no man's land. I had no idea where these phenomena had been sequestered the moment before the switch, which had caught me completely by surprise. In addition, I was totally mystified in my efforts to infer or imagine how this condition had developed. Where were the structures of DID/MPD when they were not overt and obvious? Were there childhood forms of DID/MPD? Was there a developmental process by which the DID/MPD phenomena gradually took shape, or did they emerge fully-developed, like Athena from the brow of Zeus?

Determining the natural history of DID/MPD and searching for the childhood antecedents of this condition became a major preoccupation of my clinical research efforts in the 1970s and early 1980s. I was determined to solve these mysteries and embarked on a number of research projects. I did not think that the task of finding dissociative children would be difficult, because I had discovered the work of Antoine Despine, Sr., in Henri Ellenberger's encyclopedic *The Discovery of the Unconscious* (1970), and was reasonably sure that Despine's case of "Estelle," apparent classic DID/MPD in an 11-year-old girl, could not be unique.

In June of 1836, Despine undertook the treatment of "Estelle," a Swiss youngster believed to be paralyzed by a spinal cord lesion. Incapacitating pain, paralysis, hallucinations, and visions were among her symptoms; at times she lost track of her surroundings and seemed withdrawn, in a world of her own. After some months, Estelle's mother revealed that Estelle claimed to be comforted by "angels," and Despine began to suspect a "magnetic" (i.e., hypnotic/autohypnotic) condition. After initial reluctance, Estelle permitted hypnosis. Despine contacted a comforting angel, Angeline, the first recorded helper personality, and Angeline played a role in directing the treatment.

Within a month, Estelle in her normal state remained disabled, polite, proper, and dependent on her mother. However, under hypnosis she could walk, was more assertive, and did not like to have her mother around. Soon these states were alternating spontaneously, and gradually Estelle became able to walk in her waking state. Within months a fusion occurred and Estelle was discharged home. The publicity surrounding her recovery was intense—she was described as *la petite ressuscitee*, "the little resurrected one." Despine's original work (1840) is a rarity, but the interested reader can learn more of this case from Ellenberger (1970), Fine (1988), and Goodwin and Fine (1993).

Despine's diagnostic and treatment techniques embody many of the principles rediscovered by the modern pioneers in the treatment of DID/MPD. He considered hypnotic (dissociative) psychopathologies in his differential diagnosis, so he was prepared to look beyond the apparent organic pathology and psychotic symptom picture to consider a psychopathology that might mimic them. He kept the process of assessment open and ongoing. He was respectful and nonjudgmental. He allowed the phenomena suggesting separateness to become the subject of clinical study, neither discounting nor minimizing them. He respected Estelle's fear of the proposed treatment and worked out a therapeutic alliance with her by contracting about the conditions of the therapy. He paced the treatment and avoided power struggles and clashes with Angeline, even when she was frankly grandiose. He appreciated his patient's autohypnotic talent and utilized it well. He tolerated the less "correct" stances of both Angeline and the hypnotic Estelle, and this appears to have facilitated his young patient's negotiating her problems with dependency, enmeshment, and authority. I learned a lot from my early exposure to Despine, who actually had a series of 16 dissociative patients. His son and nephew also accumulated series, of a dozen cases apiece (Fine, 1988).

As I said, knowledge of Despine's case of Estelle convinced me that an effort to discover childhood dissociative disorder patients was worthwhile and likely to succeed. However, although my efforts to track the natural history of DID/MPD were very successful, my attempts to find childhood cases of DID/MPD were an unmitigated fiasco. For years I found nothing that resembled a childhood dissociative disorder. Nor was I successful in persuading child psychiatrists, child analysts, or child psychologists to investigate my hypothesis. I approached several, hoping to develop a research collaboration with an academic colleague and screening a large number of children with an instrument I had developed. Also, since I am not a trained child psychiatrist, I hoped such a joint venture would both improve the quality of the work that we did and enhance the credibility and acceptance of whatever we published. I was received with polite indifference at best; skeptical derision was not uncommon. However, I was convinced that the topic was of paramount importance, so I continued my efforts.

When I finally discovered a cases of classic DID/MPD in an 8-year-old boy in 1978, he had been identified not by my research protocols, but by his perceptive mother! Worse, it took her months to convince me to evaluate him. I found it difficult to believe that where my systematic efforts had failed, a lay person had succeeded simply by seeing what was in front of her. Fortunately, she ultimately succeeded in opening my eyes. To my undisguised amazement, I found myself confronted with an 8-year-old boy who spontaneously manifested a series of developed personality states. His childhood trauma was documented: a witnessed near-drowning, after which he required resuscitation by his mother, and physical abuse by his father, confessed to me by the father. Known in the literature as "Tommy," he now has been integrated for 18 years. He is married and is raising his own family.

The study of this youngster and several others seemed to complete the story of DID/MPD. Yes, there were childhood antecedents to DID/MPD. In some cases there was a clear developmental process during which the dissociative processes became more elaborated, but in others fully-formed alters were found within a week of the first episode of abuse. I thought this discovery was important, but neither scientific meetings nor professional journals shared my opinion. My attempts to communicate this discovery were rejected for presentation and publication for six years, although I noted one of the patients in passing in a 1982 publication. In 1984 I was able to publish "Multiple Personality in Childhood." In the same year Joen Fagan and Polly Paul McMahon published their classic paper on incipient multiple personality in children, and at last the dissociative disorders of childhood were represented in the contemporary literature.

It was a serendipitous and fortunate coincidence that both my work and that of Fagan and McMahon were published within months of each other. Focused on finding classic DID/MPD, my scope was too narrow to consider and encompass the wider range of dissociative psychopathology in children. Fagan and McMahon, however, had a broader perspective and raised the mental health professions' sensitivity to the wider spectrum of dissociative phenomenology that children may manifest. Yet their only youngster with fully-developed DID/MPD was an early adolescent; they did not demonstrate full DID/MPD in children. Together the papers were more persuasive than either was alone.

The Dissociative Child addresses the full range of childhood dissociative psychopathology with a depth and sophistication that is lacking in prior papers on the subject. Its publication marks the movement of the study of childhood dissociative disorders to a far more sophisticated level. Much of what is said in the book was familiar from my own clinical experience (see Kluft, 1986, 1996), but I was delighted to find that a great deal was new to me, so that reading this text has been an enjoyable learning experience.

The experience of the clinicians who have contributed to this book indicate not only that there is a broad spectrum of dissociative psychopathology in children, but that the response of dissociative children to treatment itself constitutes a spectrum of sorts. That these children do not respond with uniform rapidity to treatment is an important communication. The first reports of dissociative children in treatment (Fagan & McMahon, 1984; Kluft, 1984, 1985b; Weiss, Sutton, & Utecht, 1985) generally seemed to suggest a rapid and favorable response to treatment was both possible and likely. For years thereafter, I was approached by therapists who claimed that their own experience was far different from my own. I was perplexed, because I found it difficult to believe that therapists were having such difficulty with cases like the ones I had seen. My efforts to understand their dilemmas often focused on the failure to provide a sense of safety to the children, because I found that without this, treatment was extremely difficult. While this explained many of the cases presented to me, it could not explain all of them.

Working with a data base many times the size of my own, Silberg and Waters objectify the courses of treatment of a sizable cohort of dissociative youngsters. They demonstrate a considerable heterogeneity of response, from patients who improved as rapidly as my own few cases to those whose course was far more prolonged and fraught with more difficulty. They have begun to identify prognostic variables. It will be instructive to observe whether clinicians find that these factors are consistent with their own clinical experience. These variables have considerable research potential, because most if not all can be operationalized and researched objectively.

I am particularly delighted that this book takes a level-headed stance toward the subject of child abuse and its relationship to the dissociative disorders. In this era of turmoil and controversy over allegations of abuse by adults with dissociative disorders, it is especially important that works on childhood dissociative disorders be dispassionate and objective. Our understanding of the often convoluted accounts of mistreatment given by dissociative adults must be approached not only by studying that group of patients (e.g., Kluft, 1995), but also by building bridges toward it by studying the documented abuse of younger dissociative patients (as in this volume) and the dissociative responses of normal individuals to documented exogenous stressors (e.g., Cardena & Spiegel, 1993; Koopman, Classen & Spiegel, 1994).

Although I have had many rewarding experiences in treating patients with dissociative disorders, one of the most gratifying aspects of my practice has been the treatment of dissociative youngsters. It is a wonderful thing to watch a shattered child achieve wholeness and move on to live a normal and fulfilling life. Followups of a decade or more on many of my cases have demonstrated that almost all of them, if they can achieve a sense of personal safety, will do much better, and that many of these dissociative children will simply get well and stay well. This book offers the clinician a rich resource for work with the dissociative child and shares techniques and approaches that will enable the reader to approach such evaluations and therapies with enhanced expertise and confidence. Every child with a dissociative disorder who is treated successfully has been rescued from decades of discomfort and inner despair.

Richard P. Kluft, M.D.

References

Cardena, E., & Spiegel, D. (1993). Dissociative reactions to the San Francisco Bay Area earthquake of 1989. *American Journal of Psychiatry, 150,* 474–478.

Coons, P. M. (1994). Confirmation of childhood abuse in childhood and adolescent cases of multiple personality disorder and dissociative disorder not otherwise specified. *Journal of Nervous and Mental Disease, 182,* 461–464.

Dell, D. F., & Eisenhower, J. W. (1990). Adolescent multiple personality disorder: A preliminary study of eleven cases. *Journal of the American Academy of Child and Adolescent Psychiatry, 35,* 42–50.

Despine, A. (1840). *De l'emploi de magnetisme animal et des eaux minerales dans le traitment des maladies nerveuses, suivie d'une observation tres curieuse de neuropathie.* Paris: Balliere.

Ellenberger, H. (1970). *The discovery of the unconscious.* New York: Basic Books.

Fagan, J., & McMahon, P. P. (1984). Incipient multiple personality in children: Four cases. *Journal of Nervous and Mental Disease, 172,* 26–36.

Fine, C. G. (1988). The work of Antoine Despine: The first scientific report on the diagnosis and treatment of a child with multiple personality disorder. *American Journal of Clinical Hypnosis, 31,* 33–39.

Goodwin, J. M., & Fine, C. G. (1993). Mary Reynolds and Estelle: Somatic symptoms and unacknowledged trauma. In J. M. Goodwin (Ed.), *Rediscovering childhood trauma: Historical casebook and clinical applications* (pp. 119–131). Washington, DC: American Psychiatric Press.

Hornstein, N. L., & Putnam, F. W. (1992). Clinical phenomenology of child and adolescent multiple personality disorder. *Journal of the American Academy of Child and Adolescent Psychiatry, 31,* 1055–1077.

Kluft, R. P. (1982). Varieties of hypnotic interventions in the treatment of multiple personality. *American Journal of Clinical Hypnosis, 24,* 230–240.

Kluft, R. P. (1984). Multiple personality in childhood. *Psychiatric Clinics of North America, 7,* 121–134.

Kluft, R. P. (1985a). The natural history of multiple personality disorder. In R. P. Kluft (Ed.), *Childhood antecedents of multiple personality* (pp. 197–238). Washington, DC: American Psychiatric Press.

Kluft, R. P. (1985b). The natural history of multiple personality disorder. In R. P. Kluft (Ed.), *Childhood antecedents of multiple personality* (pp. 167–196). Washington, DC: American Psychiatric Press.

Kluft, R. P. (1986). Treating children who have multiple personality disorder. In B. G. Braun (Ed.), *Treatment of multiple personality disorder* (pp.79–105). Washington, DC: American Psychiatric Press.

Kluft, R. P. (1991). Clinical presentations of multiple personality disorder. *Psychiatric Clinics of North America, 14,* 605–629.

Kluft, R. P. (1995). The confirmation and disconfirmation of memories of abuse in dissociative identity disorder patients: A naturalistic clinical study. *Dissociation, 8,* 253–258.

Kluft, R. P. (1996). Outpatient treatment of dissociative identity disorder and allied forms of dissociative disorder not otherwise specified in children and adolescents. *Child and Adolescent Psychiatric Clinics of North America, 5,* 471–494.

Kluft, R. P., & Schultz, R. (1993). Multiple personality disorder in adolescence. In S. C. Feinstein & R. C. Marhon (Eds.), *Adolescent Psychiatry, 19* (pp. 259–279). Chicago: University of Chicago Press.

Koopman, C., Classen, C., & Spiegel, D. (1994). Predictors of posttraumatic stress symptoms among survivors of the Oakland/Berkeley firestorm. *American Journal of Psychiatry, 151,* 888–894.

Weiss, M., Sutton, P. J., & Utecht, A. J. (1985). Multiple personality in a 10-year-old girl. *Journal of the American Academy of Child Psychiatry, 24,* 495–501.

Preface

Joyanna L. Silberg, Ph.D.

      This book was inspired during a coffee break at the International Society for the Study of Dissociation Meeting in 1994 in Chicago. I was bemoaning the lack of books and resources on childhood dissociative disorders to Esther Giller, Executive Director of the Sidran Foundation.

"You need to publish one," I instructed her.

"You need to write one," she replied. When I realized she was serious, I thought of all the people I had worked with and talked to over the last few years who had a unique perspective on the topic. How could I do justice to the topic alone? The idea of an edited volume was born. The more authors I could get to share their perspective, insights, and experiences, the richer the final work. I had discovered through attending conferences over the last several years, that independent clinicians working in different geographical locations around the world were finding the same characteristics in interviewing and treating traumatized children. Independently, clinicians were evolving similar treatment and interview techniques and categories of differential diagnosis. This discovery proved to me that the dissociative phenomena I was observing in patients at Sheppard Pratt Hospital in Baltimore were not isolated idiosyncratic findings. In Chicago, North Carolina, Michigan, England, and Israel the same kinds of children were reporting elaborate inner fantasy worlds peopled with characters that helped them cope with severe trauma. Abused children in all settings had had experiences that lingered within them and affected their day-to-day behavior, causing dramatic fluctuations, trance states, forgetfulness, and dramatic self-destructive and aggressive behaviors. The validation from clinicians across the world was a powerful reinforcer of the reality of what I had been observing.

Although the professional literature was beginning to document this cross validation of findings (Hornstein & Putnam, 1992), clinicians seeking practical information for diagnosis, treatment, and management were left empty-handed and overwhelmed with caseloads of dissociative children and a dearth of professional guidelines or information. Over the past four years, they have called me from Tennessee, Washington, New Hampshire, Kansas, and Hawaii with the same questions about treatment, diagnosis, and management. "Are there any books you can refer me to?" they have wondered. In this book, my goal is to satisfy that need for practical information that can assist the dedicated clinicians, parents, foster parents, and caseworkers who are seeking suggestions for dealing with these children on a day-to-day basis.

Writing a practical book is a frightening and humbling endeavor. Many of the techniques and suggestions described here are not widely used or known by child clinicians. Yet, the contributors have invited the readership behind the closed doors of the therapy office to reveal specifics of what they say and how they engage these children. We risk criticism and perhaps even ridicule by some. Nonetheless, my co-contributors and I take this risk because our collective experience has convinced us that there are powerful interventions that can dramatically improve the quality of these children's lives. At a time when child abuse is a leading cause of mortality for children in the United States, according to the U.S. Advisory Board on Child Abuse and Neglect (*The Evening Sun,* 1995), it feels like a moral imperative to share this information with the people who work with abused children.

The world has changed since I entered graduate school two decades ago. A public attitude of sympathy for abused children and battered wives has been replaced by an atmosphere of acute suspicion for "cult-like therapists" on a rampage to brainwash unwitting people into false beliefs. The backlash movement, using the media as its sometimes unknowing co-conspirator, has successfully clouded the picture of scientific information about traumatic memory, the prevalence of child abuse, and the scientific study of dissociative disorders. The study and description of dissociative children have the potential to dispel some of this misinformation. Young children, not old enough to read, describing dissociative experiences, provide compelling evidence of the reality of these phenomena, as their presentations are untainted by media presentations or therapy artifacts. Evidence of abuse, so elusive in the study of adult dissociative disorders, is often obvious and well-documented in abused children from protective service reports, including photographs of burns, and medical documentation of genital injuries.

My personal entry into this field was skeptical, scientific, and casual, as the idea of multiple personalities seemed interesting and exotic, but unrelated to anything I had ever learned in graduate school. When I first heard Dr. Richard Loewenstein speak about multiple personality disorder

(MPD, now termed DID, dissociative identity disorder) in adulthood in 1988, I experienced acute cognitive dissonance as I wondered where the dissociative children might be if the research about DID's childhood origins was valid. As a way to satisfy my own intellectual curiosity, I asked my referral sources to send me traumatized children, children in foster care, and children of dissociative parents, so I could see for myself whether any evidence of emerging dissociative phenomena could be found in these children. My search was overwhelmingly successful, as I discovered that simple questions, openness to dissociative phenomena, and willingness to listen without prejudgment provided an environment in which children could disclose secrets about their internal fantasy that were strikingly parallel to the dissociative experiences reported by adults. At this point, both my intellectual interest and sense of personal excitement were heightened as I realized that I might be seeing adult dissociation in its developmental form and that the potential to intervene in powerful ways might be available to clinicians who work with children.

However, in those first few years, it seemed implausible to me that I had discovered something that had not been seen or reported by others working with traumatized children. My reading led me to realize that dissociative phenomena had been described by many astute clinicians and writers but had been called by other names. Special educator Torrey Hayden (1981; 1982; 1995) has described children who behave in perplexing, amnestic, and contradictory ways that defy diagnostic labels. A careful reading of her books suggests that many of her students in special education classes were dissociative. Psychoanalyst Klein (1985) described a troubled child with imaginary friends closely paralleling the child's affective states—"Happy" and "Maddy," highly suggestive of a dissociative process. Perhaps even some of Bettelheim's famous case studies of autistic children (1969) might now be better understood as dissociative: one of his case studies describes a child from a neglectful and possibly abusive home with an imaginary all good "car family" and an all bad alter-ego, "Kenrad." Developmental psychologist Singer (Singer & Singer, 1990) has been researching the emergence of imaginary playmates in childhood for many years. These fantasy embodiments of the self serve to help the child cope with various developmental crises and are the normal parallel for dissociative pathology. In *The House of Make-Believe* (Singer & Singer, 1990), the authors note the similarity between these phenomena and dissociative disorders, suggesting that "benign parental sanction" allows normal children to see these imaginary selves as playful fantasy and not reality (p.107). Thus, the field of childhood dissociation is not based on completely new discoveries, but on an expansion and reinterpretation of previous observations and on the development of new connections between the developmental literature, the literature on adult DID, and childhood case studies. These connections serve to heighten the scientific credibility of theories concerning the developmental origins of adult DID.

The contemporary artistic imagination has been influenced by the trauma-induced dissociative experiences of children, suggesting that many artists have been aware of these processes, even without the help of identified psychiatric labels. In the Broadway play *Tommy* (1993, music originally written in 1969), a young child, traumatized by witnessing a murder, and then by sexual and physical abuse, has projections of himself frozen in different time periods, associated with multiple traumatic memories. This is conveyed on stage by three "Tommys," concrete multiple identities which are clearly an outgrowth of trauma. In the Alfred Hitchcock movie *Marnie* (1964), Hitchcock depicts a young woman with constant shifts in identity. The "mystery" of her puzzling behavior is solved through discovery of the traumatic events of her childhood. In the movie *Radio Flyer* (1992), a young boy traumatized by a brutal stepfather develops an imaginary animal friend to help him cope, and there are many suggestions that this young boy has an even more pervasive dissociative process. Yet the connections between trauma, childhood imagination, and dissociative behavior, apparently so clear to artists, are often missed by established psychiatry. In Patty Duke's autobiography *Call Me Anna* (Duke & Turan, 1987), Duke readily embraces her diagnosis as "bipolar illness," yet describes clearly the traumatic childhood that led her to an internal secret identity, the underlying basis for her shifting behavior patterns. Even her famous TV show about identical cousins was inspired by the widely fluctuating presentations that her producer noted in her behavior! Was it irony or destiny that my favorite childhood music (*Tommy*) and a favorite TV show (*The Patty Duke Show*) were both inspired by childhood dissociative experiences?

For those readers who are unfamiliar with the dissociative literature, I recommend reading books about adult dissociative disorders, such as Frank Putnam's *The Diagnosis and Treatment of Multiple Personality Disorder*. Richard Kluft's *Childhood Antecedents of Multiple Personality Disorder* is a classic text and provides a basic foundation for much of the material presented here.

For those readers who feel estranged by discussions that seem to give "alters" (alternate personalities) a reality, let me assure you that the contributors to this volume understand that "alters" are metaphors for the child of walled-off affects, memories, or behaviors. The children may not always understand the metaphorical aspect of their experience, but the clinicians do. Although we may encourage children to make friends with their "Robot Man," we talk in this manner in order to communicate messages that are consistent with the children's own experience. The goal of therapy is *not* for the therapist to hold a view of the child as fragmented, but for the child to hold a view of himself/herself as unified. When the child feels understood by the therapist, the therapist gains the credibility needed to move the child beyond the feeling of fragmentation. For those still put off by discussions of "alters," envision the therapy as one long play therapy puppet show, where the child and therapist suspend disbelief in order to communicate some powerful emotions, with the knowledge that when therapy is over, the puppet show will also end. The hope is that successful therapeutic interventions with children may interrupt the intensity of the dissociative process before adulthood, during which there is significantly more investment by the patient in the separateness of the disparate parts of the self.

This volume contains an initial section on diagnosis, which includes contributions from some of the most prominent names in the dissociation field—Nancy Hornstein, Gary Peterson, Jean Goodwin. This section should acquaint the reader with the history of dissociative disorder diagnosis, familiarize the reader with assessment techniques, and help the reader understand some of the quandaries in differential diagnosis among different populations of children.

The second section deals with treatment issues, and the contributions from a variety of disciplines illustrate that treatment of the dissociative child is a team effort. The reader will be exposed to play therapy techniques (Silberg and Waters) learn practical guidelines on conducting group therapy (Brand), become familiarized with psychopharmacological interventions (Nemzer), and understand the power of art therapy techniques (Sobol & Schneider). After completing this section, the reader should feel the benefit of exposure to a wealth of case material and will undoubtedly be struck by the similarity in case presentations from varying contributors, illustrating commonality in dissociative phenomena.

Finally, in the last section of the book the authors deal with the dissociative child in other settings—home (Waters), doctor's office (Graham), and school (Waterbury). This section contains a wealth of practical information that will assist program planners, teachers, parents, and physicians who come into contact with these children.

Comprehensive though it may be, this volume leaves many topics unexplored, leaving much work ahead for those who would like to continue to contribute to this field. Discussions of treatment issues as they apply to hospitals and residential centers, the assessment of childhood memory, and the legal issues involved in working with these children need chapters or books of their own. Most importantly, controlled efficacy studies that help support (or refute) the treatment concepts proposed here, need to be conducted and results reported.

The conception, development, and completion of this book was a mammoth undertaking and I am grateful to all of those who assisted with this effort. I am grateful to Dr. Kluft who offered to write a foreword without a moment's hesitation and thus inspired the drive to forge ahead without turning back. I am grateful to the contributors who accepted my prodding to put themselves on the line and break new ground. I am particularly grateful to Fran Waters for her significant contributions based on a wealth of clinical experience. I am grateful to Esther Giller for her vision about the importance of this project and her belief in my ability to pull it off. Most importantly, I am grateful to the patients whose courage and creativity in the face of overwhelming odds are an inspiration to anyone who works with them. These children bestowed on each of the contributors the gift of "trust" which allowed us to discover the rich information described in this volume.

References

Bettelheim, B. (1969). *The Empty Fortress*. New York: Free Press.

Child abuse has reached crisis proportions in US. (1995, April 26). *The Evening Sun*. p. A24.

Donner, R. (Director) (1992). *Radio Flyer*. Columbia Pictures.

Duke P., & Turan, K. (1987). *Call Me Anna*. New York: Bantam Books.

Hayden, T. (1981). *One Child*. New York: Avon Books.

Hayden, T. (1982). *Somebody Else's Kid*. New York: Avon Books.

Hayden, T. (1992). *Ghost Girl*. New York: Avon Books.

Hitchcock, A. (Director) (1964). *Marnie*. Universal Studios.

Hornstein, N. L., & Putnam, F. W. (1992). Clinical phenomenology of child and adolescent dissociative disorders. *Journal of the American Academy of Child and Adolescent Psychiatry, 31*, 1077–1085.

Klein, B. (1985). A child's imaginary companion: a transitional self. *Clinical Social Work, 13*, 272–282.

Kluft, R. P. (1985). *Childhood Antecedents of Multiple Personality Disorder*. Washington, DC: American Psychiatric Press.

Putnam, F. W. (1989). *The Diagnosis and Treatment of Multiple Personality Disorder*. New York: Guilford Press.

Singer, D. G., & Singer J. L. (1990). *The House of Make-Believe*. Cambridge: Harvard University Press.

Townshend, P. *Tommy*. (1993) St. James Theater. New York, New York, originally released in 1969, Fabulous Music LtD.

Contributors

Joyanna L. Silberg, Ph.D., Editor, is a Senior Psychologist at the Sheppard Pratt Health System in Towson, Maryland, where she coordinates dissociative disorder services for children and adolescents. She has served as chairperson of the children's committee of the International Sociey for the Study of Dissociation. She has presented her techniques on the diagnosis and treatment of dissociative disorders nationally and internationally. Her previous publications include book chapters on dissociative disorders and research on psychological testing.

Bethany Brand, Ph.D., is a licensed clinical psychologist at the Sheppard Pratt Health System in Baltimore, Maryland. She specializes in treating patients with dissociative disorders and conducts research aimed at clarifying how psychological testing can be used to diagnose dissociative disorders.

Jean Goodwin, M.D., M.P.H., is a professor in the Department of Psychiatry and Behavioral Sciences at the University of Texas Medical Branch at Galveston. Her books include *Sexual Abuse: Incest Victims and their Families* and *Rediscovering Childhood Trauma.* She is a fellow of the American Psychiatric Association and the International Society for the Study of Dissociation and a board certified forensic psychiatrist. She has consulted to protective services and social workers around issues of child abuse since the mid-1970s.

David B. Graham, M.D., FAAP, graduated from the University of Rochester Medical School and had a residency in Pediatrics and Fellowship in School Health and Child Psychiatry at the University of Maryland School of Medicine. He is presently a behavioral pediatrician in private practice at Liberty Christian Counseling Service, Inc. and Frederick Pediatric Associates in Maryland, and consultant at Chosen, a therapeutic foster care program.

Nancy Hornstein, M.D., is Assistant Professor, Division of Child Psychiatry, University of Illinois at Chicago. She was formerly Clinical Associate at the

Southern California Psychoanalytic Institute, Los Angeles. Dr. Hornstein is a past president of the International Society for the Study of Dissociation and has published many articles in the field of childhood dissociative disorders.

Richard P. Kluft, M.D., is a psychiatrist and psychoanalyst in Philadelphia, where he is Director of the Dissociative Disorders Program at The Institute of Pennsylvania Hospital, Clinical Professor of Psychiatry at Temple University School of Medicine, and on the faculty of the Philadelphia Psychoanalytic Institute. He is Lecturer on Psychiatry at Harvard Medical School, a past president of both the International Society for the Study of Dissociation and the American Society of Clinical Hypnosis, Editor-in-Chief of *Dissociation,* and Advisory Editor of the *American Journal of Clinical Hypnosis.* The author of over 200 publications, Dr. Kluft has edited or co-edited four books: *Childhood Antecedents of Multiple Personality, Treatment of Victims of Sexual Abuse, Incest-Related Syndromes of Adult Psychopathology,* and (with Catherine G. Fine, Ph.D.) *Clinical Perspectives on Multiple Personality Disorder.*

Elaine Davidson Nemzer, M.D., is a board-certified child and adolescent psychiatrist. A graduate of the Medical College of Ohio at Toledo, she completed a general psychiatry residency and child psychiatry fellowship at Ohio State University, where she is now Clinical Assistant Professor. Dr. Nemzer consults at a preschool day treatment program and a child guidance center in Columbus, Ohio.

Gary Peterson, M.D., past president and co-founder of the North Carolina Society for the Study of Dissociation, serves as Clinical Associate Professor of Psychiatry and Research Associate Professor of Psychology at the University of North Carolina at Chapel Hill. He is the author of the forthcoming book *A Dissociation Primer,* published by American Psychiatric Press, and has published many articles and chapters on dissociative children.

Karen Schneider, M.A., is the librarian at The Phillips Collection in Washington, DC and is a practicing artist. She is the art therapy consultant at The Other Way Day Treatment Program in Rockville, Maryland, and is co-founder, with author Barbara Sobol, of Washington Art Therapy Studio.

Barbara Semionova Sobol, M.A., A.T.R., is a former editor of the *American Journal of Art Therapy.* Currently she is a child and family therapist for Montgomery County, Maryland, and a teacher in the graduate art therapy program at George Washington University, New York University, and Vermont College of Norwich University. She is co-director of Washington Art Therapy Studio, a sanctuary for making art.

Marcia W. Waterbury, M.D., is Assistant Professor in the Department of Psychiatry, Division of Child Adolescent Psychiatry, University of Maryland School of Medicine, Baltimore.

Frances S. Waters, ACSW, LMFT, is a clinical social worker in private practice in Marquette, Michigan. She has presented nationally and internationally on treatment of childhood dissociative disorders. She is a charter member of the childhood and adolescent committee of the International Society for the Study of Dissociation.

The Dissociative Child

Part One

Diagnosis

o n e

Diagnostic Taxonomy: Past to Future

Gary Peterson

Recognizing dissociation in youth gives clinicians a new dimension to consider when assessing children for emotional and behavioral problems. Yet, skepticism about the diagnosis of dissociative identity disorder (formerly multiple personality disorder) remains as outspoken psychiatrists have called the dissociative phenomenon "an individually and socially created artifact" (McHugh & Putnam, 1995).

Acceptance of the diagnosis of dissociative disorders by clinicians rests in part on the diagnostic system and how the diagnostic taxonomy is organized. Factors such as including or excluding a condition in the differential diagnosis of another disorder may determine whether a clinician feels obliged to consider a specific diagnosis. In this chapter, I summarize some of the historical events that led up to the current nomenclature, examine how *DSM-IV* (American Psychiatric Association [APA], 1994) may influence the clinician to consider a dissociative diagnosis, describe how the clinician can begin to differentiate dissociative features from other conditions, and inform the reader what is being done to better inform clinicians about diagnostic assessment and treatment for dissociative disorders in youth.

Where We Were

Case studies of dissociative disorders in youth were published (Fine, 1988) long before Janet coined the term "dissociation" near the end of the 19th century. As interest in dissociative disorders waned shortly after the turn of the century, so did awareness of childhood dissociation.

Table 1
Evolving Terminology for DID/MPD

Purpose of Criterion	DSM-III — Multiple Personality	DSM-III-R — Multiple Personality Disorder	DSM-IV — Dissociative Identity Disorder
To describe that the person experiences autonomous self-states	A. The existence within the individual of two or more distinct personalities, each of which is dominant at a particular time.	A. The existence within the person of two or more distinct personalities or personality states (each with its own relatively enduring pattern of perceiving, relating to, and thinking about the environment and self.	A. The presence of two or more distinct identities or personality states (each with its own relatively enduring pattern of perceiving, relating to, and thinking about the environment and self.
To determine that the self-states take over control of the person's behavior	B. The personality that is dominant at any particular time determines the individual's behavior.	B. At least two of these personalities or personality states recurrently take full control of the person's behavior.	B. At least two of these identities or personality states recurrently take control of the person's behavior.
To establish the nature and complexity of the self-states	C. Each individual personality is complex and integrated with its own unique behavior patterns and social relationships.	*[Nature and complexity are described in Criterion A]*	*[Nature and complexity are described in Criterion A]*
To distinguish that amnesia is present	*[No amnesia criterion]*	*[No amnesia criterion]*	C. Inability to recall important personal information that is too extensive to be explained by ordinary forgetfulness.
To rule out substance abuse or medical conditions and to exclude phenomena found in normal childhood	*[No substance, medical or developmental rule out criterion]*	*[No substance, medical or developmental rule out criterion]*	D. The disturbance is not due to the direct physiological effects of a substance (e.g., blackouts or chaotic behavior during alcohol intoxication) or a general medical condition (e.g., complex partial seizures).

In 1980, with the new classification posttraumatic stress disorder (PTSD) in *DSM-III* (APA, 1980), clinicians were confronted with the fact that trauma may be associated with significant psychopathology. Research on PTSD revealed physiological residuals in addition to psychological sequelae (van der Kolk, 1987).

In *DSM-III*, for the first time in a diagnostic taxonomy, the disorder of Multiple Personality (MP) was recognized as a separate and distinct diagnosis. The disorder was called multiple personality disorder (MPD) in *DSM-III-R* (APA, 1987) and is now dissociative identity disorder (formerly multiple personality disorder) (DID/MPD) in *DSM-IV*. See Table 1 for diagnostic criteria.

A major impetus for updating the *DSM* is to have the diagnostic system used in the United States be consistent with the World Health Organization diagnostic system, the International Classification of Disease (ICD). The *ICD-10* for mental disorders, published in 1992, included MPD as a subcategory of other dissociative (conversion) disorders, along with "Ganser's syndrome" (*ICD-10*, 1992). See Table 2 for the evolving DSM taxonomy for dissociative disorders compared to *ICD-10* classification.

For a half century, there had been speculation that multiple, "dual," or "split" personality was associated with a history of early child abuse (Ferenczi, 1955). And during the 1970s and 1980s, there was an increased recognition of child abuse in the general population. The 1980s brought an expansion of interest in dissociative disorders (North, Ryall, Ricci, & Wetzel, 1993) and a corresponding explosion in publications on the subject (Goettman, Greaves, & Coons, 1991).

DSM-III described the onset of Multiple Personality as occurring in early childhood or later, rarely being diagnosed until adolescence. This is consistent with the finding of Kluft (1985b) that only about 10% of those with MPD were diagnosed prior to age 20 and only 3% were diagnosed at age 11 or younger.

Current theories of the development of DID/MPD (Braun & Sachs, 1985; Kluft, 1984) hold that this disorder begins in childhood in an individual who has the propensity to dissociate, who is exposed to trauma in an environment that cannot absorb the trauma, and who over time develops parts of the mind that consider themselves separate and distinct from the rest of the mind (alternate identities or alters). If the stage is set for DID/MPD in childhood, why have clinicians diagnosed so few youngsters with the disorder?

There have been many hypotheses about why the diagnosis of DID/MPD is not made earlier in life. Identities (alters) in childhood are not as distinct as in adults. Regressions to young identities can be mistaken for usual childhood regression. Many children with childhood DID/MPD do not display symptoms that draw the attention of the mental health community until adulthood. The full symptoms of DID/MPD do not usually appear until the late 20s or early 30s (Kluft, 1985b). Historically, there

Table 2.

Evolving Dissociative Disorder Taxonomy

DSM-III (DSM-III-R)	DSM-IV	Corresponding ICD-10 Dissociative Disorders
Psychogenic amnesia	Dissociative amnesia	Dissociative amnesia
Psychogenic fugue	Dissociative fugue	Dissociative fugue
		Dissociative stupor
		Trance and possession disorder
		Dissociative disorders of movement and sensation
		Dissociative motor disorders
		Dissociative convulsions
		Dissociative anaesthesia and sensory loss
		Mixed dissociative [conversion] disorders
		Other dissociative [conversion] disorders
		Ganser's syndrome
Multiple personality (disorder)	Dissociative identity disorder	Multiple personality disorder
		Transient dissociative [conversion] disorders occurring in childhood and adolescence
Depersonalization disorder	Depersonalization disorder	
Dissociative disorder NOS	Dissociative disorder NOS	Dissociative [conversion] disorder, unspecified

has been a long time between a person's entry into the mental health system and diagnosis of MPD (Coons, Bowman, & Milstein, 1988; Putnam, Guroff, Silverman, Barban, & Post, 1986; Ross, Norton, & Wozney, 1989).

Many specialists in dissociative disorders in children believe that in children as in adults, the main reason that dissociative disorders are not diagnosed earlier is that clinicians do not ask the questions which will lead them towards the diagnosis. For example, we clinicians may misinterpret symptoms. When we see a child who is in trance at school and does something impulsive we begin to think of a potential attention deficit disorder. Considering the old medical aphorism "if you hear hoof beats think of horses, not zebras," for those in child and adolescent psychiatry, psychology, and social work, the "horses" are attention-deficit/

hyperactivity disorder, conduct disorder, and major depression—but decidedly *not* dissociative identity disorder.

In the mid 1980s several authors came up with various concepts to address the ambiguous presentation of dissociative disorders in children. Fagan and McMahan (1984) used the term "incipient multiple personality." Kluft (1985c) published his "predictors of MPD." Malenbaum and Russell (1987) described their patient as having "MPD in evolution." The notion of "precursors" of full-fledged MPD was also discussed (Snowden, 1988). All of these authors implied that, without intervention, these children would develop MPD in adulthood. However, there was no central theme or symptom complex to tie these concepts of incipient predictors and precursors together.

During the 1980s little was being done to increase the recognition of childhood dissociative disorders. Dissociative disorders were considered in neither childhood epidemiologic studies (Beitchmen, Kruidenier, Inglis, & Clegg, 1989; Brandenburg, Friedman, & Silver, 1990; Costello, 1989) nor longitudinal studies (Cantwell & Baker, 1989; Esser, Schmidt, & Woerner, 1990). Until 1991 there was no major child psychiatry textbook that included a chapter on multiple personality disorder in childhood (Lewis, 1991). In the 1980s there was no consideration of childhood dissociative disorders by the Child and Adolescent Work Group for the DSM-IV Task Force (Shaffer, et al., 1989). While the World Health Organization did not include dissociative disorders in ICD-10 field trials, it did include a childhood dissociative disorder in the mental disorder taxonomy (ICD-10, 1992).

In 1989 I delivered a paper in which I described a constellation of symptoms which seemed to capture the nature of dissociative disorders in childhood (Peterson, 1989). In this presentation, I described a hypothetical disorder having three categories of symptoms and a rule-out criterion: (1) amnestic or trance-like experiences, (2) marked behavior fluctuations, (3) behavioral and other symptoms, many of which are frequently seen in other disorders, and (4) not multiple personality disorder.

After that presentation on a child-specific dissociative disorder, many clinicians working with children with dissociative disorders expressed excitement to me about the prospect of having this concept formally recognized. The most common and enthusiastic support came from social workers who served in public sector mental health outpatient facilities. These clinicians described similar situations typified by "I am working with a dissociative child but I can't get the support of my child psychiatrist. When I bring up the idea of dissociative disorder in children, he says, 'Show me where it is in *DSM-III.*'"

There were sound reasons for having a childhood dissociative disorder established within the diagnostic taxonomy, including: (1) to have a more accurate clinical description; (2) to alert clinicians of the dissociative dimension in children; (3) to avoid the stigma of an MPD diagnosis; (4) to use as an intermediate diagnosis if MPD is suspected but not established in the first few sessions or months; (5) to alter the course of therapy to include the dissociative dimension; and (6) to encourage research in the area.

There were several precedents for considering diagnostic categories that had one form in childhood and another in adulthood. For instance, the *DSM-III-R* listed conduct disorder, avoidant disorder, identity disorder, and overanxious disorder. These were considered to be precursors of antisocial personality disorder, avoidance personality disorder, borderline personality disorder, and generalized anxiety disorder, respectively. However, the Task Force was seeking to limit the expansion of diagnostic categories for the *DSM-IV* taxonomy, and establishing a new diagnostic category was a daunting task. Indeed, in an effort to constrain the expanding set of diagnoses, *DSM-IV* has incorporated two *DSM-III-R* childhood anxiety disorders (avoidant disorder of childhood or adolescence and overanxious disorder) into adult diagnostic categories (social phobia and generalized anxiety disorder). Identity Disorder was relegated to the status of a V code diagnosis called Identity Problem. Where it appeared that child criteria were precursors of syndromes in adulthood, the Task Force adjusted the adult criteria to fit children.

In February of 1990, I wrote the first of many letters, sending packets of information to members of the DSM-IV Task Force and diagnostic taxonomy committees of other organizations, trying to spark interest in childhood dissociative disorders. However, in October, when I spoke with a child psychiatrist Task Force member he said he had not noticed the correspondence and that dissociation had not been discussed. With this news, I heightened my efforts with phone calls and letters to bring awareness of dissociative disorders to Task Force members.

Over the next few years numerous child and adolescent clinicians and researchers made efforts to maintain interest in a child dissociation disorder diagnosis among members of the Child and Adolescent and Dissociative Disorders Study Groups. Despite these efforts, the *DSM-IV Options Book* (APA, 1991) made no mention of child, adolescent, or youth in the dissociative disorders section.

At the 1990 Annual Meeting of the American Academy of Child and Adolescent Psychiatry, I noticed that dissociative disorders still were not being considered by the *DSM-IV* Work Group for child and adolescent disorders (Shaffer et al., 1990). Dr. Shaffer subsequently appointed me to the Disorders First Diagnosed During Infancy Childhood or Adolescence Work Group and the Dissociative Disorders Work Group to act a liaison between these two areas of focus. At that meeting, I approached DSM-IV ADHD Field Trial principal investigator B. Lahey to include questions about dissociation in his project. Unfortunately, by the time he received the information, it was too late to include the dissociation questions in the study.

In 1990, the diagnostic criteria for a child dissociation diagnosis were refined and the concept was renamed "Dissociative Disorder of Childhood (DDoC)" (Peterson & Putnam, 1992). In November, I drafted a proposed *DSM-IV* text and diagnostic criteria for the disorder and shared this informally with members of the International Society for the Study of Multiple Personality and Dissociation to refine the criteria.

By March 1991, I notified DSM-IV Task Force members about the refined criteria. In that communication, I included a proposed text, differential diagnosis, and diagnostic criteria for DDoC (Peterson, 1991b). In addition, I suggested a series of paragraphs to be included the differential diagnosis for other diagnostic categories.

During the early months of 1991, F. Putnam and I modified a field trial questionnaire for a new study, the Dissociative Disorder of Childhood Field Trial. In July 1991 I sent out the first round of questionnaires to therapists who had expressed an interest in participating in this unfunded study. The purposes of this investigation were (1) to better understand the symptoms of children and adolescents with dissociative disorders; (2) to establish whether one could distinguish youngsters with DDoC from those with MPD; (3) to understand in what ways children with DDoC would differ from non-MPD children who had a dissociative disorder but did not meet the criteria for DDoC; and (4) to determine which of the criteria best characterize DDoC cases. Over a hundred cases were submitted for inclusion in the study.

The American Academy of Child and Adolescent Psychiatry co-chairs of the Diagnostic Taxonomy Committee had given us unofficial support and awaited the data to fortify our contentions. We had hoped to have the results analyzed soon enough to influence the *DSM-IV* decision process. Responses to the field trial requests were slow to arrive, and we were not able to publish the preliminary results of the field trial until years later (Peterson & Putnam, 1994). The study indicates that DDoC criteria identify a group of subjects who do not have alter personalities but do have significant levels of dissociation, based on dissociative symptoms factors and scores on a standardized checklist for child dissociative symptoms, the CDC (Putnam, Helmers, & Trickett, 1993). DDoC cases differ from other dissociative disorder (non-MPD) cases on non-dissociative factors but not on dissociative factors (identity, dissociative symptoms, amnesia, hallucinations).

Where We Are

As child advocates for recognition of dissociative disorders, we did not accomplish our goal to influence the *DSM-IV* to establish a dissociative disorder for children. DDoC was not accepted into *DSM-IV* either as diagnostic category nor as a diagnosis in the appendix for future consideration. The Disorders Usually First Diagnosed During Infancy, Childhood and Adolescence Work Group soundly rejected my suggestions to include dissociative disorder in the differential diagnosis for several disorders commonly diagnosed in youth. However, these efforts did result in two important recognitions of dissociative disorder in youth. One was to identify children in the DID/MPD criteria, and the other was to recognize dissociative disorder in the ADHD rule-out criterion.

At the suggestion of New Zealand psychiatrist J. S. Werry (personal communication, May 11, 1992), the rule-out criterion for children with DID/MPD was added: "Note: In children, the symptoms are not attributable to imaginary playmates or other fantasy play." (See Table 1.) While giving recognition to the occurrence of DID/MPD in children, this description also raises important developmental questions about the differences between imaginary friends phenomena and pathological dissociative processes.

These questions can be partially clarified if the clinician considers cognitive development in children. In the preschool child, concrete operations have not yet been reached (Kagan, 1984). The child does not understand the concept of cause and effect. If you ask preschoolers if their imaginary companions are real, they may say "Yes" if they don't understand that they brought their perception of imaginary companion into being. If you ask a 7-year-old child who has mastered concrete operations the same question, he or she will know the imaginary companion is not real but is a projection of the child's imagination. The child will know he or she made it up. If, on the other hand, you ask a school age child with DID/MPD if the imaginary companion is real, he or she will likely answer "Yes." The child with DID/MPD does not have the awareness to know that the imaginary friend is the child's own projection. This process parallels the host alters of DID/MPD patients who cannot understand that the other alters are a part of his/her own mind (Peterson, 1995).

DSM-IV ADHD Field Trial principal investigator B. Lahey (personal communication, October 1994) suggested inclusion of the term "dissociative disorder" in the differential diagnosis and the rule-out criterion for ADHD. Criterion E for ADHD reads, "The symptoms . . . are not better accounted for by another mental disorder (e.g. Mood Disorder, Anxiety Disorder, Disorder, Dissociative Disorder or a Personality Disorder)." *DSM-IV* clarifies "not better accounted for by . . . " by stating:

> This exclusion criterion is used to indicate that the disorders mentioned in the criterion must be considered in the differential diagnosis of the presenting psychopathology and that, in boundary cases, clinical judgment will be necessary to determine which disorder provides the most appropriate diagnosis. In such cases, the "Differential Diagnosis" section of the text for the disorders should be consulted for guidance (p. 6).

Taken in the context of this definition, if the child's symptoms are consistent with ADHD and with a dissociative disorder, the clinician may make both diagnoses.

DSM-IV made moderate progress in recognizing child and adolescent DID/MPD features. The *DSM-III-R* text for MPD makes no references to children other than that onset "is almost invariably in childhood. . . ." However, the *DSM-IV* DID/MPD text includes helpful comments on youth, such as "In preadolescent children, particular care is needed in making the diagnosis because the manifestations may be less distinctive than in adolescents and adults" (p. 485), and ". . . in childhood, the female-to-male ratio may be more even . . . " (p. 486).

In summary, the effective results of efforts to influence *DSM-IV* to recognize childhood dissociation were to mention children in the DID/MPD rule-out criteria, to include dissociative disorders in the differential diagnosis and rule-out criterion for ADHD, and to include comments on youth in the text for DID/MPD. These are substantial gains towards the recognition necessary to encourage clinicians to consider the dimension of dissociation when evaluating perplexing young clients. No longer will an informed child psychiatrist order the clinician to "show me where it is in *DSM*."

Differential Diagnosis

The *DSM-IV* Task Force members chose to avoid including dissociative disorders in other categories of differential diagnosis because of their concern that dissociative disorders would be over diagnosed (Wiener et al., 1995). Because dissociative disorders are not included in the differential of other diagnoses, the following may be of help to the clinician trying to make distinctions between dissociative and other disorders.

Age-appropriate dissociation does not have the degree of amnesia or trance-like states nor the marked changes in functioning and abilities seen in DID/MPD. Children in *inadequate, disorganized, or chaotic* environments may appear to have difficulty in the area of dissociation. In such cases it may be impossible to determine whether the dissociative behavior is primarily a function of the chaotic environment or whether it is due largely to the child's psychopathology (in which case a dissociative diagnosis may be warranted).

Trance-like states can be misinterpreted as being petit mal *seizures*. Complex partial seizure episodes are generally brief (30 sec–5 min) and do not involve the complex and enduring structures of identity and behavior observed in DID/MPD. DID/MPD doesn't respond to anti-seizure medication. Visual hallucinations are common in childhood dissociative disorders.

The diagnosis of *schizophrenia* is extremely rare in childhood. Auditory hallucinations common in dissociative disorders characteristically come from inside the child's head (pseudohallucinations) and can be perceived as helpful or hurtful. Negative symptoms of schizophrenia such as occupational and social deterioration, emptiness, and loss of drive are not features distinctive of DID/MPD but may be symptoms of accompanying depression. Auditory hallucinations respond poorly to neuroleptics in DID/MPD. In schizophrenia, these voices are usually perceived as coming from outside of the head (Coons, 1984; Kluft, 1985b; Putnam, 1989; p. 62; Ross, 1989, p. 100); they are chaotic, bizarre, and irrational and cannot engage in conversation. They are associated with schizophrenic thought disorder and appear in acute phases of a psychotic illness.

In DID/MPD, most of the time auditory hallucinations are perceived as coming from inside the head (Coons, 1984; Kluft, 1985b, p. 222; Putnam, 1989, p. 62; Ross, 1989, p. 100). In DID/MPD the voices present organized ideas and may retreat when confronted or inquired about. Voices can converse either directly or through the patient. Frequently they are chronically present, even when the patient is functioning well. Frequent derailment or incoherence of speech is not supportive of the diagnosis of MPD/DID. Grossly disorganized or catatonic behavior is not typical of MPD/DID but on occasion can be observed as a manifestation of the influence of alternate identities. If the criteria for DID/MPD are met, the additional diagnosis of schizophrenia should be made only in the rare instances in which prominent delusions, hallucinations, and disorganized or negative symptoms meeting the criteria for schizophrenia can be documented.

Symptoms of anxiety are common in DID/MPD. When anxiety is due to trauma, these symptoms may be viewed as due to this disorder rather than as a separate anxiety disorder, except in the case of *posttraumatic stress disorder* (PTSD), for which an additional diagnosis should be made. Symptoms of PTSD are common in DID/MPD. Often symptoms in those with DID/MPD warrant both diagnoses. Panic attacks may be triggered by stimuli reminding the person of previous trauma (the trauma may be unconscious). *Agoraphobia* may be due to unfounded, unreasonable fears of danger stimulated by young identities. *Social phobia* may be the result of the host personality state fearing that something which is out of his or her control will happen. *Obsessive compulsive* symptoms may be part of the hypervigilance of a traumatized person or an attempt to stay organized by one who has missing blocks of time. *Acute stress disorder* has prominent dissociative symptoms. Stressors may activate the alternate identities. Overt symptoms of DID/MPD may be present during periods of severe stress, opening a window of opportunity for DID/MPD diagnosis (Kluft, 1991).

In *DSM-IV* (APA, 1994, p. 631) personality disorder diagnoses "may be applied to children or adolescents in those relatively unusual instances in which the individual's particular maladaptive personality traits appear to be pervasive, persistent, and unlikely to be limited to a particular developmental state or an episode of an Axis I disorder." Therefore, a youngster with DID/MPD who is exhibiting unpredictable, perplexing changes in attitude and behavior and is not responding to the usual therapeutic interventions may be seen as having *borderline personality disorder* (BPD). If symptoms of DID/MPD are present and the person meets the criteria of BPD, both diagnoses can be made. However, caution should be taken in making the diagnosis of BPD with DID/MPD. While many people with DID/MPD may fit the diagnostic criteria for BPD (Coons, 1984; Kluft, 1984b) relatively few may fit the dynamics (Benner & Jocelyne, 1984) or have psychological testing (Armstrong & Loewenstein, 1990) conforming to the BPD diagnosis (Marmer & Fink, 1994). In addition, if the therapist interprets the patient's behavior in the context of BPD dynamics rather than trauma based dissociation, the therapist is more likely to feel or respond in a negative manner. Using the DID/MPD paradigm, the therapist may find the solution to crises through direct negotiation with personality states, an intervention not available to the therapist working with BPD.

Eating disorders are not uncommon in DID/MPD (Putnam, Guroff, Silberman, Barban, & Post, 1986). Purging may result from one personality state trying to get rid of another self-state's food intake or may be associated with somatic memory of forced oral sex.

In *sexual dysfunctions,* sexual promiscuity may be due to a promiscuous alter. The clinician should check for memory of promiscuous behavior. The host personality may not remember promiscuous behavior by an alter. Aversion to sexual activity is common for the host personality state.

Symptoms characteristic of DID/MPD are sometimes observed in *pervasive developmental disorders.* However, in pervasive developmental disorder the fluctuations in behavioral abilities are environmentally specific, i.e. the regressive or stereotypic behavior predictability occurs with a repeated stimulus. When a pervasive developmental diagnosis is made, a diagnosis of DID/MPD is usually preempted.

In *attention-deficit/hyperactivity disorder* the persistence of developmentally inappropriate and marked inattention that is associated with this disorder is not accompanied by trance-like states, periods of amnesia, and marked fluctuations in behavior. Dissociative children are distracted by internal voices, made impulses, made behaviors. They may not follow instructions because they are attending to these phenomena.

When considering *impulse control disorders* the clinician should check for sustained interest in the pathological activity in *kleptomania, pyromania,* and *pathological gambling.* In people with DID/MPD, interest in these activities may vary depending on which alter is influencing behavior. In *trichotillomania* check for internal voices commanding "hair-pulling" (dissociative) vs. a passive self-soothing ritual (trichotillomania).

Intermittent explosive disorder is described as intermittent switching to explosive states, sometimes with amnesia for the explosive state. The clinician should investigate whether the explosive behavior is due to an unrecognized personality state.

Dissociative disorders in children have a high rate of comorbidity with other disorders (Hornstein & Putnam, 1992; Hornstein & Tyson, 1991; Peterson & Putnam, 1994). Symptoms of attention deficit disorder, *oppositional defiant disorder* (ODD), or *conduct disorder* (CD) may develop later in childhood in those with childhood dissociative disorders. Symptoms may become exacerbated at puberty and become confused with the developmental roles which are part of adolescence. If the symptoms of ODD or CD are caused by the host personality, the disruptive behavior disorder diagnosis should be made. If they are determined to be due to the switching of alters, a dissociation specific intervention may address the problem and the disruptive behavior diagnosis may be omitted.

Mood disorders and *specific developmental disorders* are diagnoses commonly associated with dissociative disorders and should be noted when present. Shifts between personality states may be confused with cyclical mood fluctuations. Specific learning disorders may fluctuate with severity of dissociative symptoms. In DID/MPD changes in knowledge and learning may be a function of the self-state which is in control of the body at the time of testing. A person's answer may be indirectly influenced by an alter.

From the description above, you can understand that it is common for children suffering from dissociative disorders to have been previously diagnosed with other disorders, as illustrated in Table 3.

The following are case examples of dissociative youngsters who present with more commonly diagnosed disorders:

Case example: presentation as depression

Fifteen-year-old Vonell presents with a 3-year history of depressive symptoms including suicidal ideation and wrist slashing resulting in a 1-month psychiatric hospitalization. Discharge diagnosis was "major depression; rule out posttraumatic stress disorder."

A few months after discharge, her depressive symptoms returned and she was again thinking of cutting her wrists. Her grades had dropped markedly. She had refused school for the last few weeks. She complains of flashbacks in which she re-experiences seeing her father beat her mother (these beatings had occurred when Vonell was three). Vonell's experimentation with stimulant and depressant illicit drugs had been of no help to reduce her emotional pain, so she stopped taking them. Recent stressors include her mother's medical problems and

Table 3.

Previous Diagnoses of Youth with Dissociative Disorders

	Peterson & Putnam, unpubl. N = 102 (%)		Hornstein & Tyson, 1991. N = 17 (%)	
	MPD	DDNOS	MPD	DDNOS
	N = 53	N = 49	N = 11	N = 6
ADHD	21	6	45	50
Opposition/conduct	9	8	55	17
Dissociative disorder			36	50
MPD	9	4		
DDNOS	4	14		
Psychotic disorder	3	6	36	50
Depression				
Bipolar	4	4		
Other depression	21	10		
PTSD	25	24	18	50
Other anxiety disorders	9	8		
Specific dev. disorder	2	4	18	-
Pervasive dev disorder	4	4		
Adjustment disorders	2	18		

the fact that her mother had reminded her of her father's abuse of Vonell during Vonell's preschool years.

On interview, Vonell explains that for the past several years she has been experiencing auditory hallucinations. These are voices that number three or four and are present in most situations. Vonell has some ability to control their presence and, when she is with other people, finds she can easily ignore them. She says that at the moment she cut her wrists all the voices immediately and totally stopped. However, she got no sense of emotional relief from cutting her wrists. The wrist-cutting did not hurt, but the pain afterwards was pronounced. She experiences all her voices as being depressed, although they cover over their depression with humor. She cannot differentiate whether they are male or female voices. They seem like high-pitched male voices, and she hears them as clearly as she hears her own voice. Sometimes her mother will hear Vonell talking to the voices and when her mother asks, Vonell will say that she is talking to the dog.

During the interview, Vonell is asked whether the voices are present. They are not present, but upon the interviewer's request, she is able to bring two voices into awareness. They are happy voices saying they are 11 years old. They say they are not either boys or girls. The younger voice describes the older as a "wussey." After several minutes, the voices decide to go away, accepting thanks from the interviewer for having come to talk. During the course of the interview, Vonell contacts the voices and gets a commitment from them not to tell her to cut her wrists.

Vonell says she has missing memory for 2 to 3 hours of class a day. She has no awareness of the voices taking control of the body. However, when asked, the voices indicate they do take control of the body at school. Vonell's peers "tell me I look dazey." Only her best friends notice this, however, especially a close friend who also has the experience of hearing voices.

On 1 month followup, Vonell reports the voices were decreased by 50% on the day after the interview; they gradually diminished and disappeared within two weeks. On 1 year followup, she has had no reoccurrence of her suicidal behaviors.

Vonell's presentation was similar to an adult with DID/MPD in that she presented as depleted and depressed and had been hearing deprecating voices for an extended period. She had symptoms consistent with Posttraumatic Stress Disorder, self-destructive behaviors, self-injury, and substance abuse. Like adult DID/MPD patients, Vonell had an abuse history. She had hidden her hallucinatory experiences and told no one of her voices, even during hospitalization for Major Depression. Voices were able to dialogue and contract with the interviewer and host alter during the session. Depressive symptoms remitted in response to hospitalization. She had missing blocks of time and dysremembered behaviors. She had no idea that the voices took over control of the body. Her friends noticed her unusual behaviors.

Vonell's presentation differs from a case presentation in an average adult with DID/MPD in that her experience of hearing voices had occurred over only a few years. It is not uncommon for an adult with DID/MPD to differentiate voices poorly on first interview; however, age range and gender for some of the voices usually can be assigned by the patient. Vonell's voices diminished rapidly after the initial interview; this is uncommon in adult cases.

My experience is that in about half the cases of dissociative disorders in children and adolescents, auditory and visual hallucinations of dissociative youngsters diminish rapidly. Why this diminution occurs is not understood. Perhaps cohesion of the self-state within the child or adolescent is so poorly developed that upon inquiry it loses coherence. Reported cases of rapid treatment of childhood MPD (Kluft, 1985b) would support that hypothesis. Perhaps the self-states decide to retreat to the internal universe and will return when there seems to be less likelihood of being identified by an outsider. Vonell was no longer in a traumatic environment, and I doubt that her dissociative symptoms would have remained abated if she had been retraumatized. In discussions with colleagues, it seems that for some child outpatients in nontraumatic environments, dissociative symptoms may dissolve without much if any direct intervention. However, many outpatients do require extensive therapy (see chapters 6–9). Therapists working in hospital settings have indicated to me that their dissociative child and adolescent patients' hallucinations do not diminish spontaneously. Perhaps these hospitalized youngsters are more severely ill, or they experience the hospital setting itself as a traumatic event and therefore maintain the dissociative hallucinations as part of their familiar defense response.

Case example: presentation as suicidal behavior

Mark is a 9-year-old boy who is brought for an emergency evaluation by school personnel because a student had turned in a suicide note which had fallen out of Mark's desk. Mark has wanted to kill himself for a very long time and has written several suicide notes. His past self-destructive behavior has included striking a match and sticking it to his finger. He has considered slicing his neck with a knife, but denies feeling depressed.

Mark has restricted affect, psychomotor retardation, poor eye contact, and speech latency consistent with depression. When asked about what goes on in his mind during the time before he answers the question, he says first he hears the question from the examiner, then he hears the question repeated in the voice of the examiner, then he hears a discussion about the answer, and finally he hears the answer he is to give. Sometimes he gives the exact answer that is stated to him and sometimes he summarizes the answer. The answer comes from a voice inside his head that sounds like his voice. The voice comes from a part of him that is 9 years old. He also hears another voice he calls his "conscience." He allows the examiner to speak directly to the voice, which states he wants to kill himself so his troubles will be over. Mark has an occasional eye roll. Motor activity shifts during the interview. When he speaks from the "9-year-old voice" point of view, he moves forward in his chair and faces the examiner directly.

After his father enters the room, he is fidgety and silly in his demeanor. He mouths words frequently while his father is talking to the examiner. He asks if the people we see here at the center are "crazy" and if the examiner thinks he is crazy.

Later his father refuses to allow the boy to enter into therapy and the therapist files a petition for medical neglect. Therapy lasts for the duration of the court order. During the next several weeks, Mark describes a system of voices. One is a 24-year-old named Daniel who "is my conscience" and tells the truth. If Mark tells a lie, Daniel will make the correction for him. The 9-year-old alter, Luke, is responsible for "having fun." Mark says only he and Luke sequentially share a room in the mind. Access to the outside world is done through a television set. A red sign on the wall commands "wait for your turn," one word at a time. When the sign dictates, Luke and Mark change places. However, neither sees the other entering or leaving the room.

The therapist is never able to get the cooperation of the parents in the therapy process. A few weeks prior to the termination of the court order, Mark reports to the therapist that he has blown up the internal world and that it no longer exists.

In this example, Mark is living with an uncooperative family. Though no abuse can be substantiated, the family would cooperate only under court order. In contrast to Vonell's case, Mark's dissociative symptoms remained throughout therapy until they were "destroyed" by the patient shortly before the termination of treatment allowed by expiration of the court order. One can speculate that Mark thought he had to "destroy" his conscious awareness of his dissociative symptoms (which originally brought him to the attention of the authorities) in order for therapy to terminate. Since he has used dissociative adaptation to cope with stress in the past, it seems likely that he will use them to cope with future trauma. Given the lack of family cooperation and the premature termination of treatment, if he presents for evaluation again, we expect he again will be exhibiting dissociative symptoms.

Where We're Going

Where we are headed in the realm of dissociative disorders in children depends on the acuity and persistence of those who have come to understand the dissociative paradigm and upon the outcome of research generated from that awareness (Putnam & Peterson, 1994). In the broad view, child dissociation will go the way of dissociative disorders in adults. If the recent backlash against awareness of abuse frightens competent clinicians from the field, our clients will suffer.

A clearer understanding of the process of memory is crucial to quell the discord which has developed between clinicians who treat traumatized clients and those who believe that history of trauma is specious and therefore not worthy of clinical intervention. Neuroscientists now have assessment tools never before available to psychology. Electronic scanning techniques can assess which parts of the brain are involved in a specific task. The puzzle of how human beings establish memory is being deciphered. Recent reports show us that how we form our memory of events depends in part on the degree of stress and the repetition of the event (van der Kolk, 1994).

It is necessary to have sound basic research, as well as to have clinicians come together and examine how we conceptualize and describe clinical conditions. *DSM-IV*, like *DSM-III*, is a categorical taxonomy of mental disorders. Most of the diagnostic categories are described using "polythetic" criteria sets in which only a few of a full list of symptoms or conditions need be met (*DSM-IV*, p. xxii).

DID/MPD (as well as MP in *DSM-III* and MPD in *DSM-III-R*) is not one the polythetic criteria sets. It is a highly simplified depiction of a very complicated condition. The condition requires that in an individual there is the "presence of . . . identities or personality states." Neither "identity" nor "personality state" is clearly defined. The choice of the term "identity" is a particularly poor one because it is a commonly used term which has many meanings depending on the context (e.g., a collective set of characteristics by which a thing is known, a set of recognizable behavioral or personal characteristics, the quality of being the same, individuality, and, in math, either an equation that is satisfied for all values of the symbols or an identity element [American Heritage Dictionary, 1992]). When preceded by the word "ego" it means "a sense of unity and continuity of ones own personality" (Dorland's, 1974). After it became clear the term "identity" was to be substituted for the *DSM-III(-R)* term "personality," I urged the Task Force to define the new use of the term "identity" to no avail.

We have an even more important distinction to make than defining "identity." In each of the last three DSM publications, the criteria call for "the presence of" this thing we used to label a personality and now call an identity. In no other mental disorder does the first criterion begin with "the presence of." The clinical criteria in *DSM-IV* usually begin with a phrase such as "a pervasive pattern," "a prominent disturbance," "five or more of the following symptoms," "a repetitive and persistent pattern of," and the like. The very essence of this opening description for DID/MPD lends a sense of mystery and intrigue for the reader. Veiled in the wording of this first criterion is the implication that the "presence of" the identity or personality (state) occurs when the diagnostician or therapist recognizes it. It is as though the clinician in collusion with the patient can generate this "presence."

In the experience of the client, the opposite is true. The client usually divulges the perceived self to the clinician, as either the client no longer has the ability to hide the segmented self-states, thereby revealing these states to the alert clinician, or the client (including, perhaps, the dissociated parts) has a sense that there will be more to gain by revealing these experiences than continuing to hide them. Therefore, it is not clinicians who determine the "presence of" the self-states, it is the individual client.

Since 1994 I have been working with clinicians and organizations to press for different wording to describe alternate personality states. The term I propose is consistent with a client generated self-observation. Rather than focusing on *observer assessment of personality state or identity*, the phrase I suggest is *self-perceived autonomous self-state*. Shortened forms of this are *autonomous self-state* or simply *self-state*. Kluft, Ross, Putnam, and others have addressed this general concept in their writings, and Kluft pressed for changing the nomenclature from "personality" to "self-state" during the *DSM-III* development process (personal communication, November 4, 1994). The "self-state" is a term without other common usage which could be clearly defined for use with DID/MPD.

Currently I am working to encourage those who were members of the *DSM-IV* Task Force to consider making minor revisions to *DSM-IV* which would prevent the misdiagnosis of schizophrenia in those with DID/MPD. According to the chairperson of the Task Force on *DSM-IV*, the Task Force felt that having DID/MPD in the differential for Schizophrenia would lead to a substantial over diagnosis of DID/MPD (Wiener, et al., 1995).

Unfortunately, the way the current criteria for schizophrenia are set out, to be eligible for the diagnosis of schizophrenia an individual has only to have hallucinatory voices talking to each other for 6 months or more. Most children and adults with DID/MPD hear voices, and often they hear the voices talking to each other. With *DSM-IV* a clinician uninformed about dissociative disorders can misdiagnose someone with DID/MPD as having schizophrenia. In addition, DID/MPD is not in the differential diagnosis for schizophrenia, and dissociation is nowhere mentioned in the discussion about hallucinations.

Misdiagnosis of schizophrenia for DID/MPD is of course a major clinical error, because the treatment of these two categories differ markedly. Given that childhood schizophrenia is extremely rare (*DSM-IV*, p. 281), the diagnostician is obliged to consider a dissociative disorder diagnosis to rule out psychosis when he/she evaluates a child with auditory/visual hallucinations. I am continuing my work on these omissions and hope these efforts will induce a change in revisions of *DSM-IV* or at least impact on *DSM-V*.

To preserve the progress that is being made, we must be continually alert for major organizational moves that affect assessment and treatment and have not addressed the dissociative paradigm. The American Academy of Child and Adolescent Psychiatry (AACAP) distributed to its membership preliminary guidelines entitled "Practice Parameters for the Assessment and Treatment of Children and Adolescents with Bipolar Disorder." In this 36-page document, there was no mention of dissociation or dissociative disorder. The principal authors, J. McClellan and J. Werry, said they could find very little information on dissociative disorders in youth, so they did not have the facts they needed to evaluate what they should include in dissociative disorders (personal communications, October 3, 1995). They graciously accepted a packet with several pertinent articles and a bibliography. At the AACAP Annual Meeting symposium where the guidelines were discussed, the principal author gave assurance that the guidelines would include an appropriate discussion of dissociative disorders (McClellan & Bernet, 1995).

The late 1980s and early 1990s marked a proliferation of helpful literature on dissociative disorders. Clinicians could better assess and treat dissociative disorders with the help of newly developed assessment tools including the Dissociative Experiences Scale (Bernstein & Putnam, 1986), the Dissociative Disorders Interview Schedule (Ross, Heber, Norton, Anderson, Anderson, & Barchet, 1989), and the Structured Clinical Interview for *DSM-IV* Dissociative Disorders (Steinberg, Rounsaville, & Cicchetti, 1990). We had many new volumes on MPD (Bliss, 1986; Braun, 1986; Putnam, 1989; Ross, 1989) and the number of journal publications expanded dramatically (Goettman, Greaves, & Coons, 1991).

Today information and research about childhood dissociation is expanding rapidly. The first book devoted to dissociative disorders in childhood was published in the mid-1980s (Kluft, 1985a). Now in the mid-1990s, many more are becoming available (Lewis, 1996; Peterson, in press; Putnam, in press; Shirar, 1996; Silberg, 1996a). Chapters on childhood dissociative disorders are now being included in major texts on child psychiatry (Lewis, 1991; Silberg, 1996b). Researchers and clinicians have developed assessment tools and techniques for evaluating problems in dissociation. These include the Child Dissociative Checklist (Putnam, Helmers, & Trickett, 1993), the Children's Perceptual Alteration Scale (Evers-Szostak & Sanders, 1992), Child/Adolescent Dissociative Checklist (Reagor, Kasten, & Morelli, 1992) and the Child Dissociation Problem Checklist (Peterson, 1991a). A new child dissociative disorder assessment instrument, the Dissociative Features Profile, using standard psychological testing is described in this volume (Chapter 5) (Hornstein & Silberg, 1995), and the new Adolescent Dissociative Experiences Scale is undergoing field trials (see Appendix A). Research projects are underway to answer some fundamental questions such as family environmental factors in dissociation and psychopathology (Nash, Hulsey, Sexton, Harralson, & Lambert, 1993), pathophysiological effects of sexual abuse (DeBellis, et al., 1994), inheritability of dissociative disorders using large scale child and adolescent twin studies, and longitudinal outcome in the study of dissociation, psychopathology and psychobiology in abused children (Putnam, Helmers, Horowitz, & Trickett, 1995).

Further acceptance of the dissociative spectrum of disorders is important in the clinical care of our children. We need to further improve our clinical descriptions (Putnam, Hornstein, & Peterson, 1996) and to develop more suitable diagnostic criteria (Peterson & Putnam, 1994). While only a small segment of the therapeutic community has become aware of and feels competent in treating dissociative disorders, clinicians are rapidly being introduced to these concepts. The field has developed a critical mass of information from which clinicians can learn and understand childhood dissociative disorders. Often in my travels people tell me how excited they are to have been exposed to the concepts of the dissociative dimension. Therapists are relieved finally to have a new way of examining difficult cases. These clinicians find that cases that befuddled them before are now making sense. They have hope and a new way to engage their clients in therapy. As the field expands and we develop a mass of critical knowledge, our hopefulness about helping children and adolescents with serious dissociative disorders will grow.

References

The American Heritage dictionary of the English language (3rd ed.). (1992). Boston: Houghton Mifflin.

American Psychiatric Association. (1980). *Diagnostic and statistical manual of mental disorders* (3rd ed.). Washington, DC: Author.

American Psychiatric Association. (1987). *Diagnostic and statistical manual of mental disorders* (3rd ed., rev.). Washington, DC: Author.

American Psychiatric Association. (1991). *DSM-IV options book: (work in progress)*. Washington, DC: Author.

American Psychiatric Association. (1994). *Diagnostic and statistical manual of mental disorders* (4th ed.). Washington, DC: Author.

Armstrong, J. G., & Loewenstein, R. J. (1990). Characteristics of patients with multiple personality and dissociative disorders on psychological testing. *Journal of Nervous and Mental Disease, 178,* 448–454.

Beitchmen, J. H., Kruidenier, B., Inglis, A., & Clegg, M. (1989). The children's self-report questionnaire: Factor score age trends and gender differences. *Journal of the American Academy of Child and Adolescent Psychiatry, 28,* 714–722.

Benner, D. G., & Jocelyne, B. (1984). Multiple personality as a borderline disorder. *Journal of Nervous and Mental Disease, 172,* 98–104.

Bernstein, E. M., & Putnam, F. W. (1986). Development, reliability, and validity of a dissociation scale. *Journal of Nervous and Mental Disease, 174,* 727–735.

Bliss, E. L. (1986). *Multiple personality, allied disorders and hypnosis.* New York: Oxford University Press.

Brandenburg, N. A., Friedman, R. M., & Silver, S. E. (1990). The epidemiology of childhood psychiatric disorders: Prevalence findings from recent studies. *Journal of the American Academy of Child and Adolescent Psychiatry, 29,* 76–83.

Braun, B. G. (Ed.). (1986). *Treatment of multiple personality disorder.* Washington, DC: American Psychiatric Press.

Braun, B. G., & Sachs, R. G. (1985). The development of multiple personality disorder: Predisposing, precipitating, and perpetuating factors. In R. P. Kluft (Ed.), *Childhood Antecedents of Multiple Personality* (pp. 37–64). Washington, DC: American Psychiatric Press.

Cantwell, D. P., & Baker, L. (1989). Stability and natural history of DSM-III childhood diagnoses. *Journal of the American Academy of Child and Adolescent Psychiatry, 28,* 691–700.

Coons, P. M. (1984). The difference of diagnosis of multiple personality: A comprehensive review. *Psychiatric Clinics of North America, 7,* 51–67.

Coons, P. M., Bowman, E. S., & Milstein, V. (1988). Multiple personality disorder: A clinical investigation of 50 cases. *Journal of Nervous and Mental Disease, 176,* 519–527.

Costello, E. J. (1989). Developments in child psychiatric epidemiology. *Journal of the American Academy of Child and Adolescent Psychiatry, 28,* 836–841.

DeBellis, M. D., Chrousos, G. P., Dorn, L. D., Burke, L., Helmers, K., Kling, M. A., Trickett, P. K., & Putnam, F. W. (1994). Hypothalamic-pituitary-adrenal axis dysregulation in sexually abused girls. *Journal of Clinical Endocrinology and Metabolism, 78*(2), 249–255.

Dorland's illustrated medical dictionary. (1974.) Philadelphia: W. B. Saunders.

Esser, G. Schmidt, M. H., & Woerner, W. (1990). Epidemiology and course of psychiatric disorders in school-age children—results of a longitudinal study. *Journal of Child Psychology and Psychiatry, 31,* 243–63.

Evers-Szostak, M., & Sanders, S. (1992). The Children's Perceptual Alteration Scale (CPAS): A measure of children's dissociation. *Dissociation, 5,* 91–97.

Fagan, J., & McMahon, P. P. (1984). Incipient multiple personality in children. *Journal of Nervous and Mental Disease, 172,* 26–36.

Ferenczi, S. (1955). Confusion of Tongues Between Adults and the Child [originally: The Passions of Adults and their Influence on the Sexual and Character Development of Children]. In S. Ferenczi, *Final contribution to the problems and methods of psycho-analysis.* New York: Brunner/Mazel. (Original work published in International Journal of Psychoanalysis 1949, Vol. 30.)

Fine, C. G. (1988). The work of Antoine Despine: The first scientific report on the diagnosis and treatment of a child with multiple personality disorder. *American Journal of Clinical Hypnosis, 31,* 32–39.

Goettman, C., Greaves, G. B., & Coons, P. M. (1991). *Multiple personality and dissociation, 1791–1990: A complete bibliography.* Atlanta: George B. Greaves.

Hornstein, N. L., & Putnam, F. W. (1992). Clinical phenomenology of child and adolescent dissociative disorders. *Journal of the American Academy of Child and Adolescent Psychiatry, 31,* 1077–1085.

Hornstein, N. L., & Silberg, J. (1995, September). Diagnostic and therapeutic issues in childhood dissociative disorders [Summary]. Paper presented at the Twelfth International Fall Conference of the International Society for the Study of Dissociation, Lake Buena Vista, FL.

Hornstein N. L., & Tyson S. (1991). Inpatient treatment of children with multiple personality/dissociative disorders and their families. *Psychiatric Clinics of North America, 3,* 631–648.

Kagan, J. (1984). *The nature of the child.* New York: Basic Books.

Kluft, R. P. (1984). Treatment of multiple personality disorder: A study of 33 cases. *Psychiatric Clinics of North America, 7,* 9–29.

Kluft, R. P. (Ed.). (1985a). *Childhood Antecedents of Multiple Personality.* Washington, DC: American Psychiatric Press.

Kluft, R. P. (1985b). Natural history of multiple personality disorder. In R. P. Kluft (Ed.), *Childhood Antecedents of Multiple Personality* (pp. 197–238). Washington, DC: American Psychiatric Press.

Kluft, R. P. (1985c). Childhood Multiple Personality Disorder: Predictors, Treatment Findings and Treatment Results. In R. P. Kluft (Ed.), *Childhood An-*

tecedents of Multiple Personality (pp. 167–196). Washington, DC: American Psychiatric Press.

Kluft, R. P. (1991). Clinical presentations of multiple personality disorder. *Psychiatric Clinics of North America 3*, 605–630.

Lewis, D. O. (1991). Multiple personality. In M. Lewis (Ed.), *Child and adolescent psychiatry: A comprehensive textbook* (pp. 707–715). Baltimore: Williams and Wilkins.

Lewis, D. O., & Putnam, F. W., Eds. (1996). *Dissociative disorders. Child and Adolescent Psychiatric Clinics of North Americas.*

Malenbaum, R., & Russell, A. T. (1987). Multiple personality disorder in an eleven-year-old boy and his mother. *Journal of the American Academy of Child and Adolescent Psychiatry, 26,* 436–439.

Marmer, S. S., and Fink, D. (1994). Rethinking the comparison of borderline personality disorder and multiple personality disorder. *Psychiatric Clinics of North America 17* (4), 743–771.

McClellan, J. M., & Bernet, W. (1995, October). Review of practice parameters: "bipolar disorder." Symposium at the Annual Meeting of the American Academy of Child and Adolescent Psychiatry, New Orleans, LA.

McHugh, P. R., & Putnam, F. W. (1995). Resolved: Multiple personality disorder is an individually and socially created artifact. *Journal of the American Academy of Child and Adolescent Psychiatry, 34,* 957–959.

Nash, M. R., Hulsey, T. L., Sexton, M. C., Harralson, T. L., & Lambert, W. (1993). Long-term sequelae of childhood sexual abuse: Perceived family environment, psychopathology, and dissociation. *Journal of Clinical and Consulting Psychology, 61,* 256–283.

North, C. S., Ryall, J. M., Ricci, D. A., & Wetzel, R. D. (1993). *Multiple personalities, multiple disorders: psychiatric classification and media influence.* New York: Oxford University Press.

Peterson, G. (1989). Assessment and diagnosis of child and adolescent multiple personality disorder: issues and procedures [Summary]. *Proceedings of the Sixth International Conference on Multiple Personality/Dissociative States,* Chicago, IL, 176.

Peterson, G. (1990). Diagnosis of childhood multiple personality disorder. *Dissociation, 3,* 3–9.

Peterson, G. (1991a). Children coping with trauma: Diagnosis of "Dissociation Identity Disorder." *Dissociation, 4,* 152–164.

Peterson, G. (1991b). Description of a proposed diagnostic category of dissociative disorder of childhood for consideration by the dissociative disorders study group of the Task Force on *DSM-IV.* Chapel Hill, NC: University of North Carolina at Chapel Hill Department of Psychiatry.

Peterson, G. (1995, September). Dissociative disorder symptoms in youth: A mosaic [Summary]. Paper presented at the Twelfth International Fall Conference of the International Society for the Study of Dissociation, Lake Buena Vista, FL.

Peterson, G. (in press). *Dissociative disorders in youth: A primer.* Washington, DC: American Psychiatric Press.

Peterson, G., & Putnam, F. W. (1992). Progress towards "Dissociative Disorder of

Childhood" [Summary]. *Proceedings of the Ninth International Conference on Multiple Personality / Dissociative States,* Chicago, IL, 15.

Peterson, G., & Putnam, F. W. (1994). Preliminary results of the field trial of proposed criteria for dissociative disorder of childhood. *Dissociation, 7,* 209–220.

Peterson, G., & Putnam, F. W. (1995, October). Childhood dissociative disorders: Assessment and treatment. Workshop at American Academy of Child and Adolescent Psychiatry Annual Meeting. New Orleans, LA.

Putnam, F. W. (1989). *Diagnosis and treatment of multiple personality disorder.* New York: Guilford Press.

Putnam, F. W. (in press). *Pathological dissociation: a developmental approach.* New York: Guilford Press.

Putnam, F. W., Guroff, J. J., Silberman, E. K., Barban, L., & Post, R. M. (1986). The clinical phenomenology of multiple personality disorder: A review of 100 recent cases. *Journal of Clinical Psychiatry, 47,* 285–293.

Putnam, F. W., Helmers, K., Horowitz, L. A., & Trickett, P. K. (1995). Hypnotizability and dissociativity in sexually abused girls. *Child Abuse & Neglect, 19* (5), 645–655.

Putnam, F. W., Helmers, K., & Trickett, P. K. (1993). Development, reliability and validity of a child dissociation scale. *Child Abuse and Neglect, 17,* 731–742.

Putnam, F. W., Hornstein, N. L., & Peterson, G. (1996). Clinical phenomenology of child and adolescent dissociative disorders: Gender and age effects. In D. O. Lewis & F. W. Putnam (Eds.), *Dissociative disorders. Child and Adolescent Psychiatric Clinics of North America.*

Putnam, F. W., & Peterson, G. (1994). Further validation of the Child Dissociative Checklist. *Dissociation, 7,* 204–209.

Reagor, P. A., Kasten, J. D., & Morelli, N. (1992). A checklist for screening dissociative disorders in children and adolescents. *Dissociation, 5,* 4–19.

Ross, C. A. (1989). *Multiple personality disorder: diagnosis, clinical features and treatment.* New York: John Wiley & Sons.

Ross, C. A., Heber, S., Norton, G. R., Anderson, D., Anderson, G., & Barchet, P. (1989). The dissociative disorders interview schedule: A structured interview. *Dissociation, 2,* 169–189.

Ross, C. A., Norton, G. R., & Wozney, K. (1989). Multiple personality disorder: An analysis of 236 cases. *Canadian Journal of Psychiatry, 34,* 413–418.

Shaffer, D., Campbell, M., Cantwell, D., Bradley, S., Carlson, G., Cohen, D., Denckla, M., Frances, A., Garfinkel, B., Klein, R., Pincus, H., Spitzer, R. L., Volkmar, F., & Widiger, T. (1989). Child and adolescent psychiatric disorders in *DSM-IV*: Issues facing the work group. *Journal of the American Academy of Child and Adolescent Psychiatry, 28,* 830–835

Shaffer, D., Campbell, M., Cantwell, D., Carlson, G., Cohen, D., First, M., A., Garfinkel, B., Klein, R., Lahey, B., Loeber, R., Newcorn, J., & Pincus, H. (1990). Progress towards *DSM-IV* [Summary]. *Scientific Proceedings of the Annual Meeting of the American Academy of Child and Adolescent Psychiatry,* 35–36.

Shirar, L. (1996). *Dissociative children: Bridging the inner and outer worlds.* New York: Norton.

Silberg, J. (1996a). *The dissociative child: diagnosis, treatment, and management.* Lutherville, MD: Sidran Press.

Silberg, J. (1996b). Dissociative disorders in children. In J. D. Noshpitz (Ed.), *Handbook of child and adolescent psychiatry*. Vol. II New York: John Wiley & Sons.

Snowden, C. (1988). Where are all the childhood multiples? Identifying incipient multiple personality in children. [Summary]. *Proceedings of the Fifth International Conference on Multiple Personality / Dissociative States, 36.*

Steinberg, M., Rounsaville, B., & Cicchetti, V. (1990). The structured clinical interview for *DSM-III-R Dissociative Disorders:* Preliminary report on a new diagnostic instrument. *American Journal of Psychiatry, 147,* 76–81.

van der Kolk, B. A. (1987). *Psychological trauma.* Washington, DC: American Psychiatric Press.

van der Kolk, B. A. (1994). The body keeps the score: Memory and the evolving psychobiology of posttraumatic stress. *Harvard Review of Psychiatry, 1* (January/February), 253–265.

Wiener, J, England, M. J., Frances, A. J., First, M. B., Wise, T. N., Holland, J. C., & Williams, J. B. W. (1995, May). *DSM-IV Update.* Symposium at the Annual Meeting of the American Psychiatric Association. Miami, FL.

World Health Organization. (1992). *The ICD-10 classification of mental and behavioural disorders: Clinical descriptions and diagnostic guidelines*. Geneva: Author.

two

Complexities of Psychiatric Differential Diagnosis in Children with Dissociative Symptoms and Disorders

Nancy L. Hornstein

The development of a reasonable diagnostic understanding of a child's psychiatric difficulties is only at its most elementary stage when dissociative symptoms are first recognized or suspected. This chapter will focus on the processes of investigation and integration that enable the clinician to identify dissociative disorders and to distinguish between the different diagnoses that can be associated with dissociative symptoms. Further, the clinician will be presented with cognitive strategies to assist in the process of sorting through the symptomatic presentation of children whose diagnosis is baffling and elusive. A review of the childhood diagnostic literature on dissociative disorders begins this chapter. Next, the relationship between diagnostic categories and dissociative symptoms will be explored. Strategies for diagnostic evaluation will be illustrated with case examples.

History of the Diagnosis of Dissociative Disorders in Children

Initial interest in identifying childhood cases of dissociative disorders (DDs) arose from clinical experience with adult MPD patients who not only recounted experiences of severe childhood trauma, but also described the childhood onset of their disorder. Kluft in 1978 and Putnam in 1981 pioneered the effort to identify childhood cases of DDs through the development of childhood MPD predictor lists (Kluft, 1984). Kluft followed with the first published description of a small clinical series of children treated for MPD (Kluft, 1984), and was joined that same year by Fagan & McMahon's description of incipient Multiple Personality Disorder in childhood (Fagan & McMahon, 1984). As it became increasingly documented that the vast majority of adult dissociative patients reported experiencing severe early childhood trauma (Chu & Dill, 1990; Coon, Bowman, & Milstein, 1988; Greaves, 1980; Putnam, Guroff, Silberman, Barban, & Post, 1986; Ross, Miller, Bjornson, Reagor, Fraser, & Anderson, 1990; Ross, Norton, & Wozney, 1989; Schulz, Braun, & Kluft, 1989; Stern, 1984), interest in this area further intensified. This resulted in an increased publication of single case reports and small case series of child and adolescent DDs (Bowman, Blix, and Coons, 1985, Dell & Eisenhower, 1990; Fagan & McMahon, 1984; Hornstein & Tyson, 1991; Kluft, 1984; Malenbaum and Russel, 1987; Peterson, 1990; Riley & Mead, 1988; Vincent & Pickering, 1988; Weiss, Sutton, & Utecht, 1985).

The publication of the first case reports added fuel to the effort to identify and treat this group of children. Particularly significant were the findings that dissociative disorders are among the sequelae of early childhood trauma, including severe, ongoing sexual abuse (Bliss, 1984; Braun, 1985, 1990; Dell & Eisenhower, 1990; Hornstein & Putnam, 1992; Hornstein & Tyson, 1991; Ludwig, 1983; Putnam, 1985; Putnam, Guroff, Silberman, Barban, & Post, 1986; Ross, Norton, & Wozney, 1989; Ross, Miller, Bjornson, Reagor, Fraser, & Anderson, 1991; Schulz, Braun, & Kluft, 1989), and that early recognition of these symptoms made intervention with the child and his or her family possible, preventing a continuation of the abuse. In addition, early, appropriate therapeutic intervention was postulated to relieve children's dissociative symptoms more rapidly than those of their adult counterparts (Kluft, 1984, 1985a, 1985b, 1986).

As the child literature began developing, objections to the apparent "newness" of dissociative disorders were not as typical among child psychiatrists as they seemingly still are elsewhere in the psychiatric community. Perhaps this is because child psychiatrists see the symptomatic sequelae of severe abuse and neglect immediately proximate to its occurrence. They may also be aware that these psychiatric conditions were clearly described in clinical reports of the nineteenth and early twentieth centuries (Bowman, 1990; Fine, 1988) or of other symptomatic descriptions that sound similar to clinical descriptions of dissociative disorder patients. For example, although dissociative defenses are not recognized and identified as such, the child development literature is replete with descriptions of children utilizing defenses readily recognizable as dissociative when experiencing extreme degrees of danger and deprivation (Barach, 1991; Main, 1990; Siegel, 1995). For an excellent example of such an article see Fraiberg's "Pathological Defenses in Infancy" (Fraiberg, 1982).

Research on dissociative disorders in childhood lagged somewhat behind the burgeoning adult DD literature. Until very recently, a low index of suspicion among child clinicians and the absence of substantiated clinical profiles of childhood DDs made it difficult to differentiate these complex polysymptomatic cases from more commonly diagnosed childhood conditions (Kluft, 1985a; Kluft, 1985b; Putnam, 1991; Hornstein & Tyson, 1991).

Other complexities were noted in identifying these children; for example, dissociation as a normative phenomenon changes enormously over the course of development. Putnam (1985) and Steinberg (1991) separately describe elements of these changes, including the shifts in attention, forgetfulness, and contextually determined sense of identity common in young children and the transient depersonalization experiences common in adolescents.

Kluft noted the inherent limitations childhood social and economic realities place on opportunities for a DID child's alternate personalities (alters) to express their separateness and that additionally, adolescent development includes the emergence of adult sexuality and a coalescence of identity, along with separation/individuation tasks, all of which may influence the symptomatic expression of DID (Kluft 1984, 1985a, 1985b).

Finally, it bears emphasizing that a child's access to the mental health system requires the involvement of parents or other guardians. Given the family dysfunction associated with the development of DDs, this factor is likely to both limit the number of cases presenting in childhood and influence the nature of the cases that do present. In an article on inpatient treatment of children with DDs, we point out that a number of cases presented for treatment through foster or residential care placements only after being removed from their homes because of documented abuse (Hornstein & Tyson, 1991).

The literature on children with DSM-IV (American Psychiatric Association, 1994) diagnoses of Dissociative Identity Disorder (DID) and those with Dissociative Disorder Not Otherwise Specified (DDNOS) now typifies them as a group uniquely presenting to the mental health system as polysymptomatic, traumatized children with difficult behavior problems (Bowman, Blix, & Coons, 1985; Dell & Eisenhower, 1990; Fagan & McMahon, 1984; Hornstein & Putnam, 1992; Hornstein & Tyson, 1991; Kluft, 1984; Malenbaum and Russel, 1987; Peterson, 1990; Riley & Mead, 1988; Vincent & Pickering, 1988; Weiss, Sutton, & Utecht, 1985), and as challenging both to diagnostic acumen and to therapeutic expertise.

Putnam and I reported the first large case series that compares systematically gathered clinical data on two separately diagnosed samples of children and adolescents with dissociative disorders (64 cases—44 MPD and 20 DDNOS) (Hornstein & Putnam, 1992). This study helped further delineate the clinical phenomenology of child and adolescent dissociative disorders. Another study followed with similar findings (Peterson & Putnam, 1994). These symptomatic profiles correspond closely to earlier predictor lists for childhood multiple personality disorder (Fagan & McMahon, 1984; Kluft, 1985a; Kluft, 1985b). This convergence of similar findings serves to strengthen the validity of dissociative diagnoses in children.

Symptoms vs. Diagnosis

In *DSM-IV* (1994), the category of "Dissociative Disorders" subsumes the diagnoses of dissociative identity disorder, dissociative amnesia, dissociative fugue, depersonalization disorder, and dissociative disorder not otherwise specified. Disorders classed in other categories where dissociative symptoms have also been described (though this is not adequately attended to in diagnostic manuals) include posttraumatic stress disorder, somatoform disorders, eating disorders, paraphilias, impulse-control disorders; and in children, reactive attachment disorder and feeding and rating disorders of infancy or early childhood. In both adults and children, dissociative symptoms are recognized to occur in the symptom category problems related to abuse or neglect. In addition, dissociative symptoms can at times be a part of any severe mental illness, such as acute psychotic disorders especially brief reactive psychoses, acute onset of severe psychosis in schizophrenia, major depression with psychotic features, and mania. In some children with pervasive developmental disorders, dissociative symptoms may occasionally be present as well.

What is the clinician to make of the presence of dissociative symptoms in patients with other primary psychiatric diagnoses? How can we determine and, if possible, treat the cause of the patient's illness? Dissociative disorders have a markedly different cause from many acute psychoses. Little has been published to date on how to differentiate between dissociative symptoms and a dissociative disorder with its accompanying primary disturbances in identity during childhood. There is also a dearth of clinical understanding of the complex psychological processes involved in "self reference," or the sense of ownership of one's own emotions, thoughts, and behaviors; the diagnostician is thus perplexed at times when faced with a patient using dissociative defenses. This is a fascinating, useful, and complex area for future research.

Clinical experience suggests that acutely stressful psychiatric dysfunction leads patients to utilize whatever defenses are available to reduce anxiety and the feelings of personality fragmentation. A number of psychiatric symptoms are therefore not diagnostically specific; for example, delusions, hallucinations, and trouble focusing attention can be seen across illnesses with diverse etiologies. The possibility that dissociative symptoms represent a dissociative disorder instead of, or in addition to, the initial diagnosis should be extensively investigated. When clear dissociative processes exist in conjunction with other diagnoses, it may be most appropriate to consider the dissociative disorder a "super-ordinate diagnosis" (Putnam, 1991) encompassing the other observed symptomatology. However, when the use of dissociative defenses is less predominant, the evaluator should consider the possibility that dissociation is a way of coping with the traumatic aspects of severe psychiatric symptoms (distorted perceptions, thoughts, extreme dysphoria, altered perceptions of the patient's significant others). If the dissociative symptoms in other psychiatric conditions are viewed as a "stress" reaction, the psychotherapeutic aspects of treatment needed for recovery of function might involve education about their condition and minimization of the psychiatric symptoms rather than attention to the dissociative defenses per se.

Preschool and early school age children in the process of personality and cognitive development are particularly apt to utilize dissociation because of the developmental lag in their elaboration of more complicated defensive possibilities (Albini & Pease, 1989; Putnam, 1991). In preschool age or younger children, the occasional use of dissociation abilities in play (imaginary companions) or times of distress (staring off into space, going to sleep) is normative. Diagnosis of a dissociative disorder in this age group is a function of the pervasiveness, frequency, degree of interference with function, and atypical features of the dissociative symptoms and requires an in-depth knowledge of developmental norms and ranges. Silberg (1994; 1996) is developing diagnostic tools to assist clinicians in making the fine distinctions between normative developmental variations and significant dissociative symptoms/dissociative disorders.

To further complicate the diagnosis of a dissociative disorder in children, there are factors that delay and interfere with the child's development of an integrative identity or reflective self-awareness. These factors can include an environmental chaos and trauma sufficient to create a level of anxiety and internal conflict that impedes full integration (Group 1) and/or congenital biophysiologic impairments or interferences in the perceptual, cognitive, and organizing abilities that are required to develop an integrated identity (Group 2). These factors, singly or in combination, produce a range of difficulties in the normative development of an integrated self.

At one end of the range are children who are reactive and avoidant beings who are unable to engage in any but the most superficial interactions and who dissociate and seem to be without any stable identity. These children are more impaired than those with stable but dissociated identities (dissociative identity disorder, DID). When their disturbance has a largely environmental basis (Group 1), these children fall into the DSM-IV diagnostic category of dissociative disorder not otherwise specified (DDNOS).

At the same time, there is another group of children in this category who are very different on a functional and prognostic level, children who exhibit extensive use of dissociative defenses and who have developed and are able to maintain a fair level of self-integration, despite the impingement of traumatic anxiety and internal conflict. Children whose disturbance in self-integration has a largely biophysiologic basis (Group 2) often most appropriately receive other psychiatric diagnoses. The "developmental psychodynamics" of aspects of their difficulties outlined above is often overlooked in favor of attention to the chemical or structural aspects of their illnesses. Clinical experience with including treatment strategies aimed at assisting the child to develop more adaptive defensive strategies and the highest level of self-integration possible have helped reduce their symptomatic functional impairments in combination with other treatment modalities. A recognition of the dissociative nature of some of their defenses can provide for a more thorough apprehension of their adaptational problems.

Careful evaluation and a resistance to closure of diagnostic questions are essential to diagnostic evaluation and treatment of children in this age range. Development proceeds at a rapid clip and basic assumptions that underly psychiatric diagnoses, such as stability over time or sustained vulnerability, are inapplicable. There are also children whose disturbance most likely comes from a combination of biophysiologic vulnerability and either overt abuse and neglect or an environment that creates more conflict and distress than they are able to handle, even though the environment would likely not cause the same level of disturbance in a child with greater internal resources. (See Chapter 3 for further discussion of this patient group.) While the complexities of diagnostic evaluation of preschool and early school age children have been emphasized above, similar principles apply to children of all ages and have been useful adjuncts for a more complete diagnostic understanding of adults with dissociative symptoms as well.

Evaluation of Dissociation in Childhood

The development of a full profile of the child's symptoms is key to accurate diagnosis. Standard psychological testing should be obtained, including IQ and educational testing. When speech and language testing is available, this is of additional benefit. Whatever testing is commonly employed by each individual clinician to delineate depressive, anxiety, attentional, and behavioral symptoms should be included as indicated by the presenting complaints of the patient (assuming the clinician is up to current standards in symptomatic evaluation).

The Child Dissociative Checklist (CDC), (Putnam, Helmers, & Trickett, 1993) should be given to all children with dissociative symptoms as the only current standardized measure for quantifying dissociative behaviors in children. Standard psychological testing should be conducted and reviewed in terms of the test markers described by Dr. Silberg in this volume and elsewhere (Silberg, 1994, 1996) to aid detection and quantification of dissociative symptoms evident during the test procedures. Dr. Silberg's work should be reviewed by all clinicians interested in child dissociative disorders, since it facilitates a thorough understanding of manifestations of dissociation and is an exciting diagnostic tool with enormous research potential. Adolescents may also be given the Adolescent Dissociative Experiences Scale (Armstrong et al.; see Appendix A.) The clinical interview and behavioral observation are also indispensable for the evaluation of dissociation.

Clinical interview

Clinical experience interviewing children about their internal world is inordinately helpful when attempting to inquire about their dissociative symptoms. The child's age and developmental level profoundly influence the ways in which they recount these experiences. Experience interviewing normal children and those with other than dissociative diagnoses is helpful for developing a clinical impression about what are or are not normative responses to questioning. I am often asked to evaluate fairly average youngsters after an inexperienced clinician became overly concerned about their active fantasy life. The child and I enjoyed ourselves, but the parents were often distraught over the implications of the referral. Children younger than preadolescence have difficulty with abstract concepts and do not place events in time, except grossly in terms of recent big events (before or after their birthday) and even in this example there is limited reliability to their account. This is one of the developmental challenges when seeking information about amnesia and "time loss" experiences. The most successful approach involves anchoring inquiry in the events of the child's daily life. I ask them whether they ever "had anything happen like . . ." and describe different experiences, such as being confused that the teacher is in the middle of writing math problems on the board when the last thing they knew she was reading them a story, or they don't remember eating lunch some days, or when they ask to do something (go to the bathroom, get a drink of water), people tell them "you just did that" but they don't remember doing it, etc. I then get the child to describe in his or her own words experiences like this he or she has had. Typically children are interested in personal things that happen and provide an experience that is clearly dissociative ("Oh yeah, like this morning, I thought we just got up and I didn't know why we didn't have breakfast before going up to school, but Cynthia [the nurse] told me we had breakfast and are going back to school *again* after the break.") or more normative ("Do you mean daydreaming? Sometimes I am embarrassed because I am thinking something else and not listening to the teacher's questions."). I may ask if they ever miss half a class, or half a day. ("No, I don't think so. No, I would definitely know that—just maybe a question or two—when my name gets called I sort of wake up.")

Differentiating dissociative experiences from motivated forgetting or "lies" presents another set of difficulties with school-age children. Asking children about positive behaviors they can't remember is a way to get less motivated distortion in recall. Asking children whether they ever got thanked or told they did something helpful that they didn't recall and getting an idea of the frequency with which this occurs can be useful information. Another interviewing "tip" is that children often have incomplete amnesia, so asking if they recall anything about a behavioral incident and to "see if when you close your eyes anything pops into your mind" often brings some useful detail about the child's dissociative process. These are the occurrences in which dissociative youngsters describe control/influence phenomenon, e.g. "my arm was just hitting him, I was saying no to my arm but it kept on going. There was a somebody telling me to butt out." "Who was telling you?" "I don't know, some man, a man's voice only, I don't know from where, in my head?" In contrast, "motivated forgetters" tend to simply "draw a blank" until they trust you not to "make them feel bad."

Children who dissociate often are amnestic for emotionally laden experiences, such as explosive outbursts, punishment, or school yard fights and may confabulate a memory based on others' reports to them about their behavior in order to "appear normal" or avoid punishment for lying. Therefore, asking children whether they remember "the whole thing" or "have blanks" and finding out if they really remember these experiences or only know what they did because someone told them afterwards can help detect dissociative experiences that may be covered up. Some highly dissociative youngsters may be surprised or confused by these questions, indicating that they always thought remembering something meant knowing what somebody else described about your behavior. A patient, inquiring attitude with careful attention to whether what the child is describing is understood correctly is an important ingredient for successful interviews.

Observing the child for signs of dissociation during the interview, such as forgetting the question, amnesia for an earlier part of the interview, suddenly staring off into space when a question is stressful or otherwise, and careful questioning about what the child is experiencing (contradictory commentary, thought fragmentation, voices) often yields additional information about dissociative experiences. (For more information on interviewing see the following chapter.)

Observational data

Observing directly the behavioral manifestations of dissociation over an extended time period provides additional diagnostic information. This can be accomplished easily during a brief inpatient stay, or alternatively, in the classroom or during after-school activities. Observation of family interaction is also recommended. Behaviors to watch for include disavowal of witnessed behavior, amnesia for activities or behaviors observed, fluctuations in apparent attentional ability, concentration, knowledge, or performance, entrance into spontaneous trance-like states in which the child is oblivious to external stimuli (often leading to evaluation for seizure activity), and learning or reading difficulties.

In children with Dissociative Identity Disorder (DID) there are "switches" between different "states of consciousness" experienced as alternate personalities (alters). As in their adult counterparts, these alters in children with DID manifest relatively stable patterns of behavior, affect, gestures, speech patterns (tone, pitch, complexity of language etc.), manner of relating, and aspects of identity (gender and role identifications, name, age, etc.), that differ from one another.

The first clue that a child inpatient had DID came when an ordinarily ultra-feminine girl, calling herself Joanne, suddenly became rough and tomboyish, exhibiting differences in mannerism and voice tone during a baseball game. She insisted upon being called "Jo" in this setting. By the time she returned to the unit, she again was feminine, calling herself Joanne. When asked about the boyish uniform she still wore, and why she asked to be called "Jo" earlier, she initially stared blankly, then she said, "Oh, I'm never really there when I have to do that boy stuff." When asked what she meant, she shrugged, later elaborating, "Oh, I think that some boy Jo that talks to me takes my place." She was asked how this works. Her reply "I don't know really, I don't remember it well" preceded her entry into a state in which she appeared dazed, then had an abrupt change in manner, saying "I don't want to talk about this shit, Doc, Joanne don't bother anybody, this ain't really none of your concern." Needless to say, this was the first dissociative "change in personality" that was witnessed in her.

In children, these "switches" between alternate personality states are frequently observable as rapid age regression, sudden shifts in demeanor or personality characteristics, or marked variations in ability and skill level. The younger the child, the less elaborated these alters are relative to the often extensive elaboration of separate "personality characteristics" seen in the alters of adult DID patients. Children may be very subtle and resourceful in the ways their "alters" attempt to assert their separate identities, requiring close attention to detail on the part of the clinician.

A nine-year-old boy reported having three separate selves, a good, bad, and regular Larry. In the process of trying to understand whether or not these "selves" represented dissociative phenomenon, he was asked if it would be possible for others to identify which self he was at a given moment. He smiled slyly and said, "Yes, but they'd have to know how to." "What would they have to know?" "Well, the good Larry is all in white and is a good Larry fairy, and the bad Larry is in red like a devil, the regular Larry is just plain skin." "Well, which Larry is speaking now?" A broad smile: "Well, I'm the bad Larry, since you're asking about all the problems, I'm wearing a red shirt and you're wearing red too." Further interviewing made it clear this boy had DID.

Children's alters often have less investment in the "separateness" of their identities, and there tend to be less rigid amnestic barriers among the different personality states. I have rarely seen children, even those with a DID diagnosis, who present with open revelations about "having different personalities." At most they complained of "hearing voices" or behaving in ways they "couldn't explain" or "couldn't remember." They were unanimous in their secretiveness and fear that talking about their subjective experiences of dissociative phenomenon made them "weirdos." They were fearful of what other children and adults would think of them if they knew about this, and in all cases one basis of the treatment alliance was their expectation that their therapist would help them have more control so that these phenomena could be even more private than they were initially. There was relatively no observable secondary gain through dramatics or attention seeking for their disorder. In several of the children, observations of dissociative symptomatology were present for some time before a diagnosis of DID could be made. For two of the children, the diagnosis could only be finalized during subsequent hospitalizations. In these cases it took some time for the children to develop a level of trust that allowed them to be open about the subjective component of their dissociative behaviors.

There are ongoing questions about the role of development in the elaboration and organization of dissociative experience into alternate personalities during childhood. Children with Dissociative Disorder Not Otherwise Specified (DDNOS) may exhibit regressions, trance states, and difficulty integrating aspects of their feelings and behaviors similar to the difficulties of DID patients. These may be children who have yet to obtain the developmental organization and structure present in those with identifiable alters, or they may be children on the road to developing further integration. Observation over time is needed to tell which direction the developmental trend is taking. It is important to maintain a high index of suspicion in children with extensive abuse histories and the presence of some dissociative symptoms before a DD is ruled out, especially when symptoms suggestive of other disorders do not respond to usual treatment approaches.

Historical Data

To obtain a history to assist in the diagnosis of children who dissociate, the information contained in a detailed and thorough year-by-year history of the child's life can guide observations and assist in developing diagnostic and dynamic formulations. Data about the child's caregivers, the nature of family stressors, details of the living environment, the child's behaviors, developmental milestones attained (or lost), emergence of symptoms, along with careful descriptions of each symptom, including precipitating and ameliorating factors, should be obtained. Descriptions of traumatic experiences should indicate the timeframes and circum-stances surrounding them. These include detailed descriptions of physi-cal and sexual abuse, hospitalizations, extensive medical treatment, wit-nessing family violence, loss or separation from caregivers (including their hospitalizations, suicide attempts, periods in drug treatment, jail, etc.). Symptoms and behaviors that may represent dissociative experi-ences should be explored in depth. Information about psychiatric symp-toms in family members, including dissociative experiences, childhood trauma/abuse,and substance abuse can also be important in directing an evaluation.

Differential Diagnosis

Once detailed information has been obtained about the patient's current and historical symptoms and an in-depth understanding of the dissocia-tive symptoms has been obtained from observation and interview, it is easier to proceed with differential diagnosis to determine (a) what is the primary diagnosis, and (b) if a dissociative disorder is either a primary or co-morbid diagnosis, what is the most accurate diagnosis.

At this juncture, it is not uncommon to continue to experience some uncertainty and confusion in cases with combinations of complex and se-vere symptomatic presentations, poor "object relations," mistrust, and a history of numerous previous diagnoses and a confusing or absent re-sponse to prior treatment (seemingly the norm in some childhood DD cases). It can be helpful to sit down and compile a list of symptoms, be-haviors, and historical information. This list is then used to formulate the differential diagnosis. Diagnostic possibilities are posed and efforts are made to fit the items on the list under each diagnostic category. The like-lihood of the diagnosis is proportional to its explanatory power in terms of the symptoms, behaviors, and history and how much is left unexplained. Diagnoses that offer great explanatory power are preferable to several co-morbid diagnoses, and effort is made to utilize as few diagnoses as possible.

It is desirable to involve the entire treatment team in this process, or, in cases of outpatient treatment with a solo practitioner, to use consul-tants to assist efforts to achieve an accurate diagnosis in cases of over-whelming complexity. This differential diagnostic process may guide fur-ther testing and examination to rule in or out diagnostic possibilities. For example, an EEG may be needed to rule out a seizure disorder as an ex-planation for staring spells in a child with DDNOS. Structured diagnos-tic interviews may help in historical exploration of symptom development and course over time to evaluate the explanatory fit of some diagnostic possibilities.

Differential diagnosis requires an awareness of the possible manifestations of a variety of symptoms and how they are expressed in dissociative children. The complicated symptomatic picture present in children with DDs is created by the interaction between their use of dissociative defenses, the symptoms arising from past traumatic experiences, and the problems they experience in regulating their affect and behavior and establishing an integrated experience of self and others. The symptomatic difficulties described are based on the findings of an earlier referenced study (Hornstein & Putnam, 1992). Following is a disucssion of some symptoms included in the presentation of childhood DDs.

Affect

Symptoms such as irritability, affect lability, depression, feelings of hopelessness, low self-esteem, self-blame, etc. are common in children with DDs. Many have suicidal ideation; some actually attempt suicide. The children with DID tend to make more serious suicide attempts. In observing DD children over time, chronic dysphoria, typically unresponsive to antidepressant medication, is often present along with a very reactive mood atypical of affective disorder. They are up when things are going well, but are exquisitely sensitive to slights, frustrations, and alterations in the mood and attentiveness of caregivers and have extreme rejection sensitivity. Following a perceived injury to their self-esteem, their mood often plummets, suicidal ideation may emerge, and they can remain dysphoric for days.

In children with DID, there are identifiable alternate personalities who are sad, hopeless, and full of self-blame for the abuse they experienced. Environmental "triggers" that in some way remind the children of their abuse frequently precipitate a switch into one of these alternate personalities. Typically DD children hold themselves responsible for abusive, neglectful behavior of others towards them, and for other difficulties they experience in relationships. Their feelings of hopelessness and worthlessness, while transitory, can lead to serious suicide attempts, such as running out in front of cars or, in the case of one young girl, attempting self-electrocution by inserting a knife in a light socket.

Anxiety / posttraumatic symptoms

DD children can be described as "sick with worry"; often they have realistic or understandable concerns about the stability of their relationships, the endurance of the regard in which others hold them, the well-being of their caregivers, and their own adequacy unlike other anxiety disorders. The classic posttraumatic stress disorder symptoms of hyper-vigilance, hyper-startle, fears, flashbacks, avoidant behaviors, and intrusive thoughts related to traumatic experiences and traumatic nightmares are usually present.

The hours before bedtime are associated for many DD children with the emergence of intrusive thoughts about abuse and can be a period in which dissociative symptoms such as spontaneous age regressions, amnesias, and switches in personality occur. For other children, use of the bathroom facilities brings on sudden reactions of terror, flashbacks, or dissociative phenomena as well. An eleven-year-old boy with DID first showed signs of dissociation when he was discovered huddling in a corner of the bathroom, disoriented as to location and the identity of a familiar caregiver. Later, it was discovered that this child had been repeatedly and violently sodomized, continued to experience pain with bowel movements related to his injuries, and had severe flashbacks whenever he attempted to use the toilet.

Conduct / behavioral problems

Temper outbursts, oppositional or disruptive behavior, and problems with aggression and fighting are typical reasons for bringing a DD child for treatment. Although often accused of lying, these children frequently have at least partial amnesia for their explosive, aggressive, disruptive behaviors. These behaviors can be sudden, unpredicted, and out of keeping with the child's usual demeanor. The triad of enuresis, cruelty to animals, and fire-setting has not been presented in cases I have seen to date.

The child's frequent misperceptions of interactions, perceived threats, and rejection hypersensitivity play a role in producing these problems. Often abrupt behavior changes are preceded by a switch in personality in children with DID. Children with DDNOS have similar alterations in perception and cognition during temper explosions although they may retain conscious recall and some ability to integrate these behaviors.

Usually, when the dissociative aspect of the child's explosions are recognized, the child can be assisted to gain better control of these behaviors, unlike neurologically based "episodic dyscontrol." Caregivers who are made aware of the kinds of perceptual and cognitive distortions that occur when these children enter a state of defensive upset are also more effective at providing appropriate reassurance to these children, preventing the familiar eruption into aggressive behavior.

Sexual Behaviors

Sexualized play, inappropriate sexual behavior, compulsive masturbation and promiscuity are frequent and some DD children, including some very young children, have perpetrated sexual assaults or abuse on other children. Children with DDs and a history of severe sexual abuse can be troubled by a variety of issues related to sexuality and their sexual identity. For some, sexual acting out is a way of compulsively reenacting their own experiences; for others it serves as a reassurance that "they were normal," allaying fears of homosexuality in boys who were molested by male perpetrators or who are attempting to affirm their attractiveness and control over relationships. For a few, there is sexual excitement in the victimization of others, and many are vulnerable to re-victimization by adults or other children.

Attention / concentration, learning problems

High levels of anxiety, posttraumatic symptoms, and dissociative trance states, amnesias, etc. frequently manifest themselves through difficulty attending to lessons and concentrating on school work. Some children have significant auditory processing difficulties, learning problems, or difficulty with reading. Again, those children who have been followed through their course of treatment have had remarkable amelioration of these difficulties as their internal disruption has been decreased. This is all the more surprising given the past history of intrauterine exposure to alcohol/drugs and past head trauma to which some of these children were exposed. Co-morbid diagnoses are of course possible but even when assumed present and treated as such, the better part of clinical wisdom is served through reevaluation as treatment progresses.

Dissociative episodes in childhood may be evident at times as perplexing variations in the child's knowledge, skill level, and performance. Different alters may have differing abilities and knowledge or may have no conscious recall of having learned something when another alter was present. Marked variations on psychological tests assessing similar abilities may be seen, or there can be enormous variations on the same test on different days as the child experiences switches in personality.

A striking example of this was a young girl who had evidence of nerve deafness on two subsequent but different examinations, but in different ears. Neurologically, her hearing was perfectly intact in both ears, but when she dissociated she had two different alters, each experiencing deafness in opposite ears. The deafness was a conversion symptom related to two separate traumatic incidents.

Hallucinations / thought process disturbances

Auditory hallucinations are present in most dissociative children. In the majority of cases the child hears a voice or voices experienced as arising internally and having distinctive characteristics such as age, gender, and personal attributes (for example, "the voice of my father telling me I'm no good"). These are similar to descriptions by adults with DID of their auditory hallucinations. Other types of hallucinations may also be experienced, such as seeing "ghosts," having visual hallucinations of alters, and less commonly, a variety of somatic and tactile hallucinations, often representing hallucinated reexperiences of a somatic or sensory element of dissociated traumas.

Frequent dissociation often leads a child to appear confused or disorganized at times. This is more common in stressful or emotion-laden situations and becomes less noticeable as treatment progresses. Apparent tangentiality can be an attempt on the part of a patient experiencing time gaps to cover up his or her symptoms. Many of the children routinely confabulate to cover up memory gaps, both to others and themselves. The apparent "thought disorder" does not persist and fluctuates with level of distress, level of conflict, and events triggering traumatic associations. Dissociative experiences of having thoughts removed from or put into the mind are present in some children with DID.

These experiences are commonly reported by adult DID patients, in addition to those with schizophrenic and bipolar illnesses (Fink & Golinkoff, 1990; Kluft, 1987; Ross et al., 1990). Passive influence experiences, e.g., made thoughts and feelings, complex bodily movements not felt to be voluntarily initiated, automatic writing, etc., are commonly reported in adult MPD (DID) patients (Fink & Golinkoff, 1990; Kluft, 1987; Ross et al., 1990). In child DID cases, the experience of involuntarily initiated body movements distinguishes them from children with DDNOS. An example of a child's description of this type of dissociative phenomenon is included earlier in this chapter.

A number of clinical variables assist the clinician to differentiate between childhood dissociation and childhood onset schizophrenia. The dissociative child displays a more normal range of affect and less prominent thought disorder linked to stress, etc.). However, much lower rates of control and influence experiences are reported in schizophrenic children, compared to those with DID, along with much higher rates of delusional phenomenon (Russel et al., 1989). (For further information on differential diagnosis, see Chapter 12).

Completing the Diagnostic Process

The information just presented is intended to assist in differentiating between symptoms that can be attributed to a dissociative disorder and those in need of alternative diagnostic explanation. When a clinician has yet to attain familiarity with the symptomatic presentation of childhood dissociative disorders and diagnostic uncertainty remains, calling on the diagnostic expertise of an expert in this area can be a helpful learning experience. The presence of an approach embracing concepts similar to those described above can be helpful in distinguishing the level of reliability of an expert's diagnostic input. A frequent area of remaining uncertainty, once the presence of a dissociative disorder is established, is whether or not DID is present, as opposed to DDNOS. In children, some uncertainty is reasonable because of the ongoing interaction between the forces of development and the child's disorder. Since direct knowledge that alternate personalities are present is necessary to make the diagnosis, time may be needed for the child to develop a sufficient level of trust to allow any clarity about this question. A diagnosis of DDNOS will suffice in these circumstances, particularly since the important issue in treatment has more to do with the dynamic underpinnings of the dissociative symptoms and identity disturbance and the child's organization of "self" in terms of affects and interpersonal relationships than it does with direct interaction with alters. As discussed earlier, each child, at a given moment in time depending on environmental and individual stressors, falls uniquely onto some point on a biaxial range of disturbance, with the degree to which their defensive use of dissociation interferes with adaptive functioning on one axis and their ability to organize and integrate affects, behaviors, and relationship experiences on the other. The organization of "alters" is often fluid and dependent on the defensive needs they serve.

At times, the best diagnostic efforts are unable to reach closure. It is best to accept this and to develop a treatment approach in keeping with the differential diagnostic possibilities, looking to the response to treatment over time to assist in distinguishing between diagnostic possibilities. This includes a trial of therapy aimed at the dissociative symptoms to determine its impact on symptoms, and, if medications are used, a careful documentation of specific symptomatic response along with periodic trials of no medication to determine if symptomatic change relates to the medication or to ongoing therapy (see Chapter 1). The best treatment plans for children where co-morbid diagnoses are thought to exist includes this systematic evaluation of response.

Conclusion

This chapter provides a context for understanding that biological, environmental, and dynamic factors impact the development of dissociative disorders. The diagnostic complexity of dissociative symptoms and the polysymptomatic phenomenology present in dissociative disorders occurring in children are also reviewed. This understanding is then used within a differential diagnostic organizational framework aimed to determine and ultimately resolve the diagnostic complexities associated with childhood dissociative disorders. An overview of diagnostic tools, interviewing and observation techniques supplements the trained clinician's tools for undertaking this task.

In concluding this chapter, it should be emphasized that diagnosis is an inexact science. A diagnosis is at best a superficial thought-organizing tool that may either enhance or interfere with a real understanding of an individual child's difficulties. It's a necessary evil for research and the furthering of understanding of prototypical conditions but must be viewed as influenced by politics and as evolving as our understandings of human beings and their psychologic makeup undergoes further development. Assumptions derived from diagnoses should not be given more weight than the individual observation of a patient in treatment. Each child with a dissociative disorder is different from every other and needs an individualized treatment approach to achieve the most benefit and to allow for the realization of his or her developmental potential.

Over time, ongoing research will help us develop better tools and deeper understandings and enhance our ability as clinicians to assist children with dissociative disorders. I look forward to a time when the cumbersome aspects of differential diagnosis of childhood dissociative disorders described in this chapter become obsolete.

References

Albini, T. K., & Pease, T. E. (1989). Normal and pathological dissociations of early childhood. *Dissociation, 2,* 14–150.

American Psychiatric Association. (1994). *Diagnostic and statistical manual of mental disorders* (4th ed.). Washington DC: Author.

Barach, P. M. (1991). Multiple personality disorder as an attachment disorder. *Dissociation, 3,* 117–123.

Bliss, E. (1984). A symptom profile of patient with multiple personalities, including MMPI results. *Journal of Nervous & Mental Disease, 174,* 197–202.

Bowman, E. S. (1990). Adolescent multiple personality disorder in the nineteenth and early twentieth century. *Dissociation, 3,* 179–187.

Bowman, E. S., Blix, S., & Coons, P. M. (1985). Multiple personality in adolescence: Relationship to incestual experiences. *Journal of the American Academy of Child & Adolescent Psychiatry, 24,* 109–114.

Braun, B. G. (1990). Dissociative disorders as a sequelae to incest. In R. P. Kluft (Ed.), *Incest related syndromes of adult psychopathology,* pp. 227–246. Washington, DC: American Psychiatric Press.

Chu, J. A., & Dill, D. L. (1990). Dissociative symptoms in relation to childhood physical and sexual abuse. *American Journal of Psychiatry, 147,* 887–892.

Coons, P., Bowman, E., & Milstein, V. (1988). Multiple personality disorder: A clinical investigation of 50 cases. *Journal of Nervous & Mental Disease, 176,* 519–527.

Dell, P. F., & Eisenhower, J. W. (1990). Adolescent multiple personality disorder. *Journal of the American Academy of Child & Adolescent Psychiatry, 29,* 359–366.

Fagan, J., & McMahon, P. P. (1984). Incipient multiple personality in children: Four cases. *Journal of Nervous & Mental Disease, 172,* 26–36.

Fine, C. G. (1988). The work of Antoine Despine: The first scientific report on the diagnosis and treatment of a child with multiple personality disorder. *American Journal of Clinical Hypnosis, 31,* 33–39.

Fink, D., & Golinkoff, M. (1990). Multiple personality disorder, borderline personality disorder and schizophrenia: A comparative study of clinical features. *Dissociation, 3,* 127–134.

Fraiberg, S. (1982). Pathological defenses in infancy. *Psychoanalytic Quarterly, 51,* 612–635.

Greaves, G. B. (1980). Multiple personality: 165 years after Mary Reynolds. *Journal of Nervous & Mental Disease, 168,* 557–596.

Hornstein, N. L., & Putnam, F. W. (1992). Clinical phenomenology of child and adolescent dissociative disorders. *Journal of the American Academy of Child & Adolescent Psychiatry, 31,* 1077–1085.

Hornstein, N. L., & Tyson, S. (1991). Inpatient treatment of children with multiple personality/dissociative disorders and their families. *Psychiatric Clinics of North America, 14,* 631–638.

Kluft, R. P. (1984). Multiple personality in childhood. *Psychiatric Clinics of North America, 7,* 121–134.

Kluft, R. P. (1985a). Childhood multiple personality disorder: Predictors, clinical findings, and treatment results. In R. P. Kluft (Ed.), *Childhood antecedents of multiple personality,* pp. 167–196. Washington, DC: American Psychiatric Press.

Kluft, R. P. (1985b). Hypnotherapy of childhood multiple personality disorder. *American Journal of Clinical Hypnosis, 27,* 201–210.

Kluft, R. P. (1986). Treating children who have multiple personality disorder. In B. G. Braun (Ed.), *Treatment of multiple personality disorder,* pp. 81–105. Washington, DC: American Psychiatric Press.

Kluft, R. P. (1987). First-rank symptoms as a diagnostic clue to multiple personality disorder. *American Journal of Psychiatry, 144,* 293–298.

Ludwig, A. M. (1983). The psychological functions of dissociation. *American Journal of Clinical Hypnosis, 26,* 93–99.

Main M., & Hesse, E. (1990). Parent's unresolved traumatic experiences are related to infant disorganized attachment status: Is frightened and/or frightening parental behavior the linking mechanism? In Greenberg, M. T., Cicchetti, D., & Cummings, E. M. (Eds.), *Attachment in the Preschool years: Theory, research and intervention,* pp. 161–182. Chicago: University of Chicago Press.

Malenbaum, R., & Russel, A. J. (1987). Multiple personality disorder in an 11-year-old boy and his mother. *Journal of the American Academy of Child & Adolescent Psychiatry, 26,* 436–439.

Peterson, G. (1990). Diagnosis of childhood multiple personality. *Dissociation, 3,* 3–9.

Peterson, G., & Putnam, F. W. (1994). Preliminary results of the field trial of proposed criteria for dissociative disorders of childhood. *Dissociation, 7,* 212–220.

Putnam, F. (1989). *Diagnosis and treatment of multiple personality disorder.* New York: Guilford Press.

Putnam, F., Guroff, J., Silberman, E., Barban, L., & Post, R. (1986). The clinical phenomenology of multiple personality disorder: Review of 100 recent cases. *J Clin Psychiatry, 47,* 285–293.

Putnam, F. W. (1985). Dissociation as a response to extreme trauma. In R. P. Kluft (Ed.), *Childhood antecedents of multiple personality,* pp, 66–97. Washington, DC: American Psychiatric Press.

Putnam, F. W. (1990). Disturbances of "self" in victims of childhood sexual abuse. In R. P. Kluft (Ed.), *Incest related syndromes of adult psychopathology,* pp. 113–131. Washington, DC: American Psychiatric Press.

Putnam, F. W. (1991). Dissociative disorders in children and adolescents: A developmental perspective. *Psychiat Clin N Am, 14,* 519–531.

Putnam, F. (1993). W. Dissociative disorders in children: Behavioral profiles and problems. *Child Abuse and Neglect, 17,* 39–45.

Putnam, F. W., Helmers, K., & Trickett, P. K. (1993). Development, reliability, and validity of a child dissocation scale. *Child Abuse & Neglect, 17,* 731–741.

Riley, R. L., & Mead, J. (1988). The development of symptoms of multiple personality in a child of three. *Dissociation, 1,* 41–46.

Ross, C. A., Miller, S. D., Bjornson, L., Reagor, P., Fraser, G. A., & Anderson, G. (1990). Structured interview data on 102 cases of multiple personality disorder from four centers. *American Journal of Psychiatry, 147,* 596–601.

Ross, C. A., Miller, S. D., Bjornson, L., Reagor, P., Fraser, G. A., & Anderson, G. (1991). Abuse histories in 102 cases of multiple personality disorder. *Canadian Journal of Psychiatry, 36,* 97–101.

Ross, C. A., Norton, G. R., & Wozney, K. (1989). Multiple personality disorder: An analysis of 236 cases. *Canadian Journal of Psychiatry, 34,* 413–418, 1989.

Russel, A. T., Bott, L., & Sammons, C. (1989). Phenomenology of schizophrenia occurring in childhood. *Journal of the American Academy of Child & Adolescent Psychiatry, 23,* 399–407.

Schulz, R., Braun, B. G., & Kluft, R. P. (1989). Multiple personality disorder: Phenomenology of selected variables in comparison to major depression. *Dissociation, 2,* 45–51.

Siegel, D. (1995, December). *Cognitive processes: Memory and Adaptation to Trauma.* Abstract of presentation at conference *Restoring Brain Function,* University of Illinois at Chicago.

Silberg, J. L. (1994, November). *Psychological Testing Features Associated with Dissociative Diagnoses in Children and Adolescents.* Presentation at the 11th International Conference on Multiple Personality/Dissociative States. Rush Presbyterian-St. Luke's Medical Center, Chicago.

Silberg, J. L. (in review) Dissociative symptomatology in children and adolescents as displayed on psychological testing.

Steinberg, M. (1991). The spectrum of depersonalization: Assessment and treatment. In Tasman, A., & Goldfinger, S. M. (Eds.), *American Psychiatric Press review of psychiatry,* pp. 223–247. Washington, DC: American Psychiatric Press.

Stern, C. R. (1984). The etiology of multiple personality. *Psychiatric Clinics of North America, 7,* 149–160.

Vincent, M., & Pickering, M. R. (1988). Multiple personality disorder in childhood. *Canadian Journal of Psychiatry, 33,* 524–529.

Weiss, M., Sutton, P. J., & Utecht, A. J. (1985). Multiple personality in a 10-year-old girl. *Journal of the American Academy of Child & Adolescent Psychiatry, 24,* 495–501.

three

━━━━

Interviewing Strategies for Assessing Dissociative Disorders in Children and Adolescents

Joyanna L. Silberg

As a graduate student in clinical child psychology, I had a recurrent dream of a therapy session with a mute and mysterious child, who suddenly whispers a profound secret, and I am transported to ecstasy by the intimacy of that moment. Unfortunately, child clinical work has not lived up to the potential of that dream. However, nothing has come closer to that remembered fantasy than communication with dissociative children. The intensity of their need to find someone with whom to share the uniqueness of their internal world is balanced by the intensity of their need to protect this secret and their fear of its disclosure. If this balance is tipped in the direction of confiding in the interviewer and extending that initially fragile bond of trust, the interviewer has the potential of promoting a powerful link to the child. This powerful connection may be the child's first lifeline out of a secret world of internal contradiction, conflict, and pain. The intensity and rarity of this connection was illustrated for me by a 6-year-old boy who travelled a long distance for a one-time consultation. The interview was unremarkable as he nodded only briefly in response to interview questions, but then 6 months later asked his foster mother, "Could you get me an appointment with the lady who knows about voices?"

This chapter will highlight interviewing techniques that I have found helpful in my consultation with child and adolescent patients whose therapists suspected a possible dissociative disorder. As a consultant to both inpatient and outpatient services at a large psychiatric hospital I have had the opportunity to interview over a hundred children for whom therapists were considering a diagnosis of dissociative disorder. Through trial and error, repeated experience, and familiarity with the child dissociative literature, I have developed a set of techniques for interviewing dissociative children that help to discriminate between more normative childhood fantasy, the spectrum of dissociative conditions, and a host of other diagnoses that may become confused with dissociative disorders.

The adult literature has offered interview schedules, the SCID-D (Steinberg, 1993) and the DDIS (Ross et al., 1989), which provide guidelines for how to interview adults for the diagnostic assessment of dissociative disorders, and these structured interviews have produced excellent reliability and validity (Steinberg et al., 1991; Ross et al., 1990). However, diagnostic interview schedules for children have not included dissociative disorders in the differential diagnosis, and this has probably contributed to the omission of dissociative disorders in child psychiatric research. Steinberg and Steinberg (1995) have piloted using the SCID-D, The Structured Clinical Interview for Dissociative Disorders (Steinberg, 1993), with adolescents with promising results. However, structured interview schedules such as this one presuppose a certain level of self-observational skill that is unrealistic to expect in most children and adolescents. Children and adolescents are not particularly good at summarizing the frequency of behaviors they have experienced, and do not have the same candidness and cooperativeness about diagnosis that an interview schedule may require. A promising interview schedule for the diagnosis of dissociative disorders in younger children which allows more flexibility in the sequencing of questions has been described by Lewis (1996). With or without a standardized interview protocol, the clinician seeking to diagnose the dissociative child or adolescent through interview must rely on wits, creativity, an empathic attitude, and a knowledge base about the often covert manifestations of dissociative conditions. In this chapter I will review some of the techniques and procedures which I have found most useful in making this important diagnostic discrimination.

As a guide before beginning the interview, the interviewer should become familiar with lists of symptoms and descriptors of dissociative children, as provided by Kluft (1985), Fagan and McMahon (1984), and Peterson (1990), or as listed on Putnam's Child Behavior Checklist (Putnam, Helmers, & Trickett, 1993). The interviewer should be familiar with categories of dissociative symptoms such as trance states, amnestic experiences, fluctuating abilities or presentations, somatic concerns, depression and suicidal feelings, sleep problems, and most importantly a feeling of dividedness, experienced as discrete alter states, hallucinated internal voices, or behavior outside the child's control. Descriptions of these categories of symptoms have been found in the preceding chapter.

Although full diagnostic assessment (as outlined by Hornstein) involves observation in multiple settings, caretaker interviews, and psychological testing (see Chapter 5), it is the one-on-one disclosure of the specific manifestations of the child's sense of dividedness that truly confirms the diagnosis of DID (Dissociative Identity Disorder) or DDNOS (Dissociative Disorder Not Otherwise Specified) in a child.

Framing the Encounter

I frame the interview as a unique and special time, so the child begins to see this session as qualitatively different from other therapeutic encounters with doctors. I establish this frame of uniqueness by asking immediately if children understand the purpose of the interview. Often children will say they are not sure why I am meeting with them. At this point, I tell them that their doctor still has some important questions about them and thought I would be the best person to help the doctor figure some things out. I tell the child that I have worked with many children like him/her, and because of this experience their doctor thought I might be the one who could best understand them. In stressing the ways that other children I have seen are like the child being interviewed, I find a non-threatening aspect of their history or symptom to relate to. For example, I may tell the child that I am an expert on children who have been in a lot of foster homes, or that I am an expert on children who have had to leave their birth families. If "hearing voices" is a prominent symptom for which the child has been referred I may tell the child that I am an expert on children who hear voices. Rarely do I say that I am an expert on dissociative disorders, unless I know that the child has expressed familiarity with these conditions previously, or unless the child actually states that the reason for the interview is to determine if he or she is dissociative. Occasionally, I may state that I am an expert on children who have had "bad things" happen to them, particularly with younger children, but I usually do not say "sexual abuse" or "physical abuse," as this can automatically raise the anxiety level and associated guardedness and does not predispose the child to honest disclosure.

At this initial stage, I try to engage the child's curiosity to learn from me about other children who have experienced similar kinds of things. This gives the child a sense of control in the interview, that he/she is there to learn about himself/herself and that I may be a resource to facilitate that process. I also stress to the child that I am also in the process of learning and understanding children and how they react to things, and that I will be very interested to learn about them so that I can increase my knowledge base. Thus, the interview setting is set up as a very non-judgmental environment, where each of us is there for learning information, and each of us may have information that the other may be interested in. This feels very different to children than the usual psychiatric interview, which involves judgment and classification. Children have often picked up on the usual style of psychiatric interviews, have noticed the cold stare and the notes on a pad that accompany disclosures of hearing voices, and many children have learned what *not* to say in these interviews.

To counter their preconceived notion that I am there to judge and classify, I often tell them about how impressed I am with the children I have met and the clever ways they have of helping themselves deal with difficult things. Thus, I begin the process of reframing their "pathology," whatever it may be, as a survival strategy and a coping strength. If the child has been referred to me because of hearing voices, I may tell him/her that many children like them have heard voices and that this is a common reaction after a lot of "bad things have happened" in their environment. I may explain to them that it is "like a broken tape recorder that gets stuck in their mind" and that many children can experience this.

Education about Dissociative Processes

Within the early part of the interview, I begin to educate the child about dissociative defenses, beginning with the description of the experience of blocking pain. I begin with this, because this is a common experience of many children and adults and does not necessarily imply a dissociative disorder. I may say to them, "There is something that children do that is really amazing. Some children do it better than others. They seem to be able to get themselves not to feel anything, even after they fall down and get hurt. It happened to me once when I broke my arm. I knew it hurt because I heard myself crying but I don't think I really felt it. It was like I went numb." This normalizing description of dissociation of physical pain usually invites the child to share information about times they have gotten hurt and how they dealt with it. At times, children will share examples of physical fighting with friends, and sometimes even examples of physical abuse. If physical abuse is brought up I inquire about other times when dissociation was used to deal with abuse and may ask the child if they ever tried so hard not to feel pain that they pretended to be someone else. This may help to develop the discussion about alter states or imaginary friends. If the child discusses peer fighting, I may now inquire about aggression and anger expression, amnesia during fights, or the feeling that "something just comes over" them when angry. Further inquiry about this feeling may lead to disclosures about angry or aggressive alter states.

Indirect Communication

Abused children may have been taught that revealing secrets of abuse may result in death, and consequently many children have a fear of telling about the abuse. This intense fear is transferred into the protection of dissociative defenses, or disclosing aspects of the dissociative system. Some children who may want to disclose about their abuse history or dissociative processes may have experienced intense directives not to "talk." This may be interpreted literally by the child, so that indirect means of communicating may be outside the taboo. I capitalize on this by encouraging children to share information with me in indirect means as well, with no talking required. Children who have trouble telling me about a feeling may be asked to draw their feelings or draw "what your mind feels like." One 8-year-old boy, who was later diagnosed with DID, taught me a hand signal language wherein each hand signal stood for a different feeling state. He spent time in the interview drawing a "dictionary" for me about the hand signals so that I would be able to understand him if I forgot what each one meant. Later I learned that communicating via hand signal was allowable by his internal dissociative system but language expression was not.

The use of tape recorders has also been useful in encouraging disclosures of difficult subjects. Children may be allowed to dictate into the tape recorder, while I close my ear or wait behind the office door left slightly ajar, and later decide whether to play the tape for me or not. Over the years, I have had only one child who did not then play the tape. However, this child safeguarded the tape and religiously brought the tape to her therapist each week, as a concrete metaphor of her ownership of this secret material, the uniqueness of it, and knowledge that the therapy environment was the place this special knowledge belonged.

One child, a 9-year-old girl with DDNOS, communicated with me through typing messages on the word processor, feeling that was safer than oral communication. She asked me to close my eyes until she had completely finished using the "delete" button, so that she retained the choice about what to share.

In helping children to deal with the fear of disclosure it's important not to promise things that can't be delivered, such as "If you tell me I can make sure you are not abused again." The therapist promises should be more reality based and less grandiose: "If you trust me enough to tell me, I promise to work with you as hard as I can so that we can figure out together how to help you get out of this mess." Tricking the child into revealing too much too early may be experienced as a betrayal and may be destabilizing to the inner dissociative system, so the interviewer must be gentle and respectful of the child's protectiveness.

Inquiring about Imaginative Processes

As a way to begin entering the imaginative world of the child, I will ask that the child bring with him/her to the interview any special dolls, blankets, or favorite toys. These transitional objects discussed by Winnicott (1953) have been viewed by developmental psychologists as the basis upon which the child first learns to make distinctions between body boundaries of the self and others. Imaginary friends are also viewed by developmental psychologists as transitional objects that are projective manifestations of the child's experimentation with aspects of the self (Singer & Singer, 1990). Adult and adolescent patients have frequently reported that imaginary friends were the first developmental manifestations which later became alter phenomena (Dell & Eisenhower, 1990; Putnam, 1991) and my experience with interviewing dissociative children has provided documentation that other more concrete transitional objects such as dolls, stuffed animals, or even blankets can harbor the first self-projections, which over time become dissociated. Fink (1993) has described this phenomenon in DID adults, but the pervasiveness of stuffed animals, or doll alters in dissociative children has not been well appreciated.

If the child brings a stuffed animal or other transitional object to the session, I will inquire as to the animal's name, how long the child has had the "special friend," and where he or she got it from. I will ask the child about how the "special friend" is used in times when comfort is needed. Does the child sleep with the object? Does the child hug the object during scary or sad moments? I will ask if the child sometimes talks to the "special friend" during special moments. Frequently, children without significant dissociative pathology will respond affirmatively to all of these questions. Then I will ask the child if the child ever hears the animal or "special friend" talk back to him. This, too, is not particularly unusual even within a normal spectrum. If the "special friend" does talk back, I will ask the child what kind of things the friend says. Are they messages of "behave yourself" or "don't be scared," or are they more complex messages? Do the messages seem to revolve around a central theme or role? If so, are there any special friends or imaginary others that have a contrasting role? When transitional objects are not brought to the interview setting, I always ask about them, and it is the rare child, no matter what the diagnosis, who cannot recall having had a "special friend" of some kind during the course of their childhood.

The fruitfulness of this line of questioning is demonstrated by the case of a 9-year-old inpatient, Tony, who was hospitalized for violent behavior, including throwing a chair out of a school window. Tony had been adopted at age four after spending his early years with a psychotic grandmother and substance abusing father. Tony's adoptive parents described him as displaying intensely fluctuating behavior from charming, intelligent, and competent to destructive and violent. When I asked Tony if he had any special dolls, toys, or stuffed animals that he had since he was little, his body moved suddenly in a physical double take, he swung his head around to look at me eye-to eye and stated emphatically, "No, I would never have had anything like that. Never. Ever. Why do you ask?"

I had the distinct sense that I was "on to something" so I explained that many adopted children took something special with them from their birth families home and that this was a normal activity. Tony then stated "Well, I do have Adam, but I'm sure that's not what you mean." I asked him to tell me about Adam. Tony told me "Adam" was a Cabbage Patch doll that he had "adopted" at the time of his own adoption and that Adam had gone through a lot with him. When I asked him if Adam ever gave him any special messages, Tony stated that Adam told him "Always be good; listen to your teachers." It then occurred to me that this sporadically violent inpatient boy was most likely hearing some competing messages to this good prosocial advice. "Are there any other 'special friends' who give you opposite advice?" I asked. Again, I noticed the visible double take and emphatic denial followed by "Well. There are those two men who come around." Inquiring about the "two men" I discovered that there was a short fat one and a slim tall one whom he could see at all times who were always looking for potential danger and advised him on when to fight. I asked if I could talk to the "men" and Tony said he would check with them. He directed his eyes to a couch across from us in the room and mumbled under his breath as he "talked" with them, and then waited a few moments before looking back at me and stated "They didn't know they were allowed to talk to doctors. They never have before." With Tony as intermediary I communicated with the "men" and discovered that they had originally come to Tony when he feared his grandmother's violent rages. They helped him fight back, usually through lifting objects and throwing them. They continued to be confused as to whether his grandmother was still around, and Tony and I spent some time educating them about how circumstances have changed since their protective role was initiated. Tony was diagnosed with DDNOS and his confusing behavior finally could be understood in context by him, his family, and the treatment team.

The disclosures elicited by Tony were new for him to share, despite the fact that he had had three previous hospitalizations and several different therapists. The dramatic self-disclosure of Tony has been repeated time and time again by children who have never realized that the content of their imaginative creations are appropriate subjects for communication with doctors and therapists. It is surprising how many latency aged boys (7 to 12) I have talked with who have "GI Joe dolls," "Ninja Turtles," or "Power Ranger" figures that have become enlivened through the child's projective fantasy. Although they are at times reluctant to disclose their lifelike projections onto these fantasy figures, they seem to experience a sense of relief when finally sharing this, particularly if they feel that the fantasy has progressed to a point outside of their control.

I always ask directly about imaginary friends that the child has now or has had in the past. I ask the same kinds of questions I would ask about other transitional objects, about their helpfulness, and their role for the child. When the child describes having imaginary friends, I ask children to describe the "friends" and to draw them. Frequently, the child can share extensive visual elaborations of the imaginary friends which make them seem more like visual hallucinations. One 10-year-old girl with DID tipped me off to her diagnosis when she looked in a small mirror in my office and made disgusted faces and noises. "What do you see here?" I inquired. "Satan-girl," she replied, sharing her sense of a dissociated evil identity for the first time. One 14-year-old girl with DID described a younger alter whom she could see entering from the window and floating into her mind when she called upon her.

When inquiring about the properties of these imaginary friends, attentiveness to the child's feeling of who has control, whether he/she feels bothered by the presence of the imaginary friend, or whether the imaginary friend influences the child's actions in ways that are ego-dystonic helps to make the differentiation between more normative "imaginary friends" experiences and dissociative experiences. (See the section of this chapter on differentiation of normal fantasy for further discussion of this topic.)

Some children are more ready to share imaginary places rather than imaginary people. Singer & Singer (1990) have called such imaginary worlds "paracosms" and describes their commonness among great literary figures who were imaginative and bright. They stress the normative and creative aspects of these fantasy creations. Dissociative children, however, may rely heavily on these inner worlds as places of comfort and safety in a turbulent environment. A 7-year-old inpatient with DID told me about a magical underwater sea world where Danielle 1, 2, and 3 lived protected from imaginary sharks that surrounded her. Several children have described imaginary castles, or special secret islands. A 5-year-old boy with DDNOS described a complex audiovisual studio in his mind with VCR machines, televisions, and tape recorders. Flashbacks and amnesia were understood by this child by relating his mind's activity to this imaginary audiovisual equipment.

If hearing voices has not been brought up in the discussion of transitional objects or imaginary friends, I always ask about them directly. Some children describe hearing the sound of their name called suddenly but have no further elaborations. I have found that this is common with non-dissociative children. However, the dissociative child can share further elaborations of the inner voices. I ask them to describe what the voice sounds like, if it sounds old or young, male or female, or similar to anyone they have ever met. If they do acknowledge these voices, I give them an opportunity to ask the "voices inside" if continuing to find out about them is acceptable. Generally, children do give permission to continue with the inquiry, but asking helps to reassure any resistant inside parts that you are respectful of them and their feelings.

If I am aware that the child has experienced a significant loss, such as the death of a friend or relative or the loss of attachment to a parent or friend, I will always inquire as to whether the child still hears the missed person's voice. I normalize this as well, explaining that the mind helps us deal with losses by making our imaginations more vivid to remember special people. Some children use this as an opportunity to tell me that they are visited by the "ghosts" of dead parents or grandparents, and some may find these experiences frightening, while others find them reassuring. Once I have learned about the child's experience with a "ghost," I will ask questions about its influence on the child, and other characteristics to determine if this is an alter or a more passive internal influence, as seen in DDNOS. I have seen many children with "dead grandparent" alters whose characteristics have evolved into being more malevolent over time, even when the child's conscious memory is of a loving grandparent.

Some children will be relieved to discuss their sense of internal conflict if they have felt persecuted or harassed by inner voices that are commanding them to do self-destructive things. However, they may be hoping that through talking about the "bad part" I will find a way to help them silence it. If this comes up in an initial interview I will try to explore with the child what the original purpose of that voice, alter, or part might have been. If direct questioning does not help uncover it, I may guess with the child other possibilities: "Does it help you to guard against telling secrets? Does it help you to act real strong?"; "Does it help to fight off enemies? Does it feel the bad abuse for you?" This begins to teach the concept that the other parts of the self have a purpose that needs to be respected.

Once we have decided together on what the purpose of that negative influencing presence may be, I ask the child to create a "thank you card" for it. Children enjoy the activity of drawing, coloring, and writing out a thank you card. These thank you cards are sometimes explicit about how the part was seen as helpful, but more often are colorfully-decorated hearts, rainbows, and clowns that express their thankful feelings (see Figure 1). After the thank you card is finished I ask the child to check and see how the other part reacted to it. Often they are surprised at how appreciative the inner part is, and a foundation may be set for beginning a negotiation, even at this early stage. Although some children or adolescents find this strange or funny, they all seem to take delight in the fact that I have acknowledged an important aspect of their development, have recognized the basic adaptive nature of their defense, and am willing to be accepting and forgiving of all aspects of themselves. This models the forgiveness and acceptance that they will need to demonstrate as they enter therapy.

This exercise of making a thank you card, which I frequently initiate in the very first interview with a child, has been reported to have very positive ongoing effects as the child enters or continues with his/her treatment. Children have proudly shared these cards with teachers, parents, and therapists, have hung them on bulletin boards and refrigerators, and

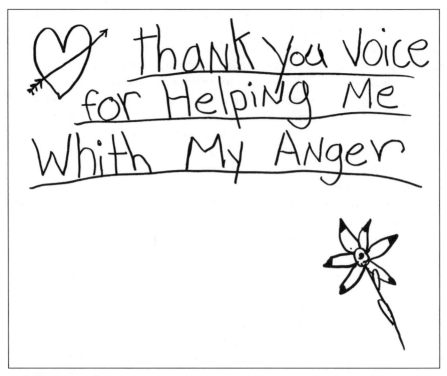

Figure 1. This "Thank you" card is typical of the gestures of appreciation encouraged during interviewing or early phases of treatment.

seem to gain a sense of mastery over their behavior by this simple act of self-acceptance. For some children whose trauma has not been as severe, and whose dissociative processes are not rigid, this simple exercise may be enough to have the child feel whole and integrated without further work directly on the dissociative system.

Sometimes when a child discloses that he/she has parts, voices, imaginary friends or special "helpers," the child requires a more concrete way to demonstrate the separateness and allow communication. We may "call up" the parts on a pretend telephone, or have them talk through puppets or dolls. Examples of using puppets or dolls to represent dissociated parts are well-illustrated in the case descriptions of McMahon & Fagan (1993). Sometimes when we are engaging in fantasy play to find out more about "inside parts" it may be difficult to tell if the child is role-playing and fantasizing or if the child is really "switching" to an alter state. Generally, in these playful interchanges with puppets, dolls, or pretend telephones, I assume that the child is not "switching." "Switching" phenomena are accompanied by confusion, momentary lapses, and discontinuity in the flow of play or conversation. In these role plays in which the child is dramatizing aspects of a voice or part, there is often continuity and engagement.

Youngsters who report the experience of influencing parts and who can dramatize them, but do not "switch," are diagnosed with DDNOS, rather than DID.

If the child has accessed communication with an internal voice I continue the conversation by talking through the child. "What does the voice part or friend think about talking to me?" is usually my first question. If communication flows easily in this manner, I will not ask to talk to the inside part directly, as I am always working with the child in an integrative manner that facilitates cohesion and memory. However, if the child feels stumped or puzzled in talking to the inside part, I may ask if that part would like to talk to me directly. Frequently, this part will spontaneously emerge if I have successfully created an atmosphere of understanding and empathy. In those cases where the child switches and presents an alternate identity, the change in developmental level of language is often the most notable difference in presentation. Changes in affect, motor activity, or level of aggressiveness may also be noted. In these cases, I consider a diagnosis of DID, particularly if I have concrete evidence regarding amnesia by history or interview.

Trance Phenomena

During the interview, the interviewer should stay alert to signs that the child is entering a trance state. Children may stare ahead of them, close their eyes for a few moments, or engage in repetitive movements while looking distracted. Frequently children have been referred, particularly outpatients, because of the complaints of teachers and parents of frequent daydreaming, staring off into space, etc. I have found it helpful to be very specific in my questions about what is going on during those "blank" moments. The child's initial response will often be "nothing" or "I don't know." I don't accept this response readily and continue to offer choices for the child to help them be more specific: "Are you spending time thinking about your favorite movie star, wondering when this interview will be over, remembering something someone told you?" I may share with the child thoughts that I have when my mind wanders—about what I had for lunch, what a friend said to me, or physiological sensations like hunger, tiredness, or having to go the bathroom. The child often laughs to realize that other people's minds may wander too. The importance of persisting with questions about daydreaming was illustrated to me by an 11-year-old youngster, Shari, who was diagnosed with DID at the initial interview. Shari's teachers had complained that she spent far too much time staring off into space. When Shari was asked what really went through her mind in school, at first she gave the typical deflective response: "nothing." When I pressed her more to help recreate her line of thinking while doing a math problem, Shari stated "I'm sometimes wondering if 'Angela' will get the problem before I do, and I get nervous." Assuming that Angela was a classmate I asked where Angela was sitting and could she see her paper. Shari responded that Angela and she shared the same paper and that Angela had no seat of her own in school. Soon it became apparent that Angela was an imaginary friend with whom Shari was very competitive; further inquiry revealed that she was an alternate identity who came out to talk to me in the course of the interview to share her point of view.

Inquiry into unusual movements may also help to elicit information about alter phenomena and trance. Toby was a 14-year-old girl with DDNOS who had strange quivering movements of her temples whenever she was quiet for a moment. When I asked Toby about this, she stated that was when her inside friend "Soldier Man" was talking to her. "Soldier Man" had come to rescue her from her abusive stepfather and continued to protect her by helping her carefully select what information she could share with others. Luckily, "Soldier Man" had given her permission to confide in me when I uncovered his covert communication style.

Amnesia

Amnestic processes are hard to uncover in children, as children are used to using the expression "I forgot" as a simple way to avoid responsibility or further conversation. The interviewer must try to elicit the child's curiosity and concern about their memory to facilitate disclosure about memory problems that the child finds truly perplexing.

Often, the child has been referred to me because the child claims to have no memory for an aggressive incident in which he or she was observed. I frequently find, even with dissociative children, that there is some ability to access a memory if questioning is persistent. When the child states they do not remember a fight, I'll ask them to show me any marks or bruises that they have from the fight and see if they can figure out how they got them. I'll ask a child to tell me all the details that they can remember, I'll write the details down, and ask the child to help me fill in what's missing. If the child still claims not to remember, I'll ask them to describe to me what other people have told them about the event and use those details to help fill in the memory. Every time I get another detail, I'll add it to an ongoing cohesive narrative that I'm creating: "So you were standing there with your blue sweater on, you saw John enter the room, and what's the very next thing that happened?"

If the child continues to deny any memory of the event, I may ask them if they think there's a part of them that may have some knowledge about it, and ask them if they are willing to try to find out about that. If they are willing, I may ask them to spend a minute with their eyes closed searching through all the different "file drawers" in their mind to see if there is some clue that can help them discover what happened. Sometimes during this process they will hear an internal voice which gives them more information that they may share with me. If no information is still forthcoming after all this questioning, it may reflect a rigid dissociative process. The child who seems truly perplexed about not having a certain memory, but has very little curiosity about what really happened, is a child for whom I am most suspicious of a DID diagnosis. They seem perfectly able to live with the contradiction of not knowing certain important information about themselves and having no strong desire to discover it. For these children dissociative barriers may be more rigid, and it may take significant therapeutic work to help them gain continuity of memory. (This, by the way, is a rare occurrence in my diagnostic work with children, happening less than 10% of the time. In most cases, even with DID patients, amnestic barriers can be dissolved rather easily.) On many occasions the interview office or therapy office may be an environment that cues memory. Several patients, in second interviews or later in treatment, have told me that when they are sitting in my office they remember things a lot better than they do outside of the office.

As a help in checking memory about childhood events, I ask the child about each grade in school, who the teacher was, and what kind of birthday party he/she had that year. These are pieces of information that most children can readily share. The years during which there is discontinuity of memory may be the years during which the child was experiencing significant trauma. I do not check memory by asking the child about abusive events in their past. However, if the topic of abuse does come up in our conversation I will ask the child how vague or specific memories of these events are, without asking them to recount the events.

School work is a neutral area in which to begin to inquire about memory processes. The interviewer might ask about forgetfulness in approaching certain kinds of math problems. Most normal children acknowledge some forgetting in this domain, but these discussions can help lead to more information about whether certain skills and abilities are sequestered into discrete states of consciousness.

If children give me information that flatly contradicts what I have been told, I check out the accuracy with them there, so that I can ask them how to make sense of the discrepancy. (For more information about interviewing for amnesia see Chapter 2.)

Fluctuations

During the course of the interview I watch the child carefully to observe if there are shifts in the child's presentation or manner, or style of relating to me. If I notice a shift, I comment: "It seemed like a moment ago you were talking to me readily and now you are very quiet; I wonder what's going on?" I ask the child if these types of shifts have happened before, and under what circumstances. This may help bring the conversation to experienced changes in consciousness that are associated with the shifts in behavior. I may ask, "Do you feel different when you're quiet like that, more relaxed, more fearful?" My noticing of these shifts and commenting on them has allowed some DID children to introduce me to different alters during this initial interview.

With younger children I have noticed dramatic shifts in their activity level during the course of an interview. One 7-year-old boy, Alex, was referred for an evaluation by the Department of Social Services after his mother had closed him in a refrigerator and he was found by a neighbor. Alex was jumpy, impulsive, and hyperactive, flitting from toy to toy in the interview room, until I began to ask him about whether he heard voices. At that moment he became still, almost motionless, made direct eye contact and began to tell me about "Handy" and "Footy"—alter states projected on to his own body, that talked to him at times of great fear and loneliness.

When asking children about their own fluctuating behavior, I may start with gentle questions about whether they have ever felt like they did something that they didn't want to do. Most children will answer "yes" to that question. My next step is to explore with them how it was that they did the thing they didn't want to do. Was it a feeling that came over them, or a bad mood? I will ask them if they felt like something or someone else was making them do it. Frequently, even non-dissociative children experience their anger as something foreign that overtakes them. I will encourage them to articulate that feeling so that I can hear for signs as to whether the foreignness of the feeling is a sign that the feeling is projected onto another presence, voice, or personality other than the self. If they have already talked with me about hearing voices I will look for connections between the voices and the feelings of lack of ownership of behavior.

One 7-year-old, Hilda, was perky, mature, and self-possessed in her interview, and I asked her about the reported rage reactions she had displayed on the patient hall. "You must have read the wrong chart," she informed me. I called the staff on the inpatient unit and they reported that they had required locked door seclusion for her on that very day. I spelled her name loudly over the phone. "H I L D A?" I asked. "Yes," the staff person replied. I asked Hilda if there was another child with her name on the hall and she said "no." I then asked, jokingly, if she might have an identical twin under her bed that might jump out and require restraint or locked door seclusion, and if that might be the source of the staff's confusion about her behavior. Hilda laughed, but still said nothing. Finally, I talked with her about how some children feel that their anger is like a jack-in-the-box that pops out when they are not expecting it to, and that lots of children felt so mad about things that have happened to them, that the only way the anger can pop out is in the "jack-in-the-box" way. Hilda became quiet, her perky demeanor changed, and she said quietly and plaintively, "That's me. Can you help me learn to deal with my anger?" I told her that her anger was like a pet bulldog that had gotten off its leash, that we wouldn't want to lose her pet, but that her pet would need to learn how to save his "attack" skills for situations of real danger. Hilda found this metaphor very useful for beginning to harness and feel owner-ship of her anger.

PTSD Symptoms, Depression, and Somatic Complaints

Sometimes the post-traumatic symptoms of the dissociative child which prompted the referral are frightening to the child but relatively easy to share. Frequently children describe nighttime visual hallucinations often of the abusers or fantasied recreations of them—monsters, devils, rob-bers. These children may describe bad dreams; I will always try to get the child to recount one of the dreams in detail, as it may provide clues to abusive figures in their life, or even alter identities. Inquiry about these symptoms is used as a lead-in to further understanding of dissociative processes.

When asking children about depression and suicidal feelings, I always get details about their belief about what will happen to them after death. Some children will describe with confidence a belief that they can rejoin a dead grandparent or parent if they kill themselves. Others may have al-ters who believe that they can survive even after the child kills him- or herself. In the interview I try to educate children gently about the final-ity of death for themselves and the alters. One 7-year-old with DDNOS explained to me her belief that if she killed herself she would die, but that her imaginary friends could live on for "about two or three weeks" with-out her. The children seem to find it reassuring that I am willing to en-gage in these frank discussions about a subject that is somewhat taboo and for which they may have erroneous and distorted information.

Children with dissociative disorders may have somatic complaints in-cluding headaches, stomachaches, pain at the site of previous injuries, or troublesome sensory experiences. One 13-year-old DID child complained of smelling a "bad smell" much of the time. This intensely unpleasant ol-factory experience appeared to be associated with a particular abusive event that took place in an abandoned dump. When asking about the child's somatic experiences, I try to get very specific language from the child about exactly what it feels like—a tight helmet on the head, a twist-ing pain, a stabbing feeling. This allows me to develop suggested metaphors that the child can use to help control the pain by imagining, for example, that the helmet is slowly being lifted, or the arm slowly untwisted. I will often introduce these exercises in the initial interview to help provide feelings of confidence to the child in being able to control the discomfort, and to assess how receptive the child is to hypnotic exercises such as these.

When Is It Not Dissociative?

In the present climate, in which there is abundant concern about over-diagnosis, people have wondered whether these approaches and techniques make every child seem dissociative. Generally, in my inpatient and outpatient consultation work, in which all patients have been referred to me because of a strong suspicion of a dissociative disorder, I find that I will confirm a dissociative diagnosis in only 75 to 80 percent of patients. A review of consults from the past year (N=40) revealed the following breakdown of diagnoses: DID (42.5%), DDNOS (37.5%), PTSD (post-traumatic stress disorder) without significant dissociative pathology (12.5%), and other diagnoses (7.5%), including developmental disorders, psychotic disorders, and normative dissociative experiences.

Over the years, I have found the children who do not receive a dissociative diagnosis have grouped themselves into several categories. Explaining these categories should shed further light on the fine discriminations in differential diagnosis that this work requires.

Children with Developmental Disorders and Psychotic Disorders

I have seen several children with autistic-like presentations who have unusual patterns of performance on psychological testing. Their fantasy and drawings may have violent themes, and their language is awkward and confusing. Sometimes they may talk about fantasy creations or imaginary friends that others can't see. These symptoms and the confusing diagnostic picture have led to the referral to rule out a dissociative disorder. I have found that these children tend to have a poor level of relatedness and do not make the good eye contact typical of the dissociative child. Their performance on psychological testing, although variable, conforms to known neuropsychological deficits, such as visual-motor or memory skills, with intact verbal or visual-spatial skills. When they do speak about imaginary friends, the content seems to constantly shift and there is a quality of "making it up as they go along."

I see these children as being neurologically impaired; their strangeness of affect, cognition, and relatedness is due to the neuropsychological deficits, suggesting a diagnosis of pervasive developmental disorder (PDD) or high functioning autism. However, there is at least some evidence that autistic or autistic-like children can develop dissociative identities as well. Donna Williams (1992, 1994) is a high functioning autistic adult who has written two books describing her experiences growing up with neuropsychological deficits in an abusive home. Williams clearly develops dissociative identity disorder in addition to the autism, illustrating that these two conditions can co-occur. Williams's books highlight that the neurologically impaired child may experience trauma simply from their brain's incapacity to process events, even when the environment appears benign. Thus, the question remains open as to whether some of the children who present with neurological and developmental deficits may be doubly handicapped and may have developed dissociative symptoms on top of their constellation of other symptoms. Similar speculations and observations are reported by Hornstein in the preceding chapter. Currently, like Dr. Hornstein, when I see a patient whose dissociative symptoms are accompanied by long-standing developmental deficits, I tend not to give a dissociative diagnosis. I believe that the treatment for these children needs to be much more structured and reality-focussed than the treatment recommended for dissociative conditions, which heavily explores metaphor and symbolic meaning, with which many of these cognitively impaired children have difficulty.

Sometimes children are referred to me who are aggressive, have borderline mental functioning, and appear to go through rapid changes of state with little awareness. Generally, these are boys from homes of chronic abuse and trauma who are currently living in residential settings. Some of them may be able to talk about influencing voices and hallucinations, sometimes vivid paranoid hallucinations involving known abusers. The cognitive confusion of these children and the lability of their affect makes them very difficult to reach. Although many dissociative features may be noted with these youngsters, they may require anti-psychotic medication to help contain the intensity of their rage, restlessness, and impulsivity. I believe that these are children who under better conditions, earlier treatment, less chronic abuse, or stronger cognitive skills might look classically dissociative. However, they have been unable to organize the perplexing array of emotions, post-traumatic symptoms, and experiences, and they look more psychotic. Dr. Hornstein refers to these children in the preceding chapter as a mixture of her "Group 1" and "Group 2." (See also Chapter 6, Cognitive Domain.)

Another group of psychotic patients looks more clearly schizophrenic, with a pattern of impaired relatedness and hallucinations that are disorganized and random. In contrast, the dissociative child's experience of voices or hallucinated visual presences is well-organized, can be articulated, and can be related clearly to a traumatic origin. However, the overlap between childhood psychotic conditions, or severe personality disorders in childhood, and dissociative disorders is certainly unclear, and there is room for much further research to assist with these discriminations. In my setting, children who may be diagnosed with dissociative disorders are frequently diagnosed with "major depression with psychotic features" before the dissociative diagnosis is made. In other settings many of these children may be labelled "borderline," as a history of physical and sexual abuse is a risk factor for this disorder as well (Gudzer, Paris, Zilkowitz, & Marchessault, 1996), and borderline children are similarly known for impulsivity and instability of affect and behavior. Hopefully, as diagnostic criteria for childhood dissociative disorders get more refined, discriminations among all of these childhood conditions can be made more accurately.

Resolving Dissociative Processes

Some patients, particularly adolescents, who have been sexually or physically abused but are now in safe environments, may describe eloquently dissociative experiences they have had of depersonalization—"I saw myself floating in the room"—or previous amnesia for trauma that they now remember, or a history of rage reactions that felt out of their control. However, they describe these experiences in the past tense, and they seem to be very clear about what happened and how they coped. These patients may get referred to me because their articulate expression of dissociative processes takes little fancy interviewing to call forth. Sometimes they still retain some post-traumatic features such as nightmares and enhanced startle reflexes. I believe these patients are in an active process of recovery and coping and have used dissociative defenses adaptively but have been able to discard them now as new developmental challenges arise. I do not diagnose these patients with dissociative disorder but instead view their symptoms as primarily post-traumatic or affective. However, these patients could be at risk for pathological dissociation if new traumatic events occur in their life. For example, a girl who has been sexually abused, coped with that experience, and then experiences a rape in her teenage years might find a reactivation of her dissociative defenses.

Other Diagnoses

Sometimes children with other diagnoses may use dissociative coping strategies to deal with the trauma of their symptoms. As discussed by Dr. Hornstein in the preceding chapter, in these cases the dissociative disorder is not the primary diagnosis. For example, a 9-year-old boy, Jonah, was referred to a school psychologist for unusual finger movements during class. Interviewing revealed that he had an elaborate ritual of counting to seven and then thirteen every time the teacher said the word "read." This obsessive-compulsive ritual developed suddenly after his mother remarried. When asked about it further, Jonah stated that he had a "little man living on his shoulder" who yelled "Count! Count!" and he could not resist this direction. This child was diagnosed with OCD (Obsessive Compulsive Disorder), and responded well to cognitive-behavioral and family therapy. In this case, the projective fantasy of the "little man" was seen as secondary to the OCD rather than as a dissociative symptom per se. In his eagerness to find an explanation to account for the intense feeling associated with the compulsion, this youngster temporarily disowned and projected the uncomfortable feeling onto this fantasy creation.

Normal Fantasy

Occasionally, a child is referred to me, particularly on an outpatient basis, who has elaborate fantasy and imaginary friends but whose history of trauma is suspected but not well-proven. Family members aware of dissociative disorders may use the child's involvement in his/her imaginary world as proof that the child was in fact abused, as they suspect. On these occasions I must make the discrimination between possibly normal fantasy projections and the pathological projections typical of DID or DDNOS.

Although the diagnostic criteria for DID include the rule-out "not attributable to imaginary playmates or other fantasy play," there has been no research available to inform a careful clinical differentiation between imaginary friends and dissociative projections. Developmental psychologists have documented imaginary friends in early childhood (Singer & Singer, 1990). They may be seen in 30 to 65% of children (Singer & Singer, 1990) and are usually found between the ages of 4 and 7, but may last up through the age of ten. Normal children use imaginary friends to cope with loneliness, to contain affects that are perceived as unacceptable, or as projections of wished for traits or abilities. The imaginary friend serves the purpose of giving the child mastery and control during a period of stress or developmental change. Children tend to feel protective of their imaginary friends and do not like interference from adults (Klein, 1985). All of these qualities could be descriptive of dissociative parts as well.

Through the course of my consultations I have developed some hypotheses about the differences between normal developmental imaginary friends phenomena and the pathological expression of this in dissociative disorders (Silberg, 1995). These hypotheses are listed below:

1. Dissociative children are more confused about whether the friend is only "pretend."
2. Dissociative children feel bossed or bothered by the friend.

3. Dissociative children feel the friend can take over their body.
4. Dissociative children feel the need to protect the secrecy of their pretend friend's identity.
5. Dissociative children believe there are conflicting imaginary friends who make him/her feel conflicted about how to behave.

To test these hypotheses, I have developed an imaginary friend questionnaire (see Appendix), a version of which has been piloted on a sample of 149 normal children in England (Frost, Silberg, & McIntee, 1996). Currently my colleagues and I are testing this measure on a clinical sample of children with diverse diagnoses and on dissociative children. Initial results suggest that 29% of the tested sample of normal children have imaginary friends, and hypotheses about the normal children's view of imaginary friends were confirmed. Initial results from a clinical sample have been promising in confirming these hypotheses as well. Trujillo, Lewis, Yeager, and Gidlow (1996) have similarly found differences between normal imaginary friends and those in a clinical population. As research in this important area progresses further, it may help with the careful clinical differentiation of normal fantasy projections from the dissociative child's pathological fragmentation.

In one of my more striking interviews Lizzy, a 12-year-old girl with DID, described the process whereby her imaginary playmates became alters. She stated that initially she created imaginary playmates named after favorite people in her environment who helped her cope with sexual and physical abuse from her father. She described how she dressed them in her mind with special clothes, pictured their faces, and invented vivid details about their life—Lizzy called this "stage 1." Next, she said, she noticed that the "friends" could talk to her, even when she had not initiated conversation. She described being surprised, though somewhat delighted that this had occurred, as their seeming autonomy was not perceived as threatening. This beginning of the separation and autonomy of the "friend" she termed "stage 2" and may be characteristic of children in early stages of DDNOS and with young normal preschoolers as well. Next, Lizzy stated that she discovered that the "friends" could take over for brief periods of time and influence her behavior without her awareness—she termed this "stage 3." She found this quite troubling as she reported that at this point (age 7), according to her memory, the "friends" initiated dangerous actions—running into the street, or trying to escape from windows. Finally, Lizzy described that the "friends" could take over her body at will and stay in her consciousness for long periods of time, including years—this was termed "stage 4." Lizzy suggested that amnesia was a common phenomenon in stage 3 and especially 4. Although Lizzy was fully aware that the initial process was under her control, she stated that she knew of no way to "go back a step." Young's (1988) descriptions of the development of alters in younger patients follows a similar sequence.

Perhaps careful research of children with dissociative disorders in various stages may help to confirm Lizzy's hypothesis. Lizzy's theory does appear consonant with child clinicians' descriptions of dissociative disorders in children as "incipient" (Fagan & McMahon, 1984) or "precursors" to the full DID picture seen in adults (Peterson, 1990). Ultimately research will continue to move forward by careful attention to the honest disclosures of patients like Lizzy, who give us remarkable insight into the private subjective reality that may underlie the development of pathological dissociation.

Summary

This chapter has discussed interviewing techniques that may be utilized to elicit frank disclosures about feelings of dividedness, fluctuations, trance states, and other imaginal processes in patients that may suggest the pathological use of dissociative defenses. Discrimination between dissociative patients' reports and those of other diagnostic groups were presented. As research continues to refine diagnostic techniques for the assessment of childhood dissociative conditions, clinicians in the future will be better equipped to make these difficult discriminations.

References

Dell, D. F., & Eisenhower, J. W. (1990). Adolescent multiple personality disorder: a preliminary study of eleven cases. *Journal of the American Academy of Child and Adolescent Psychiatry, 29,* 359–366.

Fagan, J., & McMahon, P.P. (1984). Incipient multiple personality in children. *The Journal of Nervous and Mental Disease, 172,* 26–36.

Fink, D. (1993). Observations on the role of transitional objects and transitional phenomena in patients with multiple personality disorder. In R. P. Kluft & C. G. Fine (Eds.), *Clinical perspectives on multiple personality disorder,* pp. 241–252. Washington, DC: American Psychiatric Press.

Frost, J., Silberg, J. L., McCintee, J. (1996). *Imaginary friends and clinical diagnoses* (research in progress).

Gudzer, J., Paris, J., Zilkowitz, P., & Marchessault, K. (1996). Risk factors for borderline pathology. *Journal of the American Academy of Child and Adolescent Psychiatry, 35,* 26–33.

Klein, B. R. (1985). A child's imaginary companion: a transitional self. *Clinical Social Work, 13,* 272–282.

Kluft, R. (1985). Childhood multiple personality disorder: Predictors, clinical findings and treatment results. In R. P. Kluft (Ed.), *Childhood antecedents of multiple personality* (pp. 167–196). Washington, DC: American Psychiatric Press, Inc.

Lewis, D. O. (1996). Diagnostic evaluation of the child with dissociative identity disorder/multiple personality disorder. *Child and Adolescent Psychiatric Clinics of North America, 5,* 303–331.

McMahon, P. P., & Fagan, J. (1993). Treatment of childhood dissociative disorders. In Kluft, R. P. & Fine C. G. (Eds.). *Clinical perspectives on multiple personality disorder* (pp. 253–276). Washington DC: American Psychiatric Press.

Peterson, G. (1990) Diagnosis of childhood multiple personality. *Dissociation, 3,* 3–9.

Putnam, F. W. (1991). Dissociative disorders in children and adolescents: A developmental perspective. *Psychiatric Clinics of North America, 14,* 519–531.

Putnam, F. W., Helmers, K., & Trickett, P. K. (1993). Development, reliability, and validity of a child dissociation scale. *The Journal of Child Abuse and Neglect, 17,* 731–741.

Ross, C. A., Herber, S., Norton, G., et al. (1989). The Dissociative Disorders Interview Schedule: A structured interview. *Dissociation, 2,* 169–189.

Ross, C. A., Miller, S. D., Bjornson, L., et al. (1990). Structured interview data on 102 cases of multiple personality disorder from four centers. *American Journal of Psychiatry, 147,* 596–601.

Silberg, J. L. (1995) Imaginary Friends: Precursors to Alters. Presentation at the 12th International Conference on Dissociative States. Orlando, Florida.

Silberg, J. (1996). Dissociative symptomatology in children and adolescents as displayed on psychological testing. (In review.)

Singer, D. G., & Singer J. L. (1990). *The House of Make-Believe.* Cambridge: Harvard University Press.

Steinberg, M. (1993). *Structured Clinical Interview for DSM-IV Dissociative Disorders (SCID-D).* Washington, DC: American Psychiatric Press.

Steinberg, M., Rounsaville, B., & Cichetti, D. (1991). Detection of dissociative disorders in psychiatric patients by a screening instrument and a structured diagnostic interview. *The American Journal of Psychiatry, 148,* 1105–6.

Steinberg, M., & Steinberg, A. (1995). Using the SCID-D to asses dissociative identity disorder in adolescents: Three case studies (1995). *Bulletin of the Menninger Clinic, 59* (2), 221–231.

Trujillo, K., Lewis, P. O., Yeager, C. A., & Gidlow, B. (1996). Imaginary companions of school boys and boys with dissociative identity disorder: A normal to pathological continuum. *Child and Adolescent Psychiatric Clinics of North America, 5,* 375–391.

Williams, D. (1992). *Nobody nowhere.* New York: Time Books.

Williams, D. (1994). *Somebody somewhere.* New York: Time Books.

Winnicott, D. (1953). Transitional objects and transitional phenomena. *International Journal of Psychoanalysis, 34,* 89–97.

Young, W. C. (1988). Observations on fantasy in the formation of multiple personality disorder. *Dissociation, 1,* 13–19.

four

Childhood DID:
The Male Population

Jean Goodwin

Still in the mid-1990s, two decades after the rediscovery of the dissociative disorders and their elaboration in American diagnostic manuals and textbooks, the male child or adolescent with Dissociative Identity Disorder (DID) remains a neglected rarity. As of about 1990 there were fewer than 20 published cases. A 1991 review article (Peterson) located 26 published cases of childhood DID (ages 12 and under); gender was specified in 20, and 11 of those were males. A 1990 series of 11 adolescent cases (Dell & Eisenhower) included 4 males. The largest series to date (Putnam, Hornstein, & Peterson, 1996), a collaborative study of 177 cases, includes 63 males and finds male dissociative children to be less symptomatic than their female counterparts. As studies such as this one mark a new era in the field of childhood dissociation, we may begin to identify and treat these cases more effectively.

Overall, the field of child dissociative disorders remains at an early stage, dominated by publications aimed at establishing construct validity for the syndrome in children (Hornstein & Putnam, 1992), describing phenomenology and descriptive demographics (Dell & Eisenhower, 1990; Hornstein & Tyson, 1991; Putnam, 1993), providing detailed case histories with natural history antecedents and sequalae (LaPorta, 1992; McElroy, 1992), designing psychological tests and describing test results in children (Silberg, 1996; Steinberg & Steinberg, 1995) hypothesis building and model building (Putnam, 1991), and developing criteria and instru-

Acknowledgments: David Mann, Ph.D., and Hilary Klein, M.D., contributed ideas and data through our 1994 article. Sharon Wills, Ph.D., carefully criticized and discussed this chapter.

ments for future research (Malinosky-Rummell & Hoier, 1991; Peterson & Putnam, 1994; Putnam, Helmers, & Trickett, 1993; Putnam & Peterson, 1994; Ross, Ryan, et al., 1991).

This chapter addresses each of these foundational areas, especially insofar as these preliminary studies begin to suggest clinical guidelines for the assessment of male children and adolescents who may be experiencing dissociative phenomena. Why are these diagnoses so rarely made in young males? Does this rarity reflect the true demographics of the disorder or other factors? The chapter reviews in detail the pattern of symptom presentation in five boys diagnosed with Dissociative Identity Disorder and followed by chart review for 8 to 10 years. Symptoms in this group are compared with those reported in other severely abused young males and in child and adolescent females with DID. The chapter closes with ideas about identifying and screening boys at risk for dissociation and for treating those with DID or other dissociative diagnoses.

The Rarity of Dissociative Diagnoses in Boys and Adolescent Males: Result of Victimization Rates, Gender Biology, Cultural Myths, or Obstacles to Accurate Assessment?

In adults with DID the ratio of male to female patients was reported in the two earliest large clinical surveys as 1 to 9 (Putnam, Guroff, et al., 1986; Ross, Norton, & Wozney, 1989); more recent estimates, however, are closer to 1 male to 4 females (Putnam, 1989).

Some authors have correlated this female gender preponderance with the gender ratio of childhood sexual abuse (Herman, 1992). Koss, Gidyez, and Wisniewski (1987) in a national survey of 6159 post-adolescents (ages 18–24) found that 53.7% of the women and 25.1% of the men reported some form of previous sexual victimization, with 15.4% of the women and 4.4% of the men describing having been raped. Thus, if sexual abuse is critical to the development of pathological dissociation in childhood, and if these victimization figures are accurate, young males would have only half or one-third the risk of females for developing DID. However, many types of childhood trauma other than sexual abuse have been linked to DID—physical abuse, emotional abuse, medical trauma, witnessed violence, parental illness or substance abuse, political torture or persecution—and these traumata tend to produce equal numbers of male and female victims (Perry, et al., in press).

Other biological and cultural differences could account for some of the gender difference in DID. Females are generally thought to be more suggestible than males. However, hypnotizability testing demonstrates equal capacities for hypnosis in the genders (Bliss, 1986). Particularly during the childhood years when pathological dissociation is thought to arise, about 50% of both genders are highly hypnotizable and thus probably capable of the hypnotic feats thought to be most linked with Dissociative Identity Disorder—amnesia, involuntariness, compartmentalization (such as the hidden observer phenomenon), and negative and positive hallucinations (Spiegel & Vermutten, 1994). However, at least in mainstream American culture, males may be discouraged from some forms of free-floating private reverie, from the focussed attention required in meditation or prayer, and from some repetitive automatic scripted behaviors such as household chores, all of which are optimal contexts for inducing and practicing trance states (Kirmayer, 1994). In addition to an increased cultural focus on rational thinking, self-consciousness, and executive action, males may also be under greater pressure to imagine themselves as unitary and thus resist the intimations of polypsychism that would arise if they allowed themselves to become aware of their trance capacities (Ross, 1991).

However, it remains a possibility that the gender gap in DID is entirely artifactual, based on the difficulty of identifying either victimization or dissociation in males. If one looks at gender ratios among DID patients by average age of sample, the percentage of males drops with increasing age: among child cases 50% are males (Peterson, 1991); among adolescent cases 37% are males (Dell & Eisenhower, 1991); but only 10% to 20% of adult cases are males (Putnam, 1989). A similar phenomenon is found in child sexual abuse treatment, with equal numbers of males and females present in preschool samples but very few males reported as presenting for psychological treatment in adulthood (Goodwin, 1989b).

Where do the sexually abused and dissociative males disappear to? Bliss (1986) suggested they might be diverted into the criminal justice system and thus escape diagnosis and tallying in clinical surveys. Certain differentials in male socialization clearly mitigate against complaints about victimization (Nasjleti, 1980; Kaufman, 1984; Dimock, 1988; Vander Mey, 1988) or frightening symptoms (Klein, Mann, & Goodwin, 1994). Parents, peers, and professionals may conspire to deny or minimize abuse, labeling it sexual "good luck" and minimizing consequent symptoms (Zavodnick, 1989; Briere, Evans, Runtz, & Wall, 1988). Since intrafamilial sexual abuse of males, the most traumagenic type (Finkelhor, 1985), often involves a male perpetrator, these victims face a double taboo against disclosure—incest and homosexuality (Goodwin, 1989a; Goodwin, 1989b; Watkins and Bentovim, 1992; Williams, 1988). It is also possible that certain elements of the male experience lead to amelioration of dissociative symptoms as development progresses or to partial or disguised expressions of symptoms which we are not yet capable of recognizing as dissociative or trauma-related. Some patterns of remorseless violence may someday be understood in this way (Perry, et al., in press).

In adults, the diagnosis of DID is difficult to ascertain and often delayed, with patients averaging seven years in mental health care before the diagnosis is made (Ross, 1989). The diagnostic difficulty has been even greater in children and adolescents. While adults routinely tell us retrospectively that their symptoms began in preschool years (Kluft, 1985b, 1990), only 11 percent of cases are diagnosed before age 20 (Peterson, 1990; Putnam, 1991). Assessment problems in children (Klein, Mann, & Goodwin, 1994; Kluft, 1985a) include the high levels of dissociative phenomena in normal children, the lack of separate child criteria for diagnosis (which would specify the evolving nature of symptoms), and skepticism among child psychiatrists who may not include DID in the differential diagnosis or who may choose to acknowledge in a complex comorbid case only those diagnoses which are familiar and commonplace (for example, conduct disorder). Additional facts that mitigate against recognition are the child's own unawareness of his actual history and symptoms, the fluctuating nature of the symptoms, and the hostile or malevolent environment, often requiring concealment, in which such symptomatic children find themselves. Clinicians may become so frustrated by the persistent lack of clear information in these cases that they fail to perceive that the lack of data itself may be a clue to amnesia, personality shifts, or family chaos, which should lead to screening for dissociation.

The most persistent gender differences reported in abused boys as compared to girls are increased sexual and aggressive behavior (Friedrich, et al. 1988; Watkins and Bentovim, 1992). Especially when these symptoms lead to aggressive physical or sexual victimization of others (Freeman-Longo, 1986), the diagnostic focus on the youth's uncontrolled behavior may obscure other symptom complexes. Insofar as the boy himself is trying to escape a helpless position by projecting helplessness outward onto his victims and assuming a hypermasculine stance, he may collude with authorities in defining himself as "bad" rather than "ill" or "mad." Since DID is often suspected in those adult criminals who have committed heinous offenses and whose early childhood abuse history is so grotesque as to produce incredulity, society and the courts tend to join the symptomatic criminal in refusing to consider the role of trauma-related illness (Lewis and Bard, 1991).

Hypothesis Building Using Small Samples: Characteristics of Five Child and Adolescent Males Diagnosed as Having DID

In the mid-1980s, a psychologist (D. M.) working in a rural midwestern Community Mental Health Center noticed that, in the space of two years, 5 outpatient males (ages 8 to 14) referred for routine testing switched to alternate ego states during sessions (Klein, Mann, & Goodwin, 1994). This was about 5% of the children he tested in those years. Similar percentages of new DID diagnoses have been reported on child inpatient units (Hornstein & Tyson, 1991; Silberg, Stipic, & Taghizadeh, in press). All five boys had conduct disorder diagnoses prior to the DID diagnoses, and three had juvenile records. All had substantiated prior sexual abuse and four had protective service involvement. The five boys were treated for 8 to 30 months for their post-traumatic and dissociative symptoms (definitive treatment to integration, except in Case 4, which was interrupted), and their charts were reviewed during the subsequent 8 to 10 years.

Table I summarizes the five cases along the following axes: 1) age and living arrangement at time of diagnosis and family history of dissociative disorder; 2) the nature of the child's adversity history and collateral data about abuse incidents; 3) an estimate of the delay between onset of abuse and diagnosis; 4) an outline of the child's symptoms; 5) a list of obstacles to diagnosis and treatment; and 6) the child's status at chart review followup 8 to 10 years later. Each case is described; following the cases, a composite case description is outlined.

Despite the well-substantiated sexual abuse histories (in two cases the perpetrator confessed and in one an attempt at sodomy was witnessed), there was a 1 to 7 year delay in these cases between onset of sexual abuse and diagnosis of dissociative level defenses. Three boys sustained one or more incomplete or aborted evaluations before diagnosis (cases 1, 2, and 5). This delay was time enough for one boy to be reabused (case 4) and for three to reabuse others (cases 1, 2, and 3). Even after the diagnosis was recognized, one boy was reabused (case 4), and one abused another child (case 3).

Obstacles to recognition and treatment were met with from mothers, fathers, other family members, and foster parents; such obstacles affected all 5 cases. There was resistance to believing the child had symptoms, especially sexual symptoms, resistance to believing the child had been abused, and resistance to believing in DID. In the most discouraging example (case 4) the child was kidnapped from foster care by his perpetrator after 8 months of treatment and lost to followup. Dell and Eisenhower (1990) have described a 100% treatment failure rate when DID adolescents come from profoundly abusive families and a 40% dropout rate when families are narcissistic and rejecting. The presence of a family history of dissociative disorder in three cases, while helpful as a clue to diagnosis, no doubt also contributed to ongoing chaotic information-processing and care-giving. In 3 cases other professionals—a family physician, a psychiatric inpatient unit, and two previous psychologists—contributed to delay in recognition of the prior sexual abuse and the dissociative symptoms. The boys themselves were intensely involved in keeping secret both their sexual victimization and their dissociative symptoms. In four cases the abuse history was not known to the hypermasculine host but guarded by a "secret-keeping" alter who also acted as a hypervigilant protector against further abuse. Only in Case 3 did the host know about sexual abuse and then only about one perpetrator. The host's hypermasculine defenses, which included self-isolation and an aggressive facade, also kept others at bay enough to insulate against both

Table I.

Five Child and Adolescent Males Diagnosed as Having Dissociative Identity Disorder: Demographics, Childhood Adversity, Delay in Evaluation, Symptoms, Obstacles to Diagnosis and Treatment, and Ten-Year Followup.

Case, Age at Diagnosis / Family History	Adversity	Delay	Symptoms	Obstacles	Ten-Year Follow-Up
1. Brad, 8 Living with divorced mother then foster care after protective services report. Mother diagnosed with major dissociative disorder.	Disclosed ongoing sexual abuse during Rorschach. Extrafamilial perpetrator arrested and confessed.	Sexual abuse onset 1 year prior to evaluation and disclosure.	Violence to others at school. Vivid imaginary friend. Runaway; lost after sessions. Sexually abused another child. Rapid shift to different appearance, voice tone, accent, and drawing style. Loses time. Different named identities give different abuse histories.	Symptoms episodic (e.g. Wisc-R FSIQ's, 87 and 144). Mother withdrew him from therapy when protective service report was made. Family M.D. said "boys are never molested." His sexual abuse of another child returns him to treatment.	Mother judged negligent of Brad and younger siblings, continues in treatment. Brad involved in substance abuse, criminally charged at 18, now in court-mandated treatment.
2. Bob, 14. In foster care after being charged with sexual abuse.	Describes sexual abuse by male babysitter at age 6. Records show protective services substantiation.	Sexual abuse substantiated at age 7 not connected to his psychiatric symptoms until evaluation at age 14.	Charged with sexual abuse of younger child. Two prior psychiatric hospitalizations at 7 and 10 for schizophrenia. Hostile, uncooperative. At times does not seem to recognize office or therapist. Sudden shift to frightened confused, silent state. Says he is 6 years old. Different named identities give different abuse histories.	Parents refuse to believe he was sexually abused or that he has sexually abused others.	Foster care. Treatment until he enters technical college at age 18. No further contact.

3. Jack, 12. In foster care placement, which becomes adoptive home after termination of parental rights.	Removed to foster care after substantiated sexual abuse by older brother and one year plus of chronic truancy.	Described sexual abuse by multiple family members for several years prior to removal.	Caught attempting to sodomize younger child in foster home. Sudden switches to markedly immature behaviors. Loses time and memories for sessions. Uses different names. Different named identities, describe the abuse history for each named perpetrator.	Parents denied sexual abuse. Adoptive parents "did not believe in MPD."	Parents' rights terminated. Adopted by foster parents. Withdrawn from therapy by adoptive parents. Convicted at age 18 of sexual abuse of a 13-year-old. In prison.
4. Chip, 8. In foster care. Mother, who lives elsewhere, diagnosed and treated for major dissociative disorder.	Placed in foster care because of physical abuse by father and uncontrolled truancy and runaways. Victim of witnessed attempt at sodomy by foster sibling (case 3).	Discloses sexual abuse by uncle which preceded removal by many years.	Denied witnessed incident of being sexually abused in foster care. Sleepwalking. Sudden shifts to somnambulistic frightened, angry state with inability to speak except in neologisms. Only his unnamed somnambulistic state describes either recent witnessed or past abuse.	After 6 months, kidnapped from foster care by alleged perpetrator.	Lost to followup.
5. Rick, 9. Lives with divorced father. Mother and paternal grandmother diagnosed and treated for major dissociative disorders.	Father awarded custody when Rick was 7 because of sexual abuse by custodial mother and her friends since divorce at age 2. Mother confessed.	Describes sexual abuse since age 2 and symptoms since age 7.	School says he "spaces out," refuses work, and has no friends. Describes two named alter identities who he thinks have the knowledge about his abuse that he lacks. Father concerned that Rick steals.	Symptoms episodic. (Two sets of psychological tests by two psychologists markedly different.) Rick denied abuse until treated. Father repeatedly removed him from treatment.	Returned to therapy when he began dating. Outstanding wrestler in high school. No further contact after graduation.
Combined profile. Grade school age. Lives with single parent or in foster care. At least one caretaker has a dissociative diagnosis.	Sexual abuse substantiated by child protection or criminal prosecution. Court determined custody.	1–7 year lag between onset of sexual abuse and dissociative diagnosis.	Participates in physical or sexual attacks. Problems with truancy, runaways, or stealing. Denies witnessed events. Trance, confusion, amnesia. Witnessed shifts, often to immature behavior.	Caretakers deny abuse events, and symptoms, and tend to remove prematurely from treatment.	Treatment after adolescence may be necessary. Later criminal involvement in 2 of 5.

Table 2.

Hypermasculine, Secret-Keeping Subtype: Summary of Mental Status Findings

	Behavior	Affect	Sensation	Cognition
FEAR	Hyperactive Sexualized Uses substances Counterphobic	Numbed, restricted Fears emerge in play, projective tests, drawing	Stoic Robotic	Hypervigilant Amnestic and hypermnestic Gaps in trauma narrative Variable concentration and IQ; learning problems
ANGER	Violent fights Aggressive Reenacts in identification with aggressor	Rageful High hostility Explosive temper Irritable	Images of self and others distorted by power/combat focus	Distrusts authority and caretakers Expects betrayal
SADNESS	Sleeping problems	Anhedonic Shame prone	Occasionally "low" body image, energy	Actively avoids painful memories
DISSOCIATION	Self-isolation Trance withdrawal Runaways Spontaneous age regression	Sudden mood shifts	Hallucinatory imaginary companions	Dense childhood amnesia Amnesia for (denial of) recent events State shifts determine skills, memories Awareness that internal others know and handle things may not be experi- enced as "voices"

open communication and intimacy triggers to traumatic material. This response has been termed by Salter (1995) "intimacy allergy."

Diagnosis was obvious once the therapist observed a named alter identity (with markedly different characteristics) take control of the child's behavior. In retrospect, using the Child Dissociative Checklist (Putnam, Helmers, & Trickett, 1993), which was not yet published in 1985, these boys would have scored as positive on 16 of the 20 items: denies known traumatic experiences, described by teachers as "spaced out," shows rapid changes in personality, forgets things he should know (such as who the therapist is), loses time, shows marked variations in knowledge or skill (such as drawing style), has difficulty learning from experience (impervious to discipline), continues to deny even witnessed behaviors, refers to self in third person or insists on being called by a different name, unusually sexually precocious, has vivid imaginary companions, has intense outbursts of anger, sleepwalks frequently, has unusual nighttime experiences, and has two or more distinct personalities that take control of behavior. Two of the remaining non-positive items involve hearing the voices of imaginary companions and talking to oneself using different voices. Although all these boys were aware that other internal entities held knowledge and at times handled problems, the secrecy priority seemed to preclude talking out loud even internally (Kluft, 1991). Likely a full query about Schneiderian symptoms would have helped uncover this sense of silent internal dividedness (Kluft, 1985b, 1987). The two items clearly not present in any of these children were self-injury and rapidly changing physical complaints. Self-injury seems to exacerbate after adolescence (Dell & Eisenhower, 1990) and the lack of complaints involving body sensation may relate to the intense stoicism of this group. Both symptoms have been reported in other samples of severely symptomatic male child sexual victims (Frederick, 1986) and in adult males with dissociative disorders (Goodwin, 1993a). Recent analysis of 177 child and adolescent DID cases found somatic symptoms more frequent in girls and more frequent in older patients (Putnam, et al., 1996).

Table II summarizes the mental status findings in this small group. The table looks at four core emotions—anxiety, anger, sadness, and, instead of joy, dissociation, which might be conceptualized as a preserver of the capacity for joy in extreme situations. Manifestations of each core emotion are then mapped as they appear on four axes of observation—behavior, affect, sensation, and cognition. It is probable that this group, given its subcultural homogeneity, represents only one possible presentation of DID in boys. The rural midwestern subculture in which they live probably supports a hypermasculine style of behavior and cognition as well as rigorous secret-keeping about both prior victimization and symptoms, especially those in the realm of fear and sadness. The profile is remarkably unchildlike, emphasizing not only "masculine" traits but those found in adult males of a certain "heroic" type. This may reflect the dominance of alters older than the chronological age of the host (Steinberg & Steinberg, 1995).

How does this picture differ from that seen in uncomplicated conduct disorder? And how can we distinguish the presence of dissociation when evaluating a boy with conduct problems? In both conditions one would expect positive sexual and violence histories. However, only if one asks in detail about past traumatic experiences is it possible to see, in the boys with dissociation, amnestic and hypermnestic (flashback) gaps appearing in the narrative along with the emergence of spontaneous age regressions. If one can engage the boy in play or drawing, one may see the clustering of different attitude and skill sets as different ego states predominate (Snow, et al., 1995). Projective testing led to disclosure and switching in one case. In two cases there were marked differences in standard nonprojective test results. Trancing out and somnambulism were witnessed behaviors that pointed to a dissociative problem. As therapy progressed beyond the assessment stage, one could observe lost time and amnesia in sessions and begin to describe the child's internal imaginative world, including imaginary companions.

How is this picture different from that typically observed in adolescent girls or young women with DID? In the boys, fear and sadness tend to be avoided by counterphobic behaviors and cognitions rather than manifested as surface panic, misery, anguish, suicidality, or phobias. Identification is with aggressor or rescuer elements in the fantasied abuse triangle rather than with the victim. These boys seem to try to experience and re-experience the world from a "power" viewpoint. Many of the symptoms they lack are those connected with re-experiencing from a victim viewpoint—hearing the voice of the abuser, feeling the pain of the abuse, feeling the terror in ways that interfere with eating, reenacting the abuse through self-mutilation. If one thinks about the basic limbic system responses to the distress caused by attack and abandonment, these boys seem to be trying to emphasize the "fight" response rather than the "freeze" response seen in more phobic or manifestly depressed children (Perry, 1994). Their dissociative amnesia and dissociative switching is often in the service of facilitating active aggressive behavioral outlets for their distress. In many of the female cases amnesia and switching are more in the service of allowing emotional outbursts or perceptual distortions to become briefly manifest. This tendency for males to dominate aggression measures while females predominate in depression categories is a common finding, not limited to trauma-dissociative populations (Ross & Norton, 1989). Perry, et al. (in press) speculate that the predominance of the "freeze" response in women and children may have evolved as an adaptation to warfare patterns in which these noncombatants were kidnapped, raped, and enslaved and thus might have had a better chance to survive utilizing the "freeze" mode than in "fight/flight" activation.

What can we understand from the outcome data available in these cases? Two of the boys (Table I) have left treatment and are apparently well; both had returned to treatment briefly during high school years after the initial DID diagnosis and treatment. Two of the boys are now in the prison/probation system. The boy who was kidnapped by his perpetrator may be dead or living a criminal or marginal lifestyle. It is unlikely that any of these five would define himself as DID or seek voluntary treatment. Thus, this subpopulation may be essentially non-overlapping not only with other child DID populations (those identified in inpatient settings or dominated by female cases or cases involving other subcultures), but this subgroup also may be non-overlapping with adult cases. This is an important feature to note, because there is a tendency to see child DID as more "pure" than adult cases since children are closer in time and space to the chaotic childhood experiences that so dominate the dissociative patient's internal world as it emerges clinically. Thus, Coons (1994a; 1994b) expects to find a frequency of child protective involvement in adults with "true" DID similar to that found in adolescent DID. This is probably not a realistic assumption, since most child and adolescent cases, like these five boys, do not come to treatment voluntarily because of painful or frightening inner experiences, but are brought in by caseworkers, foster parents, new custodial or adoptive parents, or school or law enforcement officials, in some of these cases because of sexual or aggressive misbehavior.

Conclusions and Recommendations

In 1989 the author (Goodwin, 1989a) listed four types of indicators that should trigger screening for dissociative symptoms in cases where childhood abuse or neglect is recognized. These included:

1. *Psychopathology in a parent* especially *dissociative disorders,* because of the possibility of genetic or intergenerational transmission (Braun, 1985; Kluft, 1984; Malenbaum & Russell, 1987), but screening should also encompass other severe psychopathology in the caretaker, especially those conditions placing the child at risk for severe abuse, such as *substance abuse, antisocial personality, sexual paraphilias,* and *manic, paranoid, or impulsive disorders*;
2. *Medical* and *physiological indicators* in the child, including severe *physical sequelae of trauma* requiring medical care or *hospitalization,* precocious onset of *sexual paraphilias* or other *sexual disorders,* and *pain syndromes, conversion symptoms, eating* and other *somatoform disorders* (including *night terrors* and *somnambulism*);
3. *Family and social indicators,* including *extreme abuse* of any type, *excessive secrecy* and *isolation,* a *malevolent* or *sadistic environment* (Goodwin, 1993b), and patterns of *"multiplicity,"* such as *multiple*

abusers, *multiple types of abuse, multiple generations* involved, *multiple family problems,* and *multiple contextual shifts* for the child, making integration of traumatic experience difficult.

4. *Psychological symptoms* in the child, such as *amnesia, accusations,* especially of *lying, active fantasy life* (O'Brien, 1985), *trancelike states, multiple ego states, episodic extreme behaviors* which may be flash-back reenactments, and *runaways,* especially those with *fugue-like* qualities.

5. Other *comorbid psychological features,* including extreme *depression* or *self-harm* syndromes, the presence of *multiple diagnoses* or *diagnostic puzzlement,* and the presence of moderate or severe symptoms of *Post-traumatic Stress Disorder* or other *severe anxiety.*

The five male cases described in this chapter conform to these recommendations. Three involved a family history of major dissociative disorder (cases 1, 4, and 5); four involved either precocious sexualization or somnambulism (cases 1, 2, 3, and 4); three involved multiple sexual and/or physical abusers (cases 3, 4, and 5) and the other two involved adjudicated parental negligence around a single extrafamilial sexual abuser; and all 5 involved excessive secrecy and multiple living contexts for the youngster. As described above, all had the dissociative symptoms diagnostic of DID—presence of amnesia and witnessed switches among multiple ego states, two had runaways (cases 1 and 4), and a third (case 3) had chronic truancy. Three were diagnostic puzzles (cases 1, 2, and 5), for whom many diagnoses had been considered. The remaining two were caught in a characteristic dissociative denial—participating in a sexual assault which both perpetrator and victim denied and apparently did not remember. Kluft (1985a) has described a similar episode where the mother who physically abused one child, the child who had been abused, and a second witnessing child all denied and were apparently oblivious to the abusive episode the psychiatrist had witnessed during a family session.

The findings in males suggest that screening for dissociation should be a consideration for child therapists other than those working specifically in child protection (James, 1990). Like the five boys described here, other delinquent and sexually perpetrating boys, as well as runaways and truants, may come to therapeutic attention because of symptomatic behaviors rather than child abuse complaints. Even in the three boys in the sample who were already removed from known child abuse or neglect perpetrators before evaluation, additional previously unknown perpetrators and abuses were disclosed once the dissociative defenses were understood. Better understanding of post-traumatic and dissociative defenses as they exist in boys may be necessary for accurate violence histories to be collected in males both in symptomatic groups and in the general population. In the five cases reported here, Putnam's Child Dissociative

Checklist would have been an effective screening tool. This 20-item instrument can be filled out by a parent, teacher, or therapist in 5 to 10 minutes (Putnam, Helmers, & Trickett, 1993; Putnam & Peterson, 1994). (See Appendix A.)

Case reports repeatedly urge early recognition of dissociative symptoms and describe rather rapid relief in children once treatment is commenced (Putnam, 1993). However, longterm followup of this small group shows at least 40% with criminal convictions in young adulthood: this approaches the catastrophic outcomes for child conduct disorder (Rutter et al., 1994). The proneness to relapse and the extreme resistance to treatment found in this sample should encourage us to develop more acceptable and effective adjunctive treatment models for boys. Some of the models that might bypass obstacles to treatment and treatment resumption include brief interventions with planned long-term reassessment and followup; treatment that is home-based or involves the family; treatment that engages the boy himself as self-rater, monitor, or student of his symptoms; treatment that involves the major motor behaviors that are most involved in symptoms, perhaps therapeutic sports teams, wilderness experiences, or building projects (Goodwin & Talwar, 1992); and treatment that engages artistic outlets, such as music, drama, and the plastic arts.

References

Bliss, E. L. (1986). *Multiple personality, allied disorders, and hypnosis.* New York: Oxford University Press.

Braun, B. G. (1985). The transgenerational incidence of dissociation and multiple personality disorder: A preliminary report. In R. P. Kluft (Ed.), *Childhood antecedents of multiple personality* (pp. 127–150). Washington, DC: American Psychiatric Press.

Briere, J., Evans, D., Runtz, M., & Wall, T. (1988). Symptomatology in men who were molested as children: A comparison study. *American Journal of Orthopsychiatry, 58* (3), 457–461.

Coons, P. M. (1994a). Confirmation of childhood abuse in child and adolescent cases of multiple personality disorders and dissociative disorder not otherwise specified. *Journal of Nervous and Mental Disease, 182,* 461–464.

Coons, P. M. (1994b). Reports of satanic ritual abuse: Further implications about pseudomemories. *Perceptual and Motor Skills, 78,* 1376–1378.

Dell, P. F., & Eisenhower, J. W. (1990). Adolescent multiple personality disorder. *Journal of the American Academy of Child & Adolescent Psychiatry, 29,* 359–366.

Dimock, P. (1988). Male sexual abuse: An underreported problem. *Journal of Interpersonal Violence, 3*(2), 203–221.

Finkelhor, D. (1985). *Child sexual abuse: New theory and research.* New York: Free Press.

Frederick, C. J. (1986). Post-traumatic stress disorder and child molestation. In A. W. Burgess & C. R. Hartman (Eds.), *Sexual Exploitation of Patients by Health Professionals* (pp. 133–142). New York: Praeger.

Freeman-Longo, R. E. (1986). The impact of sexual victimization on males. *Child Abuse & Neglect, 10,* 411–414.

Friedrich, W. N., Berliner, L., Urguiza, A. J., & Beilke, R. L. (1988). Brief diagnostic group treatment of sexually abused boys. *Journal of Interpersonal Violence, 3* (3), 331–343.

Goodwin, J. (1989a). Recognizing dissociative symptoms in abused children. In J. Goodwin (Ed.), *Sexual abuse: Incest victims and their families* (pp. 169–181). Chicago: Yearbook.

Goodwin, J. (1989b). *Sexual abuse: Incest victims and their families.* Chicago: Yearbook.

Goodwin, J. (1993a). *Rediscovering childhood trauma: Historical casebook and clinical applications.* Washington, DC: American Psychiatric Press.

Goodwin, J. (1993b). Sadistic abuse: Definition, recognition, and treatment. *Dissociation, 6,* 181–187.

Goodwin, J. & Talwar, N. (1989). Group psychotherapy for incest victims. *Psychiatric Clinic of North America, 12* (2), 279–293.

Herman, J. (1992). *Trauma and recovery.* New York: Basic Books.

Hornstein, N., & Putnam, F. W. (1992). Clinical phenomenology of child and adolescent dissociative disorders. *Journal of the American Academy of Child & Adolescent Psychiatry, 31,* 1077–1085.

Hornstein, N. & Tyson, S. (1991). Inpatient treatment of children with multiple personality and their families. *Psychiatric Clinics of North America, 14* (3), 631–648.

James, B. (1990). The dissociatively disordered child. *The Advisor, 3* (4), 8–10.

Kaufman, A. (1984). Rape of men in the community. In I. Stuart and J. Greer (Eds.), *Victims of sexual aggression: Treatment of children, women and men* (pp. 156–179). New York: Van Nostrand/Reinhold.

Kirmayer, L. J., (1994). Pacing the void: Social and cultural dimensions of dissociation. In D. Spiegel (Ed.), *Dissociation: Culture, mind and body* (pp. 91–122). Washington, DC: American Psychiatric Press.

Klein, H., Mann, D. R., & Goodwin, J. M. (1994). Obstacles to the recognition of sexual abuse and dissociative disorders in child and adolescent males. *Dissociation, 7,* 138–144.

Kluft, R. P. (1984). Multiple personality disorder in childhood. *Psychiatric Clinic of North America, 7,* 121–134.

Kluft, R. P. (1985a). Childhood multiple personality disorder: Predictors, clinical findings, and treatment results. In R. P. Kluft (Ed.), *Childhood antecedents of multiple personality* (pp. 167–196). Washington, DC: American Psychiatric Press.

Kluft, R. P. (1985b). The natural history of multiple personality disorder. In R. P. Kluft (Ed.), *Childhood antecedents of multiple personality* (pp. 197–238). Washington, DC: American Psychiatric Press.

Kluft, R. P. (1987). First-rank symptoms as a diagnostic clue to multiple personality disorder. *American Journal of Psychiatry, 144,* 293–298.

Kluft, R. P. (1990). Thoughts on childhood MPD. *Dissociation, 3* (1), 1–2.

Kluft, R. P. (1991). Clinical presentations of multiple personality disorder. *Psychiatric Clinics of North America, 14* (3), 605–629.

Koss, M. P., Gidyez, C. A., & Wisniewski, N. (1987). The scope of rape: Incidence and prevalence of sexual aggression and victimization in a national sample of higher education students. *Journal of Counseling and Clinical Psychology, 55,* 162–170.

LaPorta, L. (1992). Childhood trauma and the multiple personality disorder: The case of a 9-year-old girl. *Child Abuse & Neglect, 16* (4), 615–620.

Lewis, D. O. & Bard, J. S. (1991). Multiple personality and forensic issues. *Psychiatric Clinics of North America, 14* (3), 741–756.

Malenbaum, R., & Russel, A. J. (1987). Multiple personality disorder in an 11-year-old boy and his mother. *Journal of the American Academy of Child and Adolescent Psychiatry, 26,* 436–439.

Malinosky-Rummell, R. R., & Hoier, T. S. (1991). Validating measures of dissociation in sexually abused and nonabused children. *Behavioral Assessment, 13,* 341–357.

McElroy, L. P. (1992). Early indicators of pathological dissociation in sexually abused children. *Child Abuse & Neglect, 16* (6), 833–846.

Nasjleti, M., (1980). Suffering in silence: The male incest victim. *Child Welfare, 59* (5), 269–179.

O'Brien, P. (1985). The diagnoses of multiple personality syndromes: Covert, covert and latent. *Comprehensive Therapy, 2,* 59–66.

Perry, B. (1994). Neurobiological sequelae of childhood trauma: PTSD in children. In M. Murburg (Ed.), *Catecholamine function in posttraumatic stress disorder: Emerging concepts* (pp. 233–255). Washington, DC: American Psychiatric Press.

Perry, B., Pollard, R., Blakely, T., Baker, W., & Vigilante, D. (in press). Childhood trauma: The neurobiology of adaptation and use-dependent development of the brain. How states become traits. *Infant Mental Health Journal.*

Peterson, G. (1990). Diagnosis of childhood multiple personality disorder. *Dissociation, 3,* 3–9.

Peterson, G. (1991). Children coping with trauma: Diagnoses of "Dissociation Identity Disorder." *Dissociation, 4,* 152–164.

Peterson, G., & Putnam, F. W. (1994). Preliminary results of the field trial of proposed criteria for Dissociative Disorder of Childhood. *Dissociation, 7,* 212–220.

Putnam, F. (1989). *Diagnoses and treatment of multiple personality disorder.* New York: Guilford Press.

Putnam, F. W. (1991). Dissociative disorders in children and adolescents: Developmental perspective. *Psychiatric Clinics of North America, 14,* 519–532.

Putnam, F. W. (1993). Dissociative disorders in children: Behavioral profiles and problems. *Child Abuse & Neglect, 17,* 39–45.

Putnam, F. W., Guroff, J. J., Silberman, E. K., Barban, L. & Post, R. M., (1986). The clinical phenomenology of multiple personality disorder: A review of 100 recent cases. *Journal of Clinical Psychiatry, 47,* 285–293.

Putnam, F. W., Helmers, K., & Trickett, P. K. (1993). Development, reliability and validity of a child dissociation scale. *Child Abuse & Neglect, 17,* 731–741.

Putnam, F. W., Hornstein, N. & Peterson, G. (1996). Clinical phenomenology of child and adolescent dissociative disorders: Gender and age effects. *Dissocia-*

tive disorders: Child and Adolescent Psychiatry Clinics of North America, 5, 351–360.

Putnam, F. W., & Peterson, G. (1994). Further validation of the Child Dissociative Checklist. *Dissociation, 7,* 204–211.

Ross, C. (1991). The dissociated executive self and the cultural dissociation barrier. *Dissociation, 4,* 55–61.

Ross, C. A. (1989). *Multiple personality disorder: Diagnosis clinical features, and treatment.* New York: John Wiley & sons.

Ross, C. A. & Norton, G. R. (1989). Differences between men and women with multiple personality disorder. *Hospital and Community Psychiatry, 40,* 186–188.

Ross, C. A., Norton, G. R., & Wozney, K. (1989). Multiple personality disorder: An analysis of 236 cases. *Canadian Journal of Psychiatry, 34,* 413–418.

Ross, C. A., Ryan, L., Anderson, G., Ross, D. & Hardy, L. (1989). Dissociative experiences in adolescents and college students. *Dissociation 2,* 239–242.

Rutter, M., Harrington, R., Quinton, D., & Pickles, A. (1994). Adult outcome of conduct disorder in childhood: Implications for concepts and definitions of patterns of psychopathology. In R. D. Ketterlinus & M. E. Lamb (Eds.), *Adolescent Problem Behaviors* (pp. 57–80). Hillsdale, NJ: Erlbaum.

Salter, A. (1995). *Transforming trauma. A guide to understanding and treating adult survivors of child sexual abuse.* Thousand Oaks, CA: Sage.

Silberg, J. (In review). Dissociative symptomatology in children and adolescents as displayed in psychological testing.

Silberg, J., Stipic, D., & Taghizadeh, F. (in press). Dissociative disorders in children and adolescents. In J. Noshpitz (Ed.), *The Handbook of Child and Adolescent Psychiatry.* New York: J. Wiley and Sons.

Snow, M. S., White, J., Pilkington, L., & Beckman, D. (1995). Dissociative identity disorder revealed through play therapy. *Dissociation 8,* 120–123.

Spiegel, D., & Vermutten, E. (1994). Physiological correlates of hypnosis and dissociation. In D. Spiegel (Ed.), *Dissociation: Culture, Mind and Body* (pp. 185–210). Washington, DC: American Psychiatric Press.

Steinberg, M., & Steinberg, A. (1995). Using the SCID-D to assess dissociative identity disorder in adolescents: Three case studies. *Bulletin of the Menninger Clinic, 59* (2), 221–231.

Vander Mey, B. J. (1988). The sexual victimization of male children: A review of previous research. *Child Abuse & Neglect, 12,* 61–72.

Watkins, B., & Bentovim, A. (1992). Male children and adolescents as victims: A review of current knowledge. In G. C. Mezey & M. B. King (Eds.), *Male victims of sexual assault,* (pp. 27–66). New York: Oxford University Press.

Williams, M. (1988). Father-son incest: A review and analysis of reported incidents. *Clinical Social Work Journal, 16* (2), 165–178.

Zavodnick, J. M. (1989). Detection and management of sexual abuse in boys. *Medical Aspects of Human Sexuality,* January, 80–90.

five

Psychological Testing with Dissociative Children and Adolescents

Joyanna L. Silberg

The sparse literature on dissociative children is a testimony to the historical difficulty in diagnosing these elusive patients. Reasons for this difficulty have been offered by Kluft (1985) and include the secretiveness of the children, clinicians' unfamiliarity with the diagnosis, and the symptomatology which mimics other well-known diagnostic entities. The development of specificity in diagnostic evaluation of these patients is key for the establishment of more widespread acceptance of the diagnosis. As discussed by Putnam (1995), the development of measurement tools for adult patients have been essential for establishing the diagnostic credibility of adult DID (dissociative identity disorder, formerly MPD) (Carlson et al., 1993; Steinberg, Rounsaville, & Cichetti, 1991). If dissociative disorders in children are to be identified, treated, and researched, the diagnostic criteria must be unique, discriminating, and specific.

In fact, so far the research on formal diagnostic assessment of dissociative children has been promising, enhancing the validity of dissociative diagnoses in a children's population. Putnam's Child Dissociative Checklist (Putnam, Helmers, & Trickett, 1993) has received the most study. This 20-item parent report questionnaire is a screening tool which covers observed trance states, behavioral fluctuations, sexual precocity, attentional lapses, and a sense of divided identities found in dissociative child patients. This instrument has reliably discriminated between dissociative disorder not otherwise specified (DDNOS), MPD, and a variety of other psychiatric diagnoses for children (Putnam & Peterson, 1994).

The research described in this chapter was supported by a grant from the Sidran Foundation and the Samuel Novey Memorial Fund at the Sheppard-Pratt Hospital.

Armstrong and colleagues are developing the A-DES, a version of the Dissociative Experience Scale, appropriate for use with 11–17-year-olds. This 30 item self-report scale taps the dissociative dimensions of depersonalization experiences, amnesia, and hallucinatory experiences in language appropriate for teenagers. Initial research suggests that the test has good reliability and can discriminate between some diagnostic groups and among patients with and without an abuse history (Armstrong, personal communication).

However, individually administered psychological testing remains the premier modality for description of patients' psychopathology in child clinical work. Whether in schools, hospitals, or outpatient settings, psychological testing is heavily relied upon to establish a profile of patients' strengths and weaknesses and to provide a comprehensive evaluation. By providing an environment with both structured and unstructured features, the psychological testing setting serves to mimic a variable patient environment, providing a barometer on which to gauge a wide range of coping strategies. Observational and self-report measures are limited in their power to reveal the dynamics of underlying psychopathology. Psychological testing has often been used for uncovering hidden, covert pathology. If a dissociative inner world is the child's protected secret, as Kluft (1985) and others have suggested, psychological testing would seem a natural way to uncover diagnostic information covertly. Clinical experience suggests that child dissociative patients constitute a unique diagnostic group. Hence, it would stand to reason that a unique and discriminating pattern of test responses would be discernible.

Using this reasoning, I began to collect psychological testing protocols of child and adolescent dissociative patients in 1990. Test protocols included Wechsler Scales (WISC-III or WPPSI-R), the Rorschach Test, Thematic Apperception Test (TAT) or Child's Apperception Test (CAT), the Sentence Completion Test, and Draw-A-Person Test. I examined the responses of my first 10 cases, searching for any unique or unusual responses that I had not heard commonly in my years of testing children with diverse diagnoses. I reasoned that existing categories of responses may not be particularly productive for discrimination, as dissociative children had never been identified in large numbers through psychological testing, so I looked for new and unusual ways to look at the testing protocols. Initially, I noted a host of comments in the margins of the test protocols describing unusual behaviors during the testing procedures. These were children who seemed to be highly stimulated by the testing materials as their interactions, attitude, movements, and use of language during the testing was noted in frequent comments in margins of the test protocols. Initially, as a guide to categorize unusual test behaviors, I relied on established categories of dissociative characteristics described by Kluft (1985) and Peterson (1990). I looked for ways to operationalize the features of amnesia, trance states, fluctuations, emotional reactivity, and the sense of dividedness which characterize these children. I looked for instances in which patients could not remember questions asked of them, or responses they had given signifying amnesia. I inferred trance states from staring spells or odd repetitive movements. Observations of changes in language, appearance, skills, or attitudes as the testing session progressed tracked fluctuating behavior during testing. I inferred emotional reactivity from spontaneous comments of fear or anger in response to test stimuli. Feelings of dividedness were deduced from instances in which patients gave several conflicting responses.

After cataloguing these unusual test behaviors, I began to focus on the test responses themselves, particularly responses on projective testing, which might describe dissociative defenses, dissociative experiences, or traumatic experiences that might be unique to a dissociative population. I developed an initial list of these categories of responses, which included responses of dissociative coping, intensely morbid imagery, signs of multiplicity, and fantasy projections of magical transformations. I reported these results in an initial exploratory study (Silberg, 1991).

I continued to refine these lists of test behaviors and test responses while collecting additional cases until I had 25 complete test protocols. These test protocols were from dissociative children and adolescents, ranging in age from 5 to 17, who had been diagnosed by an experienced clinician outside of the test setting. After training a research associate to identify these characteristics, I asked her to score these test protocols along with the test protocols of 25 consecutive admissions to our psychiatric hospital who were not dissociative. Identity and diagnosis of these patients were disguised. These results (Silberg, 1994) showed that this list of behaviors and responses had impressive potential for diagnostic discrimination. These behaviors and test responses occurred infrequently in non-dissociative patients, but were remarkably common in the dissociative group. Testing on a larger sample continued to confirm the validity of these variables for assessing dissociative patients (Silberg, 1996). Discriminant analysis showed that a combination of these behavioral and response variables was able to select correctly 93% of 30 dissociative patients, while falsely identifying only 3% of non-dissociative patients. This research adds to the mounting data which support the validity of dissociative diagnoses in children, highlighting the uniqueness of symptom profiles (Peterson & Putnam, 1994; Putnam & Peterson, 1994) and the cross-validation of findings between settings (Hornstein & Putnam, 1992).

Currently, I have developed a test measure based on these significant test behaviors and test responses termed the Dissociative Features Profile (DFP).[1] The DFP can be used along with any standard test battery (if at least two standard psychological tests have been administered) and

---

[1] For ordering information on a preliminary research copy of this instrument see Appendix A.

serves as a way to classify, record, and score dissociative features. Scores for the features have been assigned based on their weights in the original discriminant analysis. The measure has two parts, test behaviors and test responses (termed "markers"), and a patient is assigned a score for each part of the test. Below I will describe in more detail the findings on psychological testing which were significant for the dissociative patients (Silberg, 1996) and are now included on the DFP. Even without the formal scoring provided by the DFP, psychologists can review psychological testing of dissociative children with an eye towards these features which appear atypical of psychiatric patients in general. Several of the described features overlap with known psychological test variables studied in the adult literature or with descriptors of psychological testing in the sparse child literature.

Behavioral Variables

During the course of psychological testing, a patient is prone to display multiple aspects of his/her psychopathology through approach to the tasks, relationship to the examiner, and interactions with or reactions to the test material. These behaviors tend to occur rarely with non-dissociative patients and in the formal DFP scoring are weighted heavily. These behaviors suggestive of a dissociative diagnosis will be described below so that they can be readily identified by evaluators.

Amnesia

This quality is manifested by patients who deny knowledge of a question, deny familiarity with instructions that have just been stated, or deny familiarity with an answer they have given or with any aspect of the test experience. For example, during the Inquiry Phase of the Rorschach the patient is asked "Where did you see the image and what made you see it that way?" At this point, the patient may deny that he/she saw the image reported, e.g. "I don't remember saying butterfly. That wasn't me." The denial often appears sincere, rather than defensive or belligerent as seen with oppositional adolescents.

On two occasions, patients who had met the examiner in a previous test session denied memory of having ever seen the examiner before.

Amnesia as defined above was not seen in any of the control group patients and appears to be highly diagnostic for dissociative disorders.

Barach (1986) studying adult dissociative patients similarly reported a frequency of "denials" signifying amnesia. Friedrich (1990) describes denials on the Rorschach responses of dissociative, sexually abused children which he interpret as amnesia as well.

Staring Episodes

The dissociative patient can be observed having periods of staring vacantly into space over the course of a lengthy testing session. These staring episodes were remarkable enough that examiners noted this behavior in the margins of test protocols, even when the dissociative diagnosis was not apparent to them. These staring episodes might precede marked fluctuations in functioning and may suggest that the patient is entering a trance state.

Odd Movements

Many of these patients engaged in odd, repetitive movements that might have served as a subtle form of trance induction. Movements included repetitive shaking of the legs, facial tics or grimaces, or subtle jaw movements. When asked about the jaw movements, one DID youngster replied, "That's what happens when the voices are talking to me."

Odd tics and gestures have also been reported by Steinberg & Steinberg (1995) during their interviews with three dissociative adolescents. Although odd movements may also be found in children with Tourette's syndrome, or various attentional disorders, peculiar and repetitive behaviors should at least alert the astute clinician to consider a dissociative diagnosis as well.

Behavioral Fluctuations

The typical testing session that may span 2 to 4 hours provides an opportunity for the patient's defenses to be challenged, and a fluctuation in behavior may signal alter interferences which are called upon to adapt to the challenges at hand. Language changes may be the first to be noted. Language complexity may shift from cultured and adult-like to clang associations or "baby talk," which may signify interference from younger alters. LaPorta (1992) similarly describes a 9-year-old MPD (DID) patient's test language as fluctuating from "age-appropriate vocabulary to whiny and immature" (p. 617). Relationship to the examiner may fluctuate from cooperative to oppositional or frankly belligerent. The change often appears dramatic and out of context when compared to the changing response styles of non-dissociative children and adolescents, who may get bored or exasperated during the course of testing. The frustrated non-dissociative patient shows more gradual changes in behavior that appear to be more in context with increasingly challenging test demands.

Actual changes in dress or name, signifying clear-cut switching of the DID patient, was less common in this patient sample than these more subtle interferences.

Affective Reactivity

Affective expressions, predominantly anger and fear, during the course of testing may signify post-traumatic reactions to the test stimuli. For example, in response to a Rorschach card, one dissociative child stated "I hate that one. Get that monster away from me." This type of loss of distance from test materials is particularly common in young dissociative children and may be seen in general with trauma victims.

Somatic Complaints

Dissociative children are known to have an abundance of shifting somatic complaints (Putnam et al., 1993). Interestingly, even on psychological testing the presence of somatic complaints was a factor that could differentiate a dissociative from non-dissociative patient sample. Patients complained of headaches or stomachaches during the course of testing or had unusual complaints that might have signified the activation of somatic memories of trauma: "You're torturing me with this one . . . it hurts my neck." One 11-year-old patient diagnosed with DID grimaced, screamed, and made a stabbing gesture to his abdomen every time he saw a new Rorschach card, suggesting intense post-traumatic associations.

Internal Dividedness

Finally, the dissociative child or adolescent may reflect their sense of themselves as divided by referring to parts, other selves, or voices during the course of the testing. In our setting, we have found that it is often in the psychological testing session that the patient is able to disclose the experience of having "parts" even if they have never described this elsewhere. This disclosure is facilitated by asking questions after noted changes in behavior or response style. For example, the examiner might ask "I notice you are having trouble making up your mind. What's going on?" This process questioning is based on an approach described by Armstrong (in press) in testing adult dissociative patients.

Alternate competing responses may also appear in answer to objective questions on the Wechsler IQ Test. However, these answers are to be distinguished from simple self-corrections or changing one's mind. In the case of the dissociative child or adolescent, the change often appears abrupt or out of context and may represent a shift in developmental level as well.

A sentence completion test where the child completes a sentence stem such as "I am happiest when" easily elicits the conflicting aspects of self seen in a dissociative youngster. In one dramatic example of conflicting response, a 10-year-old girl with suspected DID confirmed her diagnosis when she wrote two contrasting answers for each sentence completion stem, one in mature script and another in block printing. Drawing tasks may tend to induce "switching" to younger alter states and may create a situation where conflict in response styles is particularly evident.

Additional evidence for the sense of dividedness may come from conflicting perceptions to the same projective stimulus. Particularly on the Rorschach Test, those patients may vacillate—"a pig, a baby, I mean a pig." At times, one of the two responses may later be denied. Because of its suggestiveness and non-specific, unstructured quality, the Rorschach more than any other test may pull for this internal conflict over which answers to give.

In summary, the astute clinician may uncover clues regarding a patient's internal dissociative process by attentive observation of the patient during psychological testing procedures. These clues may include amnestic episodes, evidence of self-induced trances, odd movements, fluctuations in language and relatedness, affective reactivity, somatic complaints, and evidences of internal conflict. Some tests such as the Rorschach, sentence completion, or drawing tasks are particularly susceptible to elicitation of alter interferences.

The research shows (Silberg, 1996) that, using the behavior variables alone, the discriminant validity is 83%. Adding the categories listed below, the discriminant validity significantly improves to 93%.

Response Variables (Markers)

The initial categories of responses, developed in 1991, have been revised and refined through continuous research (Silberg, 1994; Silberg, 1996) and nine variables remain on the DFP to categorize dissociative responses on testing. These response variables have good content validity, as they clearly depict various aspects of dissociative experience that are familiar to those who work with dissociative patients. These variables are called dissociative "markers," as they are rarely seen in non-dissociative patients and their presence is highly suggestive of a dissociative process. These are features that can be found on a variety of tests—story-telling tasks such as the CAT or TAT, the Rorschach, drawing tasks, or sentence completion tasks. Once familiar with these markers, it's surprising how readily one can describe and identify these features in the test protocols of dissociative patients. I have read many psychological reports on dissociative patients sent to me from other settings, in which a response is mentioned which highlights one or several of these categories. Rarely has the patient been previously identified as dissociative, despite the intriguing nature of the unusual response highlighted in the psychological test report. My hope is that more widespread awareness of these dissociative categories of response will alert clinicians to the diagnosis earlier in the treatment process.

Multiplicity

"Multiplicity" denotes any doubling, tripling, or other multiplication of images that should be single. Many-headed people or animals with too many appendages often seen on the Rorschach show this quality. In addition, descriptions of twins or triplets or of people attached by cords or strings to one another are also scored under this category. Dissociative youngsters have drawn pictures of themselves with two heads, four arms, or other multiple appendages or body parts. This feature is common in reported cases of psychological testing in the literature on dissociative children. Jacobsen (1995) describes a DID youngster who drew a "double" face with two halves expressing different emotions. Weiss, Sutton, and Utecht (1985) describe a 10-year-old patient with MPD who responds on the Rorschach, "there are three different animals in one" (p. 498), clearly portraying the multiplicity feature.

Labott, Leavitt, Braun, and Sachs (1992) describe a similar response characteristic of adult dissociative patients who portray "images of things dividing." They term this test characteristic "a splitting response," but I believe that the term "multiplicity" is more descriptive and less confusing, as the word "splitting" more commonly relates to psychodynamic defensive features, which may or may not be reflected in the multiple images these children describe. (Two other response variables listed below, "emotional confusion" and "extreme categories," more closely relate to the psychodynamic understanding of "splitting.")

The multiplicity dimension appears to readily capture the multiple, overlapping, often competing senses of self and the feelings of body diffusion with which these children struggle.

Dissociative Coping

The most common feature found in the dissociative protocols studied is the dissociative coping marker, found in 20 of the 30 patients studied. This feature refers to any attempts to cope with traumatic events through fantasy, wishing, dreaming, pretending, sleeping, or forgetting. This dimension is most often seen on projective story-telling tasks. One 6-year-old DDNOS patient told the story of a child being chased by monsters. As the story progressed, the child stopped suddenly and said "My mind is going blank," reflecting the sudden emergence of a dissociative defense.

Other stories told involve people facing conflict or violence, who "go to sleep for a hundred years" or "forget that bad things are there." One adolescent with DDNOS told the story of a blind woman who "wishes herself" into seeing. The dissociative coping response clearly reflects the child's defensive style of using well-developed fantasy in the face of trauma. No feature depicts the dissociative defense as clearly as this one.

Malevolent Religiosity

Malevolent religiosity is scored whenever references to Satan or religious ceremony involving witches or devils are alluded to in the test protocol. We know that these children come from abusive families in which concepts of God and good and evil are often severely distorted. Perhaps this feature reflects familiarity with these distorted beliefs, or perhaps these images suggest exposure to sadistic practices in which images of evil are used to terrorize children. A high percentage of dissociative children have these images (52%). Examples include: Rorschach Card V—"This could be a picture of evil"; Card II—"This is a picture of 2 witches sacrificing a child"; or TAT Card 15—"A demon plotting to possess a girl's brain." One 5-year-old DDNOS patient responded to an intelligence test question to define the word "ancient" by stating "Satan is ancient." Although the internal associations that prompted this unusual answer are unclear, the marker for malevolent religiosity is clearly evident.

Emotional Confusion

The feature of emotional confusion conveys the internal conflict of feeling in these youngsters. This feature is scored whenever affect in a response shifts suddenly and without logical justification. For example, on Card I of the CAT, a 5-year-old child with DDNOS states, "These are the hungry children watching for their mommy, so hungry, so hungry that they laugh." This sudden shift of affect shows the child's primitive attempt to cope with a dysphoric feeling by changing it or undoing it. In fact, this type of feature, primitive in its defensive style, is found more frequently in the protocols of the younger patients. The sentence completion stem: "I am happiest when" when completed with the answer "I am sad" again illustrates this feature.

Extreme Categories

The dichotomy of feelings is captured in the response feature which is termed "Extreme Categories." Responses significant for this feature portray extreme "goodness" or "badness," juxtapose witches with angels or display other dramatic contrasts within an image or story. For example, a 10-year-old DDNOS patient told a TAT story "about a very nice girl and her evil twin sister." It is this dimension which more closely captures the psychoanalytic concept of "splitting."

Violent Imagery

Painful memories of violent abuse are often activated by the psychological testing, particularly with more open-ended tasks. It is not surprising that these children with their histories of extreme violence will allude to violent imagery in psychological test responses. As pointed out by Armstrong & Loewenstein (1990) and Armstrong (in press), traumatic associations are common in adult dissociative testing protocols and are best viewed as trauma-related rather than "primitive." Images of mutilation involving loss of body parts or severed limbs are not uncommon. One 8-year-old DDNOS patient said that Card IV of the Rorschach looked like "a boy with a rocket through his butt." The violent content on this response seems suggestive of sexual abuse; the intensity of fear and pain seem obvious. Images of frank torture are also frequent in the children's protocols, e. g. "This is a child. The bad man is telling him he'll cut his throat so he won't tell the secret." Clinicians hearing stories about characters who are undergoing threats of torture for fear of disclosure should attend particularly carefully to what the child may be trying to communicate indirectly.

Magical Transformation

The category of magical transformation describes a response in which one thing turns into something else. Examples might include a person who turns from a helpful friend to a "bad witch" or a "bunny" who transforms into a "snake." The transformational nature of fantasy characters in children's imaginations has been boosted by cartoon characters that "morph" or transform into other things, so that the contemporary childhood imagination is familiar with such imagery. Nonetheless, it is with the dissociative child that this imagery seems to resonate most deeply. Nearly half of the dissociative children had such images in their protocols, while only two control patients had these. This marker for changeability may be a metaphor for the children's concept of their chameleon-like capacities or may express the child's familiarity with the contrasting abusive and nurturant aspects of their environment. Transformation is a powerful concept to these children, as it evokes magical escape. The belief in transformation may be a testimony to these children's enduring optimism and belief that escape is possible even from the inescapable. Images of transformation towards health and wholeness of self can be used in therapy so that transformation can be seen as adaptive.

Depersonalized Images

Finally, the feature of depersonalization refers to humans who have become depersonalized as robots, aliens, shadows, ghosts, or inanimate objects that have become enlivened. One 8-year-old boy with DID told a story on the TAT of a "blank piece of paper taking a walk," projecting human aspects onto a piece of paper while denying the human reality of his percept. Images of shadows, aliens, or other quasi-human entities portray these children's profound alienation and sense of dehumanization.

In summary, dissociative children display common features on their psychological test protocols that depict their struggle with developing a cohesive self, their internal conflicts, their preoccupation with violence, and their use of dissociative defenses to deal with trauma. Sensitivity to the expressions of these psychological dimensions on testing can alert the clinician to a dissociative disorder even when the child has not disclosed this information directly.

Further research on the DFP and its role in diagnosis of dissociative children is proceeding. Currently a sample of 40 dissociative children is being evaluated with this instrument and plans are under way for comparisons with varying diagnostic groups as well as a non-patient population. Research is being conducted with a revised version of this instrument for adults (Bethany Brand, personal communication).

Further Psychological Testing Recommendations

Psychological testing experiences with dissociative children and adolescents has led me to modify my usual procedures to improve the sensitivity and utility of psychological testing for this patient population.

Psychological testing often has significant political power in school settings or in legal settings as the determining factor in the child's eligibility for special service or placement issues. Therefore, it is important that the psychological testing be accurate and communicate recommendations clearly. The dissociative child, who so frequently presents a diagnostic quandary, may be subject to repeated testings and evaluations, often with contradictory findings. Contradictory findings may result from patient fluctuations as differing alter states present for the testing, as well as from controversies among the evaluators concerning what to make of the child's odd behavior. To make the testing as comprehensive as possible, the evaluator should try to explain discrepancies in previously reported data, rather than just offering an additional opinion. Credibility of the findings will be much stronger if past assessments are taken into account, interpreting previously depressed IQ scores, for example, as reflections of other dissociated states.

The battery of individually administered tests should include an intelligence measure and a variety of projective tasks including a drawing task. During the evaluation, the evaluator should try to sample the child's behavior across a variety of types of tasks and elicit information from caretakers concerning how the child presents in multiple settings. Including a formal assessment of the child's behavior at home using the Child Dissociative Checklist as a guide for interviewing the primary caretaker is essential. Other established caretaker report instruments, such as the Achenbach Child Behavior Checklist, have not yet been standardized for use in a dissociative population and results may be equivocal and hard to interpret.

In orienting the child to the testing procedures, I mention to the child the importance of doing the best job possible, using all available potential. For example, "In order for us to see how well they can do, it is important that children show all of their skills and feelings during the testing. Some children feel like they are good at math sometimes but not others, and we want to be sure that this is one of the times you do as well as you can." If the child has already disclosed a feeling of having "parts" of the mind or "voices," I suggest to the child that he or she let all parts participate in the testing so that we can understand the "whole child." This instruction is adapted from instructions for testing adult dissociative patients, outlined by Armstrong (in press). After this orienting instruction, the psychologist may ask questions when switches or subtle interferences occur. These questions might include "I noticed this part seemed easier for you than the other. I wonder why that was?" The child might then use this as an opportunity to discuss the help of a more skilled alter. We have found that for patients who are not dissociative using these gentle instructions is not particularly suggestive, as all children feel that sometimes they're good at some things and other times good at others. It is only for the clearly dissociative children that this instruction has particular and specific meaning. For dissociative children, the instruction may serve to allow them to feel more free in allowing alternate states that have not been used to participating in psychological testing before to come forward. Thus, rather than invalidating results by this instruction, it may serve to counter the invalidating preconceived approach that the dissociative child may have already adopted to the test procedures—that is, "Do it easily with one part and get it over with."

The effect of this instruction was well-illustrated by a 13-year-old girl, Martha, with DID, who stated "In all previous testings, my school part, Jean, took the psych testing, but because you told me to let us all participate I allowed Annie out." In fact, Martha's performance on Digit Span increased by five scale points from the previous testing. Martha explained that "Jean," who had always done the testing, had a very poor memory, but was assisted by "Annie" to help with the Digit Span subtest this time. Apparently, the orienting instruction stated above assisted in improving the validity of this testing.

The fluctuating cognitive picture of the dissociative child has been stressed repeatedly (Hornstein, this volume; Putnam, et al., 1993; Fagan & McMahon, 1984), but evaluators must be cautious not to overgeneralize from wide fluctuations in performance and always assume that the patient has greater ability than the test score shows. Varying skill levels could indicate alter interference of different developmental levels, but may also reflect learning disabilities or developmental weaknesses which remain part of the child's cognitive profile even after treatment. I have had referrals of patients who had tested in the retarded range and then were diagnosed with DID. Evaluators were suspecting that the new IQ would be significantly higher. However, these patients on retesting, even with sensitivity to the switches and elicitation of the best possible functioning, continued to test in the retarded range. One patient, an 11-year-old girl with DID, had a 64 IQ, but counselors stated they had observed her reading a Stephen King novel. During the consultation, the patient and I took a walk to the hospital library where I tested the accuracy of this observation after meeting "Jimmy," the 16-year-old boy alter who liked horror books. I discovered that "Jimmy" deduced plot lines through book cover pictures, movies seen on TV, and the patient's traumatic memories. The reading level of this patient did not fluctuate from a second grade level, whatever alter state presented.

The most dramatic cognitive fluctuations I have seen are within the higher levels of cognitive functioning with patients who are bright and may test as high average, superior, or very superior, depending on alter influences. In cases where children have been in extremely deprived conditions, IQ scores may tend to slowly increase over time as their environments stabilize and improve, but this happens with both dissociative and non-dissociative children. Intelligence test scores can be viewed as a barometer of the child's adaptive coping potential. As dissociative defenses develop as a way to cope, adapt, and master the surroundings, one might expect that dissociative defenses would be utilized during testing to maximize the child's coping with the challenge of the testing, and IQ scores derived be largely representative of the child's ability.

I have found no pervasive patterns of strengths and weaknesses that the patients display on testing, although there is a slight trend towards stronger verbal skills in DID as compared to DDNOS youngsters (Silberg, 1996). This may reflect the DDNOS patient's lack of skill in reporting on his dissociative system, or may suggest that there is a group of DDNOS children who lack the verbal skill to successfully elaborate on fantasy projections and are precluded from achieving the elaborated self-system characteristic of DID. Hornstein (chapter 2, this volume) has identified similar patient groups whose cognitive deficits prevent development of an organized dissociative system.

The psychologist writing up test results for the dissociative patient should be careful not to make sweeping statements that could be misquoted out of context. For example, the psychologist may write "No evidence of dissociation was found on testing," and this statement might follow the patient even after a definitive diagnosis of DID has been made. It would be more advisable to say, "Although during this testing the child showed no features associated with a dissociative disorder, these disorders are frequently secretive and hidden and more dissociative pathology might express itself over time."

Similarly, if dissociative features are found on testing, this should be expressed with caution as well, leaving open the importance of continued assessment and reevaluation of the patient that must take place in a therapeutic setting where the full dimensions of the dissociative disorder will express itself.

The techniques and recommendations described here are preliminary and need to be replicated and studied over time. As instruments continue to be developed that assist in the diagnosis of dissociative disorders, clinicians will be better equipped in the future to research how dissociative children and adolescents present in testing and these recommendations can be modified.

It is hoped that the formal classification of the DFP features will assist clinicians in the diagnosis of dissociative disorders when psychological testing data are available. Adding these categories of psychological testing to results from patient-report measures and parent-interview screening tools will help give clinicians increased confidence in making this important diagnostic assessment. It is hoped that continued research on psychological testing with dissociative patients will serve to enhance clinical sensitivity outside of formal testing as well and provide insights that improve our understanding of these children's psychological functioning.

References

Armstrong, J. (in press). Psychological testing. In J. Turkus, (Ed.), *Dissociative Identity Disorder: Stage-oriented Treatment*. Northvale, NJ: Jason Aronson.

Armstrong, J. G., & Loewenstein, R. J. (1990). Characteristics of patients with multiple personality and dissociative disorders on psychological testing. *Journal of Nervous and Mental Disease, 178*, 448–454.

Armstrong, J., Carlson, E., Putnam, F. W., & Libero, D. (Data in preparation). Reliability and validity of an adolescent dissociative experiences scale.

Barach, P. (1986). *Rorschach signs of Multiple Personality Disorder in MPD and non-MPD victims of sexual abuse.* Paper presented at Third International Conference on Multiple Personality/Dissociative States, Chicago.

Carlson E. B., Putnam, F. W., Ross, C. A., Torem, M., Coon, P., Dill, D. L., Loewenstein, R. J., & Braun, B. G. (1993). Validity of the dissociative experiences scale in screening for multiple personality disorder: A multicenter study. *American Journal of Psychiatry, 150,* 1030–1036.

Fagan, J., & McMahon, P. P. (1984). Incipient multiple personality in children. *Journal of Nervous and Mental Disease, 172,* 26–36.

Friedrich, W. N. (1990). *Psychotherapy of sexually abused children and their families.* New York: Norton.

Hornstein, N. L., & Putnam, F. W. (1992). Clinical phenomenology of child and adolescent dissociative disorders. *Journal of the American Academy of Child & Adolescent Psychiatry, 31,* 1077–1085.

Jacobsen, T. (1995). Case Study: Is selective mutism a manifestation of dissociative identity disorder? *Journal of the American Academy of Child and Adolescent Psychiatry, 34,* 863–866.

Kluft, R. (1985). Childhood multiple personality disorder: Predictors, clinical finding and treatment results. In R. P. Kluft (Ed.), *Childhood antecedents of multiple personality,* Washington, DC: American Psychiatric Press.

Labott, S. M., Leavitt, F., Braun, B. G., & Sachs, R. G. (1992). Rorschach indicators of multiple personality disorder. *Perceptual and Motor Skill, 75,* 147–158.

LaPorta, L. D. (1992). Childhood trauma and multiple personality disorder: The case of a 9-year-old girl. *Child Abuse & Neglect, 16,* 615–620.

Lovitt, R., & Lefkof, G. (1985). Understanding multiple personality with the Comprehensive Rorschach System. *Journal of Personality Assessment, 49,* 282–94.

Peterson, G. (1990). Diagnosis of childhood multiple personality. *Dissociation, 3,* 3–9.

Peterson, G., & Putnam, F. W. (1994). Preliminary results of the field trial proposed criteria for dissociative disorder of childhood. *Dissociation, 7,* 212–219.

Putnam, F. W. (1995). Resolved: Multiple personality is an individually and socially created artifact. Negative rebuttal. *Journal of the American Academy of Child and Adolescent Psychiatry, 34,* 960–961.

Putnam, F. W., Helmers, K., & Trickett, P. K. (1993) Development, reliability, and validity of a child dissociation scale. *Journal of Child Abuse and Neglect 17,* 731–741.

Putnam, F. W., & Peterson, G. (1994) Further validation of the child dissociative checklist. *Dissociation, 7,* 204–209.

Silberg, J. L. (1991, November). *Differential diagnosis of dissociative disorders in children.* Paper presented at the 8th International Conference on Multiple Personality/Dissociative States. Rush Presbyterian-St. Luke's Medical Center, Chicago.

Silberg, J. L. (1994, November). *Psychological testing features associated with dissociative diagnoses in children and adolescents.* Presentation at the 11th International Conference on Multiple Personality/Dissociative States. Rush Presbyterian-St. Luke's Medical Center, Chicago.

Silberg, J. (In review). Dissociative symptomatology in children and adolescents as displayed on psychological testing.

Steinberg, M., Rounsaville, B., & Cichetti, D. (1991). Detection of dissociative disorders in psychiatric patients by a screening instrument and a structured diagnostic interview. *American Journal of Psychiatry, 148*, 1105–625.

Steinberg, M., & Steinberg, A. (1995). Using the SCID-D to assess dissociative identity disorder in adolescents: Three case studies. *Bulletin of the Menninger Clinic, 59*, 221–231.

Weiss, M., Sutton, P. J., & Utecht, A. J. (1985). Multiple personality in a 10-year-old girl. *Journal of the American Academy of Child and Adolescent Psychiatry, 24*, 495–501.

Part Two

Treatment

s i x

Factors Associated with Positive Therapeutic Outcome

Joyanna L. Silberg and Frances S. Waters

As pointed out by Friedrich (1996), child psychotherapy outcome literature is a poorly developed field which has produced only minimal research. Child psychotherapy techniques are rarely tested in controlled studies despite the efforts of Kazdin (1988) and others to develop a more scientifically rigorous approach to measuring outcome.

However, the psychotherapy outcome literature for children does give us some clues as to what to look for in a successful psychotherapeutic approach and may shed some light on preferred characteristics of child dissociative treatment. Approaches emphasizing cognitive behavioral interventions have been shown to be effective for the treatment of a variety of child psychiatric disorders (Kazdin, 1990) and specifically for post-traumatic stress symptoms (Deblinger, McLeer, & Henry 1990). Although psychotherapeutic techniques for children have often emphasized a passive nondirective approach, trauma therapists believe that more directive approaches work better with traumatized children (Gil, 1991; James, 1994), and at least one outcome study confirms that a directive approach compared to a nondirective approach relieved symptoms more successfully among sexually abused preschool children (Cohen & Mannarino, 1996). Research has increasingly demonstrated that involving the family in treatment improves outcome for a variety of child and adolescent disorders (Diamond, Serrano, Dickey, & Sonis, 1996) and for sexually abused children in particular (Cohen & Mannarino, 1996). Intuitively, it seems clear that psychotherapeutic approaches for children should focus on mastery

The authors would like to thank Diane Brandt for her research assistance and Dr. Bethany Brand for her contributions.

and growth towards increasingly developmentally appropriate behavior.

Extrapolating from the above criteria, therapy for dissociative children should involve cognitive techniques that help the child learn how to cope with the aftereffects of trauma, directive approaches in dealing with traumatic content, sensitivity to the family context, and emphasis on the child's need for mastery of developmentally appropriate tasks. The cognitive aspects of the treatment might involve helping the child understand dissociative processes and post-traumatic phenomena. The therapist's directiveness might be evidenced in keeping goals clear, addressing the traumatic content and working explicitly towards unity of the personality. The dissociative therapy must recognize the major struggles of the dissociative child in a family and developmental context and be sensitive to multiple domains of the child's experience.

The therapeutic approach described in more detail in the following chapters of the book incorporates the above principles and has been used with dissociative children in two geographically different settings by the authors. This chapter will review the setting and characteristics of dissociative patients treated by the authors, and present some preliminary research findings on factors affecting positive outcome.

Just as the field of outcome research for child psychotherapy is in a preliminary stage, outcome information for children treated for DID and DDNOS is limited to a few case reports (LaPorta, 1992; Weiss, Sutton, & Utecht, 1985) and a few case series (Dell & Eisenhower, 1990; Fagan & McMahon, 1984; Kluft, 1985). Many therapists are just learning identification skills for this patient population and do not have sufficient length of experience or caseloads to establish a track record of success. As many of the treatment techniques are not well-known, the presentation of some baseline treatment outcome information is beneficial in giving credibility to the work in this expanding field.

The Settings

Author JS

This setting is within a large not-for profit psychiatric hospital (Sheppard-Pratt) in a large metropolitan area which is often seen as a tertiary referral site, accepting patients for whom diagnosis is unclear or who have been resistant to treatment in other settings. The hospital provides a continuum of services for children and adolescents including outpatient, inpatient, and day hospital. Several of the patients in this sample participated within many of the levels of care within the hospital system. Inpatients treated in short term hospitalization alone for under two months were not included in this study, as it was assumed that this short a treatment duration would not have a significant effect on outcome. Patients who were seen in consultation only and treated in other settings primarily also were not included. Inpatients were referred from a wide geographical area but outpatients came from Maryland. The author's specialization in treatment of child and adolescent dissociative disorders has been communicated through conferences, and hospital-sponsored lecture series producing a wide referral base.

Author FW

Author FW's case load has been exclusively outpatient in a small town rural setting, within a community mental health center, as well as a private practice. The author has been specializing in childhood trauma within the same town for over 15 years and her reputation as a specialist in abuse and dissociation is widely known in the community and surrounding counties. Affiliations with protective services, the courts, and foster care organizations have lead to a wide referral base of traumatized children, particularly those for whom protective services have questions about appropriate living arrangements. Some of author FW's patients were also treated in other levels of care such as residential or hospital during the course of treatment, but not directly by the author. Patients for whom chart information was not retrievable or for whom diagnosis was unclear were not included in this study.

The Patients

These 34 patients (11 from author JS and colleagues; 23 from author FW) ranged in age at the outset of treatment from 3 to 14, with 22 girls and 12 boys. All of them had documented histories of severe abuse, including physical, sexual, emotional, ritual,[1] and severe neglect, and many had more than one perpetrator of abuse. The severity of abuse was described on a 3-point scale that took into account the number of perpetrators, that seemed to closely correlate with the numbers of types of abuse:

1. One perpetrator (less than 3 types of abuse).
2. Two perpetrators (3 types of abuse).
3. More than two perpetrators (more than 3 types of abuse).

For this sample of traumatized children, onset of abuse was early—between the ages of 0 to 5. Some of the patients lived in birth family homes and some resided within adoptive or foster placements. All patients had been diagnosed with either DID (MPD) or with DDNOS (dissociative disorder not otherwise specified). Diagnosis was established through careful assessment including diagnostic interviews, caregiver reports and observation, and ongoing therapy in which dissociated aspects of the self were revealed.

[1] Ritual abuse refers to any physical or sexual abuse in the context of ritualized or ceremonial practice.

Treatment Characteristics

Length of treatment varied from 3 months to 7 years; the length was determined by a variety of factors including patient continuing in ongoing treatment, completion of treatment, the family moving, the child moving to another more restrictive treatment setting, or precipitous discontinuation of therapy by the parents. The stage of treatment reached was assessed on a 5-point scale that parallels the authors' 3-phase treatment model described in Chapters 8 and 9:

1. Assessment and identification of personality system (Phase I)
2. Building Internal Cooperation (Phase I)
3. Processing trauma (Phase II)
4. Integration (Phase III)
5. Post-unification treatment (Phase III)

Family Characteristics

These patients came from a wide variety of families that spanned the range of social class and family stability. Nineteen lived in their birth families during the course of treatment and 15 lived in foster or adoptive homes. Nine patients had a parent with a diagnosed dissociative disorder. The family environments were assessed based on the degree of continuity, availability, and consistency they provided for the child or adolescent:

1. *Consistent home:* At least one parent, a foster parent, or other parental figure was consistently available to the child during the course of treatment. Disruptions or crises were short-lived and able to be resolved.
2. *Moderately Consistent:* At least one parent, foster parent, or other parent figure had some availability to the child during the course of treatment. However, this availability was inconsistent due to parental illness or psychopathology, separations, divorce, or death.
3. *Inconsistent:* There was little parental consistency during the course of treatment. In these cases, the child either changed settings frequently or was an inpatient awaiting foster placement, or parental figures were largely unavailable.

Five of these patients were re-traumatized during the course of treatment; these patients were grouped to determine what effect this re-traumatization might have on outcome.

Outcome Measure

To assess the children's response to treatment, a 5-point scale was developed that reflected the degree of symptom improvement that the patient demonstrated. The resolution of dissociative pathology was not used as the outcome measure per se, but age-appropriate coping skills and reduction of symptomatology were assessed. Many of these patients have not terminated treatment; therefore, this assessment reflects "outcome so far" rather than the true final outcome of treatment.

1. No symptom reduction or worsening of symptoms.
2. Mild symptom improvement.
3. Moderate symptom improvement.
4. Significant symptom improvement.
5. Achievement of age-appropriate coping.

Results

Univariate analysis of variance looked at each factor to assess its relationship to the outcome measure. Multivariate analysis of variance assessed the relative weights of each factor as predictors of outcome. The results lead us to the following conclusions that may impact our therapeutic work with children and adolescents.

1. All patients except two had some symptom reduction through the course of treatment.

Twenty-six percent of the patients showed moderate improvement (3) and another 26% showed significant improvement (4 or 5). This finding gives general support to the benefit of this therapeutic approach, even for patients who were not able to receive a complete course of treatment (see Table 1).

2. Stage of treatment correlates significantly with outcome.

This finding gives general support to the sequential treatment phases described in Chapters 8 and 9. As patients moved through the therapeutic phases they responded with increased symptom reduction and gradual improvement. Those patients with less opportunity to move through the complete phases of treatment showed less symptomatic improvement. Clearly the patient's symptomatic progress and the treatment stage reached were by no means independent measures. These were closely interwoven barometers of the ongoing progress of treatment as the therapist judged when to move on to a subsequent stage of treatment by evaluating the patient's symptomatic improvement.

3. Length of treatment predicts positive therapeutic outcome.

The positive correlation between length of treatment and outcome success further supports the sequential treatment model and the value in persisting in treatment after initial symptom relief. It is important to note that optimum treatment outcome was for patients in treatment between 12 and 24 months; this time period was associated with the best outcome (see Table 2). The group in treatment over 2 years may be a self-

Table 1

Number of Patients Showing Varying Outcomes to Treatment

Outcome	Mean length of treatment	# of patients	# of patients at stage				
			1	2	3	4	5
1	4 mo.	2	1	1			
2	20 mo.	6		3	3		
3	22 mo.	13		3	5	2	3
4	14 mo.	5		1	1	1	2
5	19 mo.	8			1	2	5

selected group of more difficult patients with a poorer prognosis. It is an optimistic finding that effective and consistent treatment can serve to reverse or mitigate the damaging effects of even a devastating background. This message of reassurance to families who care for these children may go a long way towards boosting morale as they navigate through the sometimes stormy course of a lengthy treatment.

However, the patients with the poorest outcome were those for whom treatment was precipitously interrupted during the early stages. The therapeutic lesson one might learn from this is to recognize that the early stage of treatment with a dissociative child is a period with some potential danger, as dissociative barriers are revealed and disclosures about abuse may first surface. The therapist must give significant support to families during this early stage and assess their commitment to treatment so that treatment is not interrupted suddenly just as the child has entered an even more fragile state as dissociative barriers are uncovered.

It will be important for further research to help answer the question of how to match patient needs with optimum treatment length. Some research has shown that relief of anxiety and depression in sexually abused children can occur from shorter term treatments (Lanktree & Briere, 1995) but longer treatment may be required for problems of sexual acting out and aggression (Friedrich, Luecke, Beilke, & Place, 1992). This study supports the idea of varying treatment lengths matched to patient needs; a shorter course of treatment may be appropriate for some patients, such as DDNOS girls (see Table 4).

4. Consistent parenting is the most important factor in the prediction of successful outcome of therapy for dissociative children and adolescents.

This finding is consistent with findings of Fagan and McMahon (1984) and Dell and Eisenhower (1990), who also determined that the level of parental participation and involvement in therapy affected outcome of both children and adolescents. The therapist working with the dissociative patient should take it as a challenge to involve the family, support

Table 2

Mean Outcome for Patients with Varying Lengths of Treatment

Length of Treatment	N	Outcome
0–5 months	8	2.7
5–12 months	8	2.7
12–24 months	13	4.1*
More than 24 months	5	3.0

(*This value is significantly different from A & B values at p<.01.)

Table 3

	N	Mean Outcome
Consistent	14	4.1*
Moderate consistency	16	2.7
Inconsistent	4	2.7

(*This value is significantly different from other values at p<.002.)

their progress, and stay aware of their multiple needs as therapy with the child progresses.

5. Severity of abuse or age of onset of abuse, when under 5, made little difference with respect to outcome.

Although severity of abuse will certainly affect some aspects of the treatment, it did not ultimately relate to outcome in this study. Again, this result can lead to optimism in our interaction with children and their parents, as we can offer reassurance that a good treatment outcome is still possible despite a history of severe and overwhelming trauma. This finding helps reiterate the importance of treating these patients while they are still in their developing years, because the outcome potential may not be as positive for severely traumatized patients once dissociative barriers have become rigid in adulthood.

6. Dissociative children living with DID parents had outcomes just as positive as those in non-dissociative households.

This finding is consistent with that of Kluft (1987), who assessed the parental fitness of mothers with multiple personality disorder and found that 38.7% were considered particularly competent. Although not all of the dissociative parents within our study were in that selective group of exceptional parental competence, their parenting skill, consistency to the child, and participation in treatment reflected the diversity of the group as a whole. This finding is significant for those therapists who may be involved in assisting with custodial decision-making. In court, testimony is frequently presented that implies a parent should not have custody due

Table 4

Outcome and Length of Treatment by Diagnosis and Gender

Diagnosis	Gender	N	Mean Age	Length of tr.	Outcome
DID	girls	16	10	25.8	3.3
	boys	6	8	13.5	2.8
DDNOS	girls	6	8.3	8	3.7
	boys	6	7.8	18	3.5

(None of these values were significantly different.)

to their suffering from a dissociative disorder. This study supports the notion that dissociative children are equally likely to respond to treatment whether in dissociative or non-dissociative households, as long as the parent is consistent and available.

7. Although there was no overall difference in outcome between DID and DDNOS children, there was a trend for DID boys to fare worst, and DDNOS girls to fare best.

Hornstein and Putnam (1992) and Putnam, Hornstein, and Peterson (1996) have shown that DDNOS as compared to DID patients have less amnesia, are less symptomatic, and are more typically represented at younger ages. As described in earlier chapters of the book, DDNOS youngsters may be seen as spanning the range from severe to milder forms of psychopathology. The field should probably begin to pay closer attention to how to differentiate the DDNOS category across the continuum of severity. Although the values were not significantly different, the findings seem to reflect a trend suggesting that DDNOS as a diagnosis in girls is associated with milder impairment. An indirect suggestion of the lesser degree of impairment in the DDNOS girl subgroup was the trend toward shorter treatment length coupled with greater improvement. This finding lends some credence to Goodwin's hypothesis (Chapter 4) that we may need to develop new approaches to work with DID boys whose defenses against any fear or vulnerability may make them very difficult to identify or reach in therapy.

8. Re-traumatization did not affect the treatment outcome for patients in this study but did relate to length of treatment.

This finding reflects that these children are as a whole a high-risk group for traumatization. This may be due to the instability of their placements, personal characteristics that make them particularly vulnerable (aggressiveness, impulsivity, or poor judgment), or ongoing contact with known perpetrators. Given these risks, it is important for the therapist to be constantly alert to the reoccurrence of trauma in these children's lives, as it seems the longer one knows them the more likely one is to find a reoccurrence of a traumatic event in their lives. The good news is that if the therapy proceeds beyond the point of the re-traumatization, it can still be effective in helping to alleviate these children's difficulties. This finding is consistent with the case report of Kluft (1985), who described a re-traumatized youngster who still responded well to therapy despite a regression at the time of the abuse. Clearly, if re-traumatization occurs it increases the length of required treatment.

9. Treatment outcome was unaffected by whether the patient was in the birth family or foster/adoptive home.

This finding suggests that there are many family environments that may be appropriate for dissociative children; each case must be looked at individually to assess under what circumstances the child has the best access to consistent parenting. Children removed from their birth families can do equally well as children who remain in their birth families but, as described in Chapters 7 through 9, working through these attachment issues in whatever family they are with is particularly important.

Conclusions

Although this study is preliminary, it is important as an initial attempt to collate treatment outcome findings for dissociative children in two different settings. Although the outcome measure was somewhat unsophisticated and the measurement of outcome admittedly subjective, the study presents some important trends worthy of tracking in future, more rigorous outcome studies. The factors of parental consistency and length of treatment as predictors of outcome were important findings that have implications for clinical interventions with dissociative patients. This study gives support to the 3-phase treatment approach described in this book and supports the treatment concepts described in the following chapters, in which parental involvement is encouraged, education regarding dissociative processes is given, and children are encouraged to achieve developmentally appropriate behavior and personality unity. It is hoped that future research can build on these preliminary findings by assessing outcome with pre- and post-treatment measures (Becker et al., 1995) and providing longitudinal tracking of at-risk children.

References

Becker, J. V., Alpert, J. L., Bigfoot, D. S., Bonner, B. L., Geddie, L. F., Henggeler, S. W., Kaufman, K. L., & Walker, C. E. (1995). Empirical Research on child abuse treatment. Report by the child abuse and neglect treatment working group, American Psychological Association. *Journal of Clinical Child Psychology, 24,* 23–46.

Cohen, J. A., & Mannarino, A. P. (1996). A treatment outcome study for sexually abused preschool children: Initial findings. *Journal of the American Academy of Child & Adolescent Psychiatry, 35,* 42–50.

Deblinger, E., McLeer, S., & Henry, D. (1990). Cognitive behavioral treatment for sexually abused children suffering post-traumatic stress: Preliminary findings. *Journal of the American Academy of Child and Adolescent Psychiatry, 29,* 747–752.

Dell, D. F., & Eisenhower, J. W. (1990). Adolescent multiple personality disorder: A preliminary study of eleven cases. *Journal of the American Academy of Child and Adolescent Psychiatry, 29,* 359–366.

Diamond, G. S., Serrano, A. C., Dickey, M., & Sonis, W. A. (1996). Current status of family-based outcome and process research. *Journal of the American Academy of Child and Adolescent Psychiatry, 35,* 6–16.

Fagan, J. & McMahon, P. P. (1984). Incipient multiple personality in children. *Journal of Nervous and Mental Disease, 172,* 26–36.

Friedrich, W. N. (1996). An integrated model of psychotherapy for abused children. In J. Briere, L. Berliner, J. A. Bulkey, C. Jenny, & T. Reid (Eds.), *APSAC handbook on child maltreatment* (pp. 104–117). Thousand Oaks, CA: Sage Publications.

Friedrich, W. N., Luecke, W. J., Beilke, R. L., & Place, V. (1992). Psychotherapy outcome of sexually abused boys: An agency study. *Journal of Interpersonal Violence, 3,* 331–343.

Gil, E. (1991). *The Healing Power of Play.* New York: Guilford Press.

Hornstein, N. L., & Putnam, F. W. (1992). Clinical phenomenology of child and adolescent dissociative disorders. *Journal of the American Academy of Child and Adolescent Psychiatry, 31,* 6.

James, B. (1994). *Handbook for treatment of attachment-trauma problems in children.* New York: Lexington Books.

Kazdin, A. E. (1988). *Child Psychotherapy.* Elmsford, NY: Pergamon Press.

Kazdin, A. E. (1990). Psychotherapy for children and adolescents. *Annual Review of Psychology, 41,* 21–54.

Kluft, R. P. (1985). Hypnotherapy of childhood multiple personality disorder. *American Journal of Clinical Hypnosis, 27,* 201–210.

Kluft, R. P. (1987). The parental fitness of mothers with multiple personality disorder: A preliminary study. *Child Abuse & Neglect, 2,* 273–280.

Lanktree, C., & Briere, J. (1995). Outcome of therapy for sexually abused children: A repeated measures study. *Child Abuse & Neglect, 19,* 1145–1155.

LaPorta, L. D. (1992). Childhood trauma and multiple personality disorder: The case of a 9-year-old girl. *Child Abuse & Neglect, 16,* 615–620.

Putnam, F. W., Hornstein, N., & Peterson, G. (1996). Clinical phenomenology of child and adolescent dissociative disorders: Gender and age effects. *Dissociative disorders: Child and Adolescent Psychiatry Clinics of North America, 5,* 351–360.

Weiss, M., Sutton, P. J., & Utecht, A. J. (1985). Multiple personality in a 10-year-old girl. *Journal of the American Academy of Child and Adolescent Psychiatry, 24,* 495–501.

seven

The Five-Domain Crisis Model: Therapeutic Tasks and Techniques for Dissociative Children

Joyanna L. Silberg

Although treatment techniques for adult dissociative patients have been discussed, debated, and refined over the past 15 years, treatment literature on child and adolescent cases remains scarce. Kluft (1984) and Fagan and McMahon's (1984) initial observation that childhood dissociative patients can be integrated rapidly and easily has given way to appreciation of the multiple stages of childhood treatment (Hornstein & Tyson, 1991; McMahon & Fagan, 1993) and unpredictable outcomes of treatment, particularly with adolescents (Dell & Eisenhower, 1990). However, numbers of treatment cases described have been few (Laporta, 1992; Malenbaum & Russell, 1987; Snow et al, 1995; Weiss et al, 1985) and a detailed description of therapeutic approaches are just beginning to appear (McMahon & Fagan, 1993; Shirar, 1996).

It is interesting that, despite the large numbers of books and articles on treatment of child abuse (Donovan & McIntyre, 1990; Friedrich, 1990, 1996; Jones, 1986; Sgroi, 1982) the treatment of dissociation and dissociative disorders is alluded to only marginally in these writings. Jones (1986) emphasizes treating the "process" of dissociation rather than the "content," but gives a striking example of a 4-year-old child who may indeed have dissociative identity disorder. Several writers emphasize the importance of attending to the onset and triggers of dissociative defenses as observed in therapy and using that information to help the child identify the dissociative process (Friedrich, 1990; Gil, 1991). Friedrich (1990) has emphasized the use of hypnosis to help dissociative children manage self-destructive behavior but is skeptical of the frequency of true multiple personality disorder among traumatized children. Donovan & McIntyre (1990a; 1990b) discuss dissociative processes in children at length but view the play therapy itself as a dissociative experience in which the child uses imagination to resolve crises on a metaphorical level. They advise against making metaphoric interventions explicit on a verbal level and do not discuss interacting with or addressing alternate states directly. James (1994) and Gil (1991) have been alone among trauma therapists in addressing the content of dissociated material in traumatized children. Gil (1991) describes a 10-year-old girl with DID whose art work revealed five alters. Therapy took the form of encouraging expression, cooperation, and clarification of their roles. James (1994) advises the therapist to identify and process all split off parts to make them more "user-friendly."

Putnam (1994) has pointed out that it remains an open question as to what approaches to treating dissociative children are most effective, cautioning that children may be particularly susceptible to "shaping and reinforcing influences." The increasing backlash against "recovered memories" and adult dissociative disorders has perhaps prompted an increased cautiousness among child therapists who do not want to be accused of the iatrogenic creation of disorders as have adult therapists (Mersky, 1995). Cautions against over-diagnosis or possible iatrogenesis of dissociative conditions in children have been expressed by Friedrich (1990) and Donovan & McIntyre (1990b). Hacking (1995), who has reviewed the psychotherapy literature from a philosophical perspective, scoffs at a portrayal of therapy for children that seems to give credence to the child's belief in the reality of dissociated identities. Although not a trained psychotherapist, Hacking may be picking up on the zeitgeist of the current child therapy mainstream that would rather dissociate itself from the intense criticisms polarizing adult psychiatry.

This reluctance, cautiousness, and fear about addressing dissociated parts directly is very familiar to me in my speaking and consulting in a wide variety of child clinical settings. Clinicians have challenged the notion that there could be a totally "new" kind of child psychotherapy differing significantly from what has been taught historically by the great masters. However, I believe that the new insights gleaned from the juxtaposition of child developmental literature, psychoanalytic play therapy literature, and adult dissociative treatment provide a framework for treatment of child dissociation that is wholly in keeping with the spirit of established psychotherapeutic approaches. In fact, the adult psychotherapeutic technique of addressing alter states directly, which is a kind of sustained metaphorical communication, is more closely aligned with conventional child play therapy than with adult psychotherapy techniques. Psychotherapy with children has always stressed entering the child's imagination, world of play, and symbolic expressions. The suspension of disbelief for enacting play scenarios that deal with important psychological themes is common practice in traditional play therapy where puppet shows, role-plays, and dramatic doll play are commonplace. The techniques described for child therapy with dissociative children stress the same fantasy play components (McMahon & Fagan, 1993; Shirar, 1996).

Communications that temporarily accept a child's imaginative creations are accepted among lay people as well. Psychoanalyst Bruce Klein (1985) describes a commonplace scenario in which a richly imaginative preschooler attributes blame for his broken toys and oppositionality to his imaginary friend, a horse named "Alexander." The child playfully asks "What can we do about Alexander?" The parent responds "Maybe Alexander just had a bad day," briefly entering and acknowledging the child's imaginary world and helping him move beyond the "splitting" defense by an accepting, forgiving, reassuring, and affirming comment. It is a logical extension of this well-accepted approach to children's fantasy to readily accept the dissociative children's metaphorical communication as well, and enter into reassuring dialogue to move the dissociative child to a more sophisticated, less fragmented level of development.

What is new about the treatment techniques that directly address dissociative parts is not the entering into a child's fantasy creations; psychotherapists and parents alike have always engaged in this kind of dialogue with children. What *is* new and different about therapeutic approaches for dissociative children is that now we know what to look for in traumatized children who have dissociated identities and other post-traumatic reactions, and we can offer more substantiated reassurance and explanations to children who may be frightened of these experiences. With the current understanding that we have, we can create a therapeutic environment of knowledge and reassurance, where the secrets of the abuse and the dissociative defensive system no longer need to be kept. The child has an opportunity to hear from a credible adult that his or her view of self is not that strange, that other kids have felt that they have separated parts of themselves as well, and that there is a way to begin to feel less fragmented in the future. If the therapist is reluctant to talk about and address the dissociative identities, the child may continue to believe that this subject is taboo and unacceptable, and the barriers rise to true disclosure.

Thus, I believe that therapeutic work with dissociative children must deal directly with the split-off parts, voices, or dissociated multiple identities that these children present, and the therapist must readily enter into therapeutic, metaphorical communications with the child to help them with more complete disclosure and to move them into an increasingly mature concept of themselves and how they have dealt with trauma. It is true, as Putnam suggests, that therapists may have the influence to "shape and reinforce" children's behavior, but I believe the therapist must knowingly use that influence to shape the child's functioning in the direction of normative and adaptive behavior. For dissociative children, the goal is to shape them into development of a cohesive sense of self. How do we best shape that cohesive self? I believe we must acknowledge their fragmented self-view and try to understand how they see themselves. The traumatized child (Donovan & McIntyre, 1990b) is engaging in an active constructive process of creating hypotheses about the nature of the world and the self just as is the normal child (Stern, 1985). The dissociative "self-system" constitutes the child's working hypothesis about their fragmented experiences and circumstances. Ignoring the child's current theory of self for fear of strengthening their dissociation may mean ignoring the central challenge of the treatment. A therapy approach that ignores the dissociative system exhibits a kind of denial that is reminiscent of dealing with a suicidal patient's wish to die by talking about happier subjects. With suicidal patients we must enter their sadness, their death wish, their demoralization, and find a way out with them, but not ignore it. To ignore the dissociative system would involve complicity with the secretiveness of this defensive style and be a shaping influence in its own way, shaping the patient not to disclose honestly and further reinforcing the need for secrecy.

However, Putnam's concern that therapists could unwittingly strengthen dissociative defenses is well-taken. To preserve the appropriateness of interventions and to avoid making the dissociative system more fragmented, the therapist must heed several cautions. When talking to or about "parts," "voices," or "alters," the therapist should try to engage them, whenever possible, through the child, and while the child is conscious and aware—but not encourage abundant switching in the course of the treatment. The therapist should assume that memory will be consolidated and support all movement towards awareness of other self-aspects. The therapist should occasionally make gentle statements of what things will be like when wholeness is obtained, providing hope and expectation that therapy will lead to this end, while not implying that the therapeutic relationship will end at this time. Recognizing the therapist's potentially powerful impact, this therapy promotes shaping influences that defeat fragmentation. The hope is to provide children with the capacity for healthy attachments and normal self-development, in order to prevent the devastation of living with a dissociative disorder as an adult.

Over the past years I have developed a set of treatment techniques that are used with dissociative children that recognize their fragmented self-view and its expression across many domains of experience. These techniques, described in this and the subsequent chapter, have produced good outcomes for the children studied (see Chapter 6). These techniques are organized around a 5-stage crisis model that crystallizes the central themes that are a focus of the dissociative child's struggle for healing from their traumatic past. This model is sensitive to the developmental growth of the child and highlights the pitfalls of the child's inability to resolve the crisis. Each domain encompasses therapeutic tasks that all traumatized children must master, and appropriate techniques to facilitate this mastery for dissociative children are suggested.

The Five Domains

The traumatized child is seen as having his or her experience of the world shattered through many modalities of experience. The child has cognitive distortions due to what has intentionally been taught by abusive parents (that the child is bad or blameworthy), what he/she has learned indirectly (that he/she is weird, possibly crazy) and what the child has deduced about himself/herself and the world—both are seen as fragmented, diverse, and inexplicably unpredictable. These contrasting cognitive schemata add to the child's fragmentation. The child's emotional experience and capacity for expression have been damaged as feelings (rage and fear) have been too intense to process or too contradictory, leading to dissociated feeling states. The child's physical self has been harmed through physical trauma, confusing sexual arousal, and the experience of overwhelming physical pain, for which the child may have used dissociative defenses for survival, separating off painful aspects of physical experience. Interpersonally, the child's potential for trust, interpersonal safety, and intimacy has been damaged, while family expectations of love, attachment, and obedience may be strong, creating dissonance and contradiction in their relatedness. Spiritually, the child has been demoralized and bereft of belief in God, his/her own worth, or human worth in general, while cultural messages preach self-esteem and human worth and more mature self-aspects of the child strive for this experience. These domains—the cognitive, affective, physical, interpersonal, and spiritual—each a battleground of contradiction and fragmentation, need to be addressed for the child to resolve the damage of his/her early experience and the fragmented self-view that these experiences have created. The remainder of this chapter will describe each of these domains and describe therapeutic tasks and techniques that focus the dissociative child's movement into a healthy resolution of the crisis towards a broader, more well-integrated self-view.

The Cognitive Domain: Appropriate Reality Testing versus Distortion and Confusion

The dissociative child must develop an organizing cognitive schema to account for their atypical internal and external experiences. Failure to do so effectively may lead to distortions in reality testing or cognitive distortion.

The cognitive impact of physical, sexual, and psychological trauma has been well-documented. Traumatized children may have impaired achievement in school (Egeland & Erickson, 1987; Kendall-Tackett, Williams, & Finkelhor, 1993) and a variety of other cognitive impairments that cause distortions in their beliefs about themselves and the world (Briere, 1992; Einbender & Friedrich, 1989). As children feel powerless in response to overwhelming trauma and betrayed by their caregivers, these feelings of powerlessness and betrayal become internalized in self-defeating cognitions (Finkelhor & Browne, 1985). Specific cognitive errors found in adult dissociative patients, such as dichotomous thinking, overgeneralization (Fine, 1988a), confusion of past and present, and misattribution of responsibility (Ross & Gahan, 1988), are typical of dissociative children as well. Many of these cognitive misconceptions are reflections of a more developmentally primitive thinking style, in which the traumatized child may get "stuck" as they lack information to help correct the misattributions and faulty deductions that are being shaped in their pathological environment.

In addition to the cognitive confusion that results from attempts to process the traumatic events, children may become confused and disorganized from the post-traumatic reactions themselves. Traumatized children may experience confusing dissociative episodes, flashbacks, amnesia, somatic memories, feelings of depersonalization, and auditory or visual hallucinations (Hornstein & Putnam, 1992; Putnam, Hornstein, & Peterson, 1996), all of which add to the mounting cognitive confusion of the traumatized dissociative child. Thus, a central task for the dissociative child is to develop a cognitive schema to account for the myriad of post-traumatic symptoms that affect his/her sensory and cognitive experiences. The dissociative child may become confused by his/her hallucinatory experiences, such as internal voices and commands, or visual images of past abusers that may haunt him/her, particularly at bedtime. Young children who are only in the early stages of learning to distinguish fantasy from reality may be deeply perplexed by hallucinations and internal experiences which they come to realize others do not share. As Donovan & McIntyre (1990b) have pointed out, children are in the process of actively constructing hypotheses about their world, and the post-traumatic and dissociative sensory distortions become important data on which they build their theories.

Having interviewed over a hundred of these children, I have come to appreciate the intricacy of explanations children may offer to account for unusual internal experiences that they deduce others are not experiencing. A frequent theory is that they are visited by "guardian angels" that talk and guide them, or "devils" that may steer them wrongly. Interestingly, this was also the belief of the earliest known dissociative child, an 11-year-old described by Despine in 1840 (Fine, 1988b). Other children I have interviewed have come to interpret their internal voices as ghosts, visitations from old ancestors, past life memories, alien life forms, or radio waves for which they have a unique "brain receiver." Although these theories may have a psychotic flavor, they can be better understood as the children's attempts at a logical theoretical framework to make sense of their own experiences.

However, the brighter children usually discover rather quickly that others are not particularly receptive to their theorizing about their experience, and they may be ridiculed or labeled crazy. At this point, the theories which they are trying to develop to make sense of their experience become a new source of shame and secrecy and they may try internal tricks to silence the voices, setting up further internal conflict and fragmentation.

When faced with the reexperiencing of traumatic events through sensory modalities and flashbacks, the child must make a rather sophisticated leap to appreciate that what is happening, though vivid, is not "now." To make sense of this confusion of voices and hallucinations, the child must determine what is internal versus external, and what is memory versus current reality. The dissociative child with less cognitive sophistication is truly taxed by these demands. Given this confusing barrage of post-traumatic and dissociative symptomatology, it is not surprising that so many of these youngsters appear psychotic or profoundly disoriented. I have seen hospitalized dissociative children who have not been able to achieve cognitive schema to understand hallucinated voices and they may be trying to violently harm themselves in hopes of quieting the voices. They react to staff as abusers as if unable to exit from frequent flashbacks of the abuse. These children may be put on heavy doses of major tranquilizers and spend a long time in the quiet room as their dissociative post-traumatic perceptions continue to rule their behavior.

These observations lead to the matter-of-fact conclusion that education is the primary intervention to assist children in resolving the essential cognitive task of interpreting their atypical internal experiences. These children must be taught what dissociation is and why they have internal voices that others do not hear. They must be taught what a flashback is and what a somatic memory is and begin to use more sophisticated cognitive schema to make sense out of their confusing sensory experiences. Language usage should always be shifted to the developmental level of the child but it is always possible to explain these ideas even in very simplified language. The following are some simplified explanations which can help even very young dissociative children make sense of their experiences.

Auditory Hallucinations

Some children have theorized that they have internal VCRs, computers, or tape machines that explain their memory gaps and vivid reexperiencing. In fact, this is one type of image that children can find very helpful.

"Sometimes when children keep hearing something, like someone yelling at them 'You're dumb,' it can get stuck in their mind like a broken tape and then they just keep hearing it again and again. I can help you with some tricks for fixing that broken tape."

Experiencing themselves as parts

"People's minds are made in a wonderful way (or "God made people in a wonderful way," introducing the idea of God as a positive world force that can have a healing effect over time). When things get really, really scary and hard to take, the brain has special ways of helping children. It can help children forget really bad things. Sometimes separate parts of the brain can take over so kids won't remember stuff that was really bad. It's important to stay friends with all parts of your mind so we can find out how they have helped you and how they can keep on helping you."

Flashbacks

"Usually after we think about something, we can store it away in our memory carefully, like in a special trunk or dresser drawer. Sometimes, if we try really hard to forget something, we stick it away far back in our brain too quickly without putting it away really neatly or carefully, just to get rid of it. Sometimes those memories can push themselves back out as if they're saying 'Remember me.' They come back so quick and fast that they almost seem real, not like memories at all. What we need to do is just put them away better so they don't pop out and scare you when you're not expecting them. We can work together so that I can help you to do that with your scary memories. It could be sort of like you put away a jack-in-the-box without really closing the top properly."

As treatment progresses, the central dimensions that need to be explained and re-affirmed are the difference between *then* and *now* and the difference between *what's inside* and *what's outside*. The younger the child, the more cognitively unsophisticated, and the worse the trauma, the more important it is to emphasize and reemphasize these basic distinctions. For example, I treated 6-year-old Felicity with DID, who was in foster care and heard the internal voices of her abusive parents, Candace and Philip, threatening her and telling her not to attach to her foster mother. She believed that her birth parents had actually inhabited her brain and could hear her at all times. Felicity perceived no distinction between the hallucinated voices and the real Candace and Philip. The central cognitive task here was to persuade her that these voices were not the real voices of her parents and that the real Candace and Philip could not really see and hear her. This was a difficult task which involved continual emphasis on the differences between these voices and her real parents and staged experiments to see if the internal voices knew true factual information about her that others had access to. Finally, Felicity came to the realization that the internal mother's voice came to her as it was at a moment when her actual mother had abandoned her in a homeless shelter. Thus, the internal Candace was reframed as Felicity's "first foster mother," and the distinction between the inside and outside reality was strengthened.

Ten-year-old Robert believed that an internal part, "Ghostman," could kill him at will. By challenging the ghostman, while still respecting him, Robert began to realize that Ghostman made many empty threats (like his stepfather) and did not have the power to hurt him that he feared. Internal parts may be very receptive to simple explanations that help to dramatize the differences between *then* and *now*.

Sometimes the differentiation between past and present can lead to the important task of reframing a negative alter. A 12-year-old girl, Michelle, had an alter named Vincent, who had the name of the abuser, a former preschool teacher. This alter believed that he, Vincent, might be punished and go to jail for the offense of sexual abuse. When the therapist showed Vincent a calendar with the current date and an address thousands of miles away from the incident of the abuse, this alter was convinced that he was not in current danger of arrest. Further explanations allowed Vincent to realize that he was not the actual abuser, but a helpful part that had kept 4-year-old Michelle from talking when it might have been too dangerous to talk. Now it was time to develop a new job appropriate to the new age, time, and place. Vincent decided to be "message sender" to facilitate communication between all the parts.

The central dichotomies between *then* and *now* and *inside* and *outside* may need to be emphasized and reemphasized throughout treatment as cognitive distortions continue to arise. Though this message may need reemphasis throughout therapy, it is in the early stages of therapy that orienting cognitive explanations and theories are provided which become a foundation for further communication. The risk of avoiding these educational interventions is that the child may be left in a state of confusion and distortion, with impaired reality testing that may look psychotic.

Cognitive interventions can also be used to help reorient the child's belief systems about what happened to them and why. In an effort to make cognitive sense out of their experience, they may internalize a self-view of badness as a reason for what occurred. Here our tools are more limited; we can give the children no good reason why they were abused. We can use explanations regarding their parents' lack of knowledge and information or parental sickness. Some children who are older and more sophisticated may be able to come to a view of their history as contributing to a helpful approach to other abuse survivors. The reeducation about their belief in their deserving the abuse is a longstanding process that must proceed throughout the therapy. Matter-of-fact disagreement about their perceptions is a starting ground, and the message can be reiterated over time. Continued use of expressions like "I don't believe that; I don't believe children deserve that. Your abusers were wrong when they said that" may begin the process of this reeducation. There are developmental reasons why didactic approaches may be particularly powerful for traumatized children (Friedrich, 1996).

In summary, the task of the therapist in the cognitive domain is to educate the child about his/her dissociative and post-traumatic sensory distortions emphasizing the differences between *inside* and *outside* and *then* and *now,* and to reeducate the child regarding their beliefs about their role in causing or deserving the abuse. To accomplish this, the therapist must be sensitive to the developmental level and cognitive sophistication of the child and begin slowly to educate, correct major distortions, and gradually bring the child's belief system into line with that of the therapist. This creates the common language and common basis of experience on which the rest of the therapeutic work can be based.

The Affective Domain: Expressed Ambivalence versus Uncontrolled Lability

The dissociative child must learn to accept a wide range of affective experiences which may at times feel contradictory, and learn to regulate affective expression. Failure to do so may result in uncontrolled lability.

Greenspan (1981) has described in depth the ongoing learning process of the infant and young child that allows them to learn to differentiate and regulate emotional expression. This process is a learned interactional process that can become severely dysfunctional if the child is lacking the feedback and modeling loop provided by an appropriate caregiver. Stern's (1985) notion of "affective attunement" in early infancy, wherein children learn to model and share affective states with a caring parent, may be particularly relevant for understanding affective disorders in traumatized children. The traumatized child develops clear impairments in emotional regulation, differentiation, and expression, which are likely the result of the absence of this formative early developmental learning. Cichetti, Ganiban, and Barnett (1991) have reported on four patterns of affect dysregulation disorders in children that are related to caregiver responses—developmentally and affectively retarded, depressed, ambivalent and affectively labile, and angry. The ambivalent and affectively labile pattern of affect dysregulation might most closely approximate what we see in the dysregulation of the dissociative child.

Given the affective instability of the traumatized dissociative child, it is not surprising that there is frequent co-morbidity of child sexual abuse and child dissociative disorders with affective disorders (Browne & Finkelhor, 1986; Dell & Eisenhower, 1990; Hornstein & Putnam, 1992). Clearly the rapid switching between extreme emotions associated with contrasting alter presentations can look like phases in bipolar illness. The affective instability of these children can dramatically interfere with their functioning by plunging them into dark self-destructive phases or hypervigilant, fearful modes where they are triggered into flashbacks.

The fragmentation of emotions is at the central core of the process of pathological dissociation. It is the inability of the child to reconcile extreme contrasts of emotions or tie together the extremities of emotion in a unified self-view that may initially provoke dissociation. One might speculate that in normal development emotions are modulated by soothing interventions of a nurturant caregiver: the crying baby is picked up and soon soothed into a calmer state. In the absence of this external regulation and in the face of extreme emotional provocation, the child's ability for self-regulation is severely taxed. Thus, each emotion may be compartmentalized, developing a life of its own, unchecked, without the balancing learned over time in normal development.

Some children, in fact, report feeling names—"Happy," "Fear," "Mad" —as their first description of alters. One 8-year-old with DDNOS described feeling that his behavior reflected the interference of "Mad James," "Happy James," and "Sad James." "Mad James" went into destructive, aggressive fits in which he attacked teachers and classmates, leaving "Sad James" a depressed, regressive part to take the consequences. A 16-year-old girl with a history of abuse by her father from an early age denied at first that she had DID, as she experienced that her "feelings" were fragmented, not her personality. Her rapid switching involved giggling alternating with shouting and fearful crying. These fragmented feelings had no names but were capable of communication. Her extreme lability made her appear severely mood disabled, yet she was unresponsive to Lithium. This fragmentation into discrete feeling states may be a more primitive or preliminary type of dissociative process. Yet, even when alter identities are more complex, with histories, personalities, and traits, it is their emotional tone that sets them apart most clearly.

As in approaching any disorder of affect, the eventual therapeutic goal is to stabilize the mood so that the patient is free to use cognitive skills and his or her full range of abilities. Mood is stabilized over time through allowing affective expressions of anger, fear, and grief within the context of therapy and teaching the patient an abundance of techniques for managing these intense affects when they are out of control. As emotions are expressed, the therapist encourages toleration of the feeling of ambivalence. The ability to simultaneously accept contradictory emotional experience, a hallmark of normal emotional development, needs to be encouraged in the dissociative child to defeat the emotional fragmentation.

Frequently it is the angry affect which can be accessed early particularly with boys (see Chapter 4), as the child's resistance to treatment or acting out behavior at home or school may be the precipitant for therapist intervention. The therapeutic key that provides an environment for healing is reacting to the angry part, alter, or voice in a calm, accepting manner without provoking the aggressive interaction typical of all previous encounters with this part. The dissociative child learns to compartmentalize interactions with others in the manner that he or she has compartmentalized the self. Thus, a therapist's refusal to be provoked by an angry alter is very healing. A comment such as "I know how angry you must feel about what happened. I'd be angry like you are. Any words are okay but hurting yourself and me is not" helps to validate angry feelings and interrupt the cycle of provocation. Angry feelings can be given vent in a variety of play therapy techniques described in the subsequent chapter. Over time, as feelings are shared between affect states or alters, this allows the dissolution of the barriers between affect that makes central regulation possible.

Dissociative children may have conditioned responses to specific objects that are associated with trauma. One 8-year-old boy, Chad, had a fearful, oppositional response to his toothbrush, which had been an instrument of abuse in his birth home. He refused to brush his teeth, and over time this was generalized to avoidance of the bathroom. Chad was asked to use his toothbrush as a paintbrush with tempera paints to paint a picture about the abusive event and then throw the toothbrush away following the art exercise. Chad worked diligently on his "toothbrush picture," enjoying the physical release of large sweeping motions and the clear symbolic and actual destruction of the toothbrush through the exercise. This exercise served to begin a process of desensitization to the feared object while allowing expression of the emotion associated with the trauma.

Often fearful affect is contained in frightened alter presentations, which are usually dependent, authority conscious, and easily befriended. However, it is important to befriend angry presentations as early in therapy as possible, so they do not punish the fearful alter for trusting the therapist. Sometimes fearful alters, when first encountered, feel internal pressure to disclose abuse secrets, but it's important to reach a stage of more internal cooperation before encouraging this disclosure, as there may be other parts that do not feel ready for the disclosure process (see Chapter 8). For example, 14-year-old Ann was abused by a club leader and her mother's boyfriend and was about to disclose information, but an introject of the abusive club leader threatened to hurt her. She was able to negotiate with that part to get permission to tell about the leader's acts, but only using specific words that he dictated. The part agreed not to inflict self-harm if the child used the previously agreed-on terminology.

Hypnotic strategies that allow the child to imagine a "safe place" (see Chapter 8) or deal with the intensity of affect with images suggesting modulation can be very helpful. For example, children can be asked to imagine that they have "volume" dials to turn down intense anxiety or fear.

In summary, fearful emotion can be managed by desensitization to feared objects, developing trust before secrets are revealed, and using a variety of hypnotic strategies to imagine safe, nurturing, and consoling places.

The feelings of grief associated with loss of attachment objects, even abusive ones, are perhaps the most painful emotions with which the dissociative child must deal. It's important to recognize elements of love and special attachment the child had to the abusive parent, as described in Chapter 8 (see Bereaving Alters). These feelings are particularly strong when new foster family relationships are in jeopardy or when placement decisions are pending.

Therapeutic tasks in the affective domain are to express and help to modulate emotion, desensitize to feared stimuli, and move to less fragmentation of affect. If feelings can be expressed without guilt or shame and all types and ranges of affects tolerated equally, the child can move away from the rigid compartmentalization of feelings to tolerance for ambivalence and ambiguity, a clear step towards growth for the dissociative child.

The Physical Domain: Healing versus Re-traumatization

The dissociative child must heal physical wounds and accept the soothing presence of others in this process, or the child will be bound in a cycle of inflicting harm to the body to numb feelings or seek abuse in new traumatic relationships.

These children have experienced assaults on their bodily boundaries that led to lasting impairment in their experience of their physical self. The somatic effects of early abuse may be the experience of somatic symptoms (Friedrich & Schafer, 1995) or the initiation of self-abusive behavior, including head-banging, biting, self-cutting, starving, or other attempts to injure the physical body (Green, 1978; van der Kolk, Perry, & Herman, 1991). Self-abuse may be a way for children to seek longed-for comfort, as they have learned to associate physical abuse with attention from caregivers. Research is beginning to document specific physiological sequela to abuse (see Chapter 13); this physiological damage may be responsible for the reduced sensitivity or abnormal sensory experience of pain that has been documented in abused children (Rosenthal & Rosenthal, 1984). Recent researchers have speculated that self-abuse may be a way to induce the body to release neurotransmitters that provide soothing and anesthesia (Pittman, van der Kolk, Orr, & Greenberg, 1990). My patients have described to me how the infliction of physical pain serves as a powerful distraction from ongoing emotional pain, which feels even more painful and for which defenses are weaker. The challenge in the physical domain is to learn to treat the body with respect, and to relearn normal associations between physical pain and sensation. The risk is that without the physical relearning the child will be frozen in the pattern of retraumatization and continue to seek out physical pain, self-abuse, or continuous physical danger, particularly in adolescence.

Techniques to restore appropriate physical respect for the body are to model care and concern for the body, reestablish positive connections to the body, and help the child understand the feelings of alters who feel pain. Soothing rituals, particularly when performed in conjunction with a loving foster parent, can begin to have the child appreciate the positive elements of the sense of touch (see Chapter 8). Children and parents can invent together magical healing lotions that the parent rubs on the child's arms, legs, or back, with soothing words about love and healing. As therapy progresses, sport activities, swimming, playing in the snow, and encouraging other sensory activities that heighten awareness of the senses with positive physical sensation can help the child feel mastery over his/her physical self.

Many organ systems, such as those used in eating, urinating, defecating, breathing, or swallowing, may have been assaulted during the abuse. The therapist and child will have to identify which areas of the body hold the memories of the assault and establish new positive connections with reconditioning and hypnotic strategies. Many dissociative children will have an alter that has felt the pain of the abuse, which may remain localized in the body as stomach pain or headache. I have found it useful to work with the alter, either through the child or directly, to provide visualization exercises to reduce the intensity of the pain. As discussed by Benjamin and Benjamin (1993), formal hypnosis may not be necessary with young children who become easily absorbed in the trance-like properties of fantasy play, and images of safety and healing can be suggested without formal hypnotic inductions. Images of untwisting coils or gears in the stomach, or slowly turning down "pain" volume dials for headache, may be useful. One child, who was abused in a garbage dump, had an alter with intense olfactory sensations of "bad smells." She was helped to envision in fantasy a multisensory image of a park on a breezy spring day with many allusions to abundant "fresh air" that she could "turn on" as needed.

Some children have described alters whose role or purpose is to seek out abuse by provoking adults in their environment to use physical punishments or physical restraint. Hospitalized children or adolescents with these alters have described great relief at the "hands-on" experience of being carried to the quiet room by a group of trained staff. Some will purposely break minor rules or provoke hospital staff, simply to attain that experience. These alters may require a relearning period of experiencing strong physical touch of a non-abusive variety, such as massage or playful hand-wrestling, or for younger children, periods of rocking with parents to slowly reshape the physiological experience of touch to a more positive one. Therapists can help the parents and child work out bargains such as rewards of specific physical activities in return for more control of the provocative behaviors. If the dissociative child can learn to counter the past physical conditioning of pain and abuse to the body, he/she may be able to escape from the cycle of self-abuse that is often so relentless in adult dissociative patients.

The Interpersonal Domain: Healthy Attachment versus Alienation and Victimization

The dissociative child must learn to attach to a consistent caregiver and develop trust and love. The risk of not developing attachment is that the child will be doomed to feel isolated and ultimately risk becoming a perpetrator of further victimization.

The widespread interpersonal effects of the traumatized child's victimization have been documented in research that shows that abused children are less socially competent and less trusting, have more impaired object relations, and have a higher level of behavioral and sexual disturbances (Berliner & Elliott, 1996). The children who do begin to perpetrate on others may be reenacting the qualities of the only kind of relationships with which they are familiar.

Alexander (1992) has outlined three constellations of disordered attachment—resistent, avoidant, and disorganized. Dissociative children might be seen as fitting the category of disorganized attachment, with simultaneous approach and avoidance to caregivers. This disorganized attachment pattern may be characteristic of children with parents who themselves have suffered unresolved trauma (Friedrich, 1996).

The reestablishment of positive attachment is by far the most important work that can be done for dissociative children. The complexity of this work involves the fact that the child has multiple facets with varying degrees of attachment to the original abusive caregivers and multiple facets of connection to the nonabusive parental figures in his or her life. This fragmentation of attachment results in frequent disruption and testing of any new relationships, as well as intense confusion about receiving positive nurturance. James (1994) has described the trauma bond, wherein the child is attached in a way that promotes injury-seeking behavior. The central challenge is to develop attachments that are consistent and non-conflictual. The risk if this cannot occur is that the child will go on to establish relationships that are based on victimization of the self or others. As stressed by Benjamin and Benjamin (1994), interrupting the cycle of perpetration is an essential component of the therapeutic work with dissociative patients of any age.

I believe that involving the new positive attachment model in therapy as much as possible assists with this important task of attachment. The parts that are angry or scornful of the new parent need to express their doubts in a family therapy context. These parts need to tell the parent what they are seeking and what they fear. The challenge for the new adoptive or foster parent is to try to connect without defensiveness and tolerate these expressions verbally, so that they do not have to be made by physical assaults or other negative behavior. Eventually, over time, these parts can realign their identification with the nurturing parent. They may be resentful of the new parents' intrusiveness if they have had caretaking roles (see Maternal Alters, Chapter 8) or they may be attached to the birth parents and feel loyalty (see Bereaving Alters, Chapter 8). Sometimes unattached parts may hold the angry feelings of the child and be experiencing only punishments and limits and not have an opportunity for positive attachment to the new family. One 12-year-old DID patient, Priscilla, was brought to me for consultation after she had torn up the clothes in her closet and engaged in other destructive activities against her own possessions. Consultation revealed that she had a part called "Tina," who felt jealous of all of the new things Priscilla had received in her adoptive home but felt she had never been adopted by these parents. Tina agreed to refrain from her destructiveness in a family therapy session with the adoptive mother, who emphasized that Tina too had been adopted. Priscilla was instructed to let Tina wear her clothes, and in therapy drew a picture of herself and Tina wearing the new clothes together.

The challenge is equally difficult when there is no new parent, but abuse happened within the family with whom the child remains. In these cases, it is still essential to attempt to reattach the dissociated parts to the original birth family. If abuse has happened through attendance at a day care facility or exposure to an abusive extended family member, the child must sort through the intense anger at the parent for not being protective when protection was needed. The child needs an opportunity to let the angry parts that felt abandoned during the trauma express their rage and disappointment. Parents need to be prepared beforehand for these sessions, so they can respond without being overly defensive and provide apologies as needed. To help prepare parents for this work, I may tell them that they are lucky in a way, because they have a way to go back in a sort of "time machine" and meet the child at the time of injury to express their important feelings and try to reconnect with parts that they were unable to connect with at the time of the assault.

These sessions where parents apologize to dissociated parts that have felt abandoned can be very powerful and emotionally draining but can elicit huge therapeutic strides. One such meeting took place with a mother and abandoned angry alter who had been forcibly sent to day care and had been abused there. During a family therapy session, the part accepted the mother's apology, repentance, and grief, stated "I'm not needed anymore," and was amenable to an integration ritual at that moment. Three years later, this part has not reemerged and angry affect is managed appropriately. As a note of caution, it is important before conducting these sessions to be clear about the source of the original abuse. If one of the parents was involved in the abuse and this has not been disclosed, a family therapy session like this can cause further splits in the dissociative system. The child needs to protect himself/herself from the parent "lies" about being sorry, if abuse has never been acknowledged.

The requirement to attach to an unknown person may be seen as a traumatizing event to which a dissociative child may react automatically by splitting. This appears to be a safer strategy than risking further pain and loss, in case the new family is abusive as well. One 10-year-old dissociative patient told me that he had developed a new alter for each foster placement. Each alter contained memories of abuses in each foster setting, except one who had not been abused in his latest environment. However, the other alters proceeded to test the new foster family, and these provocative tests resulted in the loss of this placement as well. If a child is in a new foster placement the need to withhold closeness at first should be respected in the child, with attempts to teach him/her that this withholding can take place without creating new dissociative barriers.

Three types of parental environments have been described by Fagan and McMahon (1984) and Dell and Eisenhower (1990). Prospects are much more positive if the child is in the highest level of environment where this kind of work can be accomplished (see Chapter 6).

In summary, the dissociative child must learn to attach to the nurturing parental object across all states. If this task can be accomplished, the prospect for healthy relationships as the child matures is vastly improved. If the child is unable to find parents for whom attachment is possible, the learning will be much slower and may be delayed until adult therapy, when the therapist must play that difficult role of being the first object for whom attachment and trust have been developed. I believe that it is this potential availability of objects of nurturing and attachment in a child's environment that makes child work potentially easier, more successful, and quicker than treatment with adult dissociative patients.

The Spiritual Domain: Faith and Optimism versus Despair and Demoralization

The dissociative child must learn to establish a sense of hope and faith in God, themselves, or human potential, or they will be caught in recurrent feelings of despair and demoralization.

The dissociative child's life experiences provide a serious threat to the development of a meaningful trust in God, religions as they are often taught, or belief in humanity and the capacity for goodness. A logical cognitive step after the child no longer blames himself/herself for what has occurred, is to attribute blame to God, or to believe that the world is random, violent and unpredictable.

In some abusive families organized religion is taught, but the basic tenets are hypocritically reversed in the child's day-to-day experience. These children will have great difficulty accepting and trusting organized religion after leaving these environments. Less hypocritical, but even more lethal are environments in which the child is taught reversals, that the Devil is all powerful and "God" too weak to be obeyed. A description of the philosophy of these sects, which is often based on rationalization and justification of their abusive behavior, has been provided by Smith (1993) and Singer (1995). Attempts by the abusive Branch Davidians to instill distorted values of mistrust, paranoia, and adult entitlement have been documented by Perry in his study of the Waco Cult children as reported by Singer (1995) and corroborated in studies of other cult children as well (Singer, 1995).

Although the widespread existence of religious sects that worship the devil is an area of continued controversy, it is my experience and that of my colleagues that children with these distorted belief systems do frequently present themselves in treatment. Having a distorted value system is not a criminal act, and because of this, the powerful messages not to tell or disclose information do not necessarily apply to discussions of belief.   Several children have told me that they believe that "Satan" is more powerful than "God" and that they know this because they have prayed and nothing happened, but they have witnessed powerful satanic forces hurting people. It may be necessary to engage in a discussion with the child about theological belief. I find it important to stay anchored in a strong faith in the belief in the human capacity for goodness, and the belief that goodness is stronger in the long run. Although this belief cannot be proven, the feeling that the therapist holds this view provides anchoring and reassurance for the child. In therapy we discuss openly what things human beings can never really know—what is God, what happens after death—and how belief systems arise to help people answer these questions. I encourage children to formulate their own beliefs and explore how various religions have assigned meaning to events.

The underlying depression that remains within these children even after intensive therapy is often related to this profound sense of loss of meaning and lack of belief. I believe in facing these issues head on, discussing them, and providing resources, books, religious figures, or classes for the older child or adolescent to find personally satisfying answers. Bowman and Amos (1993) have described using clergy with adult dissociative patients who are struggling with existential issues. Children and adolescents can also benefit from meeting with representatives of a faith who can answer their questions and reconcile contradictory information and attitudes. A priest has been helpful in attending therapy sessions with two of my dissociative patients.

One patient who had been abused by people who claimed to be Jewish had misinformation and distortions about what Judaism was. She had interpreted a 5-pointed star worn by her abusers as a Star of David. The priest was helpful in clarifying information about current Catholic ecumenicism and acceptance of all religions. On another occasion, the priest talked with a 12-year-old girl who felt estranged from all religions; he helped her find a metaphor of something beautiful in the world that she could believe in that was symbolic of the potential for beauty and hope in her world.

Some children may be adopted into families with rigid beliefs that make strong discriminations between good and evil and believe in magical use of crosses and other symbols to eradicate bad feelings or ideas. I find that these environments can encourage additional dissociative defenses in the child, who may feel that angry alters are being suppressed and unrecognized, and they may act out. When I am asked to help find adoptive or foster families for dissociative children, I believe religious non-hypocritical homes can be wonderful environments, as long as they respect the child's right to develop his or her own belief systems, do not have overly rigid views about the negative effects of expressing anger, and can handle the child's questioning and lack of belief. The anchoring faith of the adoptive parent's environment can feel very soothing if it meets these criteria.

As children work through these issues of belief and ultimate purpose, some find that adopting a mission, such as planning to become lawyers who prosecute abusers, helping to pass legislation to deal with issues of abuse, or planning to parent foster children themselves when they get older, can help them sublimate their anger and betrayal into humanistic purposes.

Summary

This chapter has presented a framework for organizing therapeutic interventions for dissociative children highlighting five central domains in which they must feel mastery and normalization. Techniques described advocate dealing directly with the child's "split-off" parts or alter presentations to assist the child in overcoming the fragmentation that the traumatic background has caused. Techniques most useful in the early stages involve educational interventions which help the child understand dissociative processes and the differences between *inside* and *outside* and *now* and *then,* and correcting cognitive errors such as misattribution of responsibility. In the affective domain the dissociative child must learn to regulate emotions and accept ambivalent feeling states. Interpersonally, the child must learn to trust and attach despite the ambivalence of emotions. The child must learn a new way of handling physical sensation so that it is not dissociated or a new cycle of abuse initiated. Finally, the child must find a way to make life meaningful again despite his/her abusive experiences. Identification of these central crises in these five domains of experience may help to provide clear goals for therapeutic intervention with dissociative children. The following table summarizes the major therapeutic tasks in these five domains.

Table 1

Therapeutic Tasks for Children with Dissociative Disorders

Domain	Task
Cognitive	understand dissociative processes
	develop a common language to communicate internal experience
	shift view of events
	reframe negative alters
	retell what happened
Affective	discharge emotion—rage, fear, helplessness
	express ambivalence
	identify commonality of feelings
	find socially appropriate channels to express emotion
	identify triggers, desensitize and interrupt automatic responses
Physical	understand the body's reaction to trauma
	reconnect physical feelings
	experience soothing for somatic pain
	learn to appreciate physical touch instead of physical pain
Interpersonal	learn to trust therapist and family
	avoid abusive reenactment
	develop healthy, consistent attachments
Spiritual	find faith, purpose, forgiveness of self and others

References

Alexander, P. C. (1992). Application of attachment theory to the study of sexual abuse. *Journal of Consulting and Clinical Psychology, 60,* 185–195.

Benjamin, L. R., & Benjamin, R. (1993). Interventions with children in dissociative families: A family treatment model. *Dissociation, 7,* 47–53.

Benjamin, L. R., & Benjamin, R. (1994). Various perspectives on parenting and their implications for the treatment of dissociative disorders. *Dissociation, 7,* 246–260.

Berliner, L., & Elliot, D. M. (1996). Sexual abuse of children. In J. Briere, L. Berliner, J. A. Bulkey, C. Jenny, & T. Reid (Eds.). *The APSAC handbook On child maltreatment* (pp. 51–71). Thousand Oaks, CA: Sage.

Bowman, E. S., & Amos, W. E. (1993). Utilizing clergy in the treatment of multiple personality disorder. *Dissociation, 7,* 47–53.

Briere, J. N. (1992). *Child abuse trauma: Theory and treatment of the lasting effects.* Newbury Park, CA: Sage.

Browne, A. & Finkelhor, D. (1986). Impact of child sexual abuse: A review of the research. *Psychological Bulletin, 99,* 66–77.

Ciccetti, D., Ganiban, J., & Barnett, D. (1991). Contributions from the study of high risk populations to understanding in the development of emotion regulation. In J. Garber & K. A. Dodge (Eds.), *The development of emotion regulation and dysregulation* (pp. 15–48). New York: Cambridge University Press.

Dell, D. F., & Eisenhower, J. W. (1990). Adolescent multiple personality disorder: A preliminary study of eleven cases. *Journal of the American Academy of Child and Adolescent Psychiatry, 29* (3), 359–366.

Donovan, D. M., & McIntyre, D. (1990a). Child psychotherapy. In J. G. Simeon & H. B. Ferguson, (Eds.), *Treatment strategies in child and adolescent psychiatry,* pp. 177–195. New York: Plenum.

Donovan, D. M., & McIntyre, D. (1990b). *Healing the hurt child: A developmental-contextual approach.* New York: Norton.

Egeland, B., & Erickson, M. F. (1987). Psychologically unavailable caregiving. In M. R. Brassard, R. Germain, & S. N. Hart (Eds.), *Psychological maltreatment of children and youth* (pp. 110–120). Elmsford, NY: Pergamon.

Einbender, A. J., & Friedrich, W. N. (1989). Psychological functioning and behavior of sexually abused girls. *Journal of Consulting and Clinical Psychology, 57,* 155–157.

Fagan, J., & McMahon, P. P. (1984). Incipient multiple personality in children. *The Journal of Nervous and Mental Disease, 172,* 26–36.

Fine, C. (1988a). Thoughts on the cognitive and perceptual substrates on multiple personality disorder. *Dissociation, 1,* 5–10.

Fine, C. G. (1988b). The work of Antoine Despine: The first scientific report on the diagnosis and treatment of a child with multiple personality disorder. *American Journal of Clinical Hypnosis, 31* (1), 33–39.

Finkelhor, D., & Browne, A. (1985). The traumatic impact of child sexual abuse: A conceptualization. *American Journal of Orthopsychiatry, 55,* 530–541.

Friedrich, W. N. (1990). *Psychotherapy of sexually abused children and their families.* New York: Norton.

Friedrich, W. N. (1996). An integrated model of psychotherapy for abused children. In J. Briere, L. Berliner, J. A. Bulkey, C. Jenny, & T. Reid (Eds.), *The AP-SAC handbook on child maltreatment* (pp. 104–117). Thousand Oaks, CA: Sage.

Friedrich, W. N., & Shafer, L. C. (1995). Somatic symptoms in sexually abused children. *Journal of Pediatric Psychology, 20,* 661–670.

Gil, E. (1991). *The healing power of play.* New York: Guilford Press.

Green, A. H. (1978). Self-destructive behavior in battered children. *American Journal of Psychiatry, 133,* 579–582.

Greenspan, S. I. (1981). *Psychopathology and adaptation in infancy and early childhood.* New York: International Universities Press.

Hacking, I. (1995). *Rewriting the soul.* Princeton, NJ: Princeton University Press.

Hornstein, N. L., & Putnam, F. W. (1992). Clinical phenomenology of child and adolescent dissociative disorders. *Journal of the American Academy of Child & Adolescent Psychiatry, 31,* 1077–1085.

Hornstein, N. L., & Tyson, S. (1991). Inpatient treatment of children with multiple personality/dissociation disorders and their families. *Psychiatric Clinics of North America—MPD, 4,* 631–648.

James, B. (1994). *Handbook for treatment of attachment-trauma problems in children.* New York: Lexington Books

Jones, D. P. H. (1986). Individual psychotherapy for the sexually abused child. *Child Abuse and Neglect, 10,* 377–385.

Kendall-Tackett, K. A., Williams, L. M., & Finkelhor, D. (1993). Impact of sexual abuse on children: A review and synthesis of recent empirical studies. *Psychological Bulletin, 113,* 164–180.

Klein, B. R. (1985). A child's imaginary companion: A transitional self. *Clinical Social Work Journal, 13,* 272–282.

Kluft, R. P. (1984). MPD in childhood. *Psychiatric Clinics of North America—MPD, 7,* 121–134.

LaPorta, L. D. (1992). Childhood trauma and multiple personality disorder: The case of a 9-year-old girl. *Child Abuse and Neglect, 16,* 615–620.

Malenbaum, R., & Russell, A. T. (1987). Multiple personality in an 11-year-old boy and his mother. *Journal of the American Academy of Child and Adolescent Psychiatry, 26,* 436–439.

McMahon, P. P., & Fagan, J. (1993). Play therapy with children with multiple personality disorder. In R. P. Kluft & C. G. Fine (Eds.), *Clinical perspectives on multiple personality disorder* (pp. 253–276). Washington DC: American Psychiatric Press.

Mersky, H. (1995). The manufacture of personalities: The production of multiple personality disorder. In L. Cohen, J. Berzoff, & M. Elin (Eds.), *Dissociative Identity Disorder.* Northvale, NJ: Jason Aronson, Inc.

Pittman, P. K., van der Kolk, B. A, Orr, S. P., & Greenberg, M. S. (1990). Naloxone-reversible analgesic response to combat-related stimuli in post-traumatic stress disorder. *Archives of General Psychiatry , 47,* 541–544.

Putnam, F. W. (1994). Dissociative disorders in children and adolescents. In S. J. Lynn & J. W. Rue (Eds.), *Dissociation: Clinical and theoretical perspectives.* New York: Guilford Press.

Putnam, F. W., Hornstein, N., & Peterson, G. (1996). Clinical phenomenology of child and adolescent dissociative disorders: Gender and age effects. *Dissociative disorders: Child and Adolescent Psychiatry Clinics of North America, 5.*

Rosenthal, P. A., & Rosenthal, S. (1984). Suicidal behavior by preschool children. *American Journal of Psychiatry, 141,* 520–525.

Ross, C. A., & Gahan, P. (1988). Cognitive analysis of multiple personality disorder. *The American Journal of Psychotherapy, 12,* 229–239.

Sgroi, S. M. (1982). *Handbook of clinical interventions in child sexual abuse.* Lexington, MA: Lexington Books.

Shirar, L. (1996). *Dissociative children: Bridging the inner and outer worlds.* New York: Norton.

Singer, M. T. (1995). *Cults in our Midst.* San Francisco: Jossey-Bass.

Smith, M. (1993). *Ritual Abuse.* San Francisco: Harper.

Snow, M. S., White, J., Pilkington, L., & Beckman, D. (1995). Dissociative identity disorder revealed through play therapy: A case study of a four-year-old. *Dissociation,* 120–123.

van der Kolk, B. A., Perry, J. C., & Herman, J. L. (1991). Childhood origins of self-destructive behavior. *American Journal of Psychiatry, 148,* 1665–1671.

Weiss, M., Sutton, P. J., Utecht, A. J. (1985). Multiple personality in a 10-year-old girl. *Journal of the American Academy of Child and Adolescent Psychiatry, 24* (4), 495–501.

eight

■

Therapeutic Phases in the Treatment of Dissociative Children

Frances S. Waters and
Joyanna L. Silberg

Several years ago the authors discovered that, working independently in different cities with no contact, we had developed similar techniques for treating dissociative children. These techniques were developed through close attention to the adult dissociative literature (Kluft, 1984; Putnam, 1989), experience and familiarity with play therapy techniques (Schaeffer, 1979), and close familiarity with family systems theory (Bowen, 1978; Karpel & Strauss, 1983). The adult dissociative literature taught us what to look for and how to interact with a fragmented personality. Our knowledge of child therapy techniques helped us adapt these approaches to a child's developmental level, and our knowledge of family systems theory influenced our emphasis on the family context to sustain positive behavioral change. Although we had each treated traumatized children before there was an awareness of dissociative disorders, we discovered that this paradigm for understanding traumatized children could have powerful therapeutic implications. Similarly, in the early years of the development of adult treatment techniques, Kluft noted that "clinical realities of MPD influenced clinicians with different backgrounds toward common approaches" (Kluft, 1984, p. 10). As increasing numbers of clinicians describe treatment techniques with children (Benjamin & Benjamin, 1993; McMahon & Fagan, 1993; Peterson, 1996; Shirar, 1996) this cross-validation of treatment methods is occurring in child therapy circles as well and stimulates increasing confidence about successful ways of approaching these patients in treatment. As described in Chapter 6, our methods have been largely successful in symptom reduction and resolution of fragmentation for those patients who have remained in treatment. However, the formal findings reported do not capture the subjective feeling of relief that so many of these children expressed in having their dissociative defenses identified and understood. The relief, trust, and hope that these children communicated served as a powerful reinforcer to us of our treatment methods. It is our hope that as the field of childhood dissociative disorders develops, large scale outcome studies can provide further validation of these approaches and provide useful clinical feedback that stimulates refinement of the techniques to improve their efficacy.

Dissociative disorders in children, defined and described in earlier chapters of this book, are understood as the mind's way of coping with brutal, traumatizing events. The child's mind internalizes memories, feelings, or behavioral schemata associated with the trauma. These segregated parts may then influence the child's thoughts, feelings, and behaviors throughout childhood and into adulthood. For the purpose of therapeutic intervention, it is most useful to conceive of this model as a metaphor that describes how children perceive their own experience. To debate the reality or unreality of alters, voices, or parts of the mind is to miss the point—that this metaphor resonates powerfully with how these children feel about themselves. By entering into this metaphorical communication, the therapist has a powerful tool for encouraging health and promoting healing and a sense of integrated identity. Whether a child has a diagnosed DID (dissociative identity disorder) with clear-cut alter states or a nondescript DDNOS (dissociative disorder not otherwise specified) with puzzling rage reactions, the techniques described here can be effective in defeating fragmentation.

Many theorists have described sequences for treatment of trauma related disorders in children and adults (Gil, 1991; Herman, 1992; Hornstein & Tyson, 1991; Jones, 1986; Kluft, 1986). Although the names and breakdowns of the exact stages vary, the basic progression is often seen as a 3-phase process. The first phase involves assessment and relationship building (internal and external), the second phase involves processing the traumatic events, and the third phase involves resolution or integration. The treatment sequence that we have found useful is based on this 3-phase model and will serve as a basis for the organization of the subsequent discussion. However, the reader should remember that the phases blend into one another, and techniques appropriate for one phase are used throughout the therapy. Although convenient for didactic purposes and organization, the reader should understand that this segmentation is somewhat artificial and therapy does not progress evenly. There can be environmental stressors, sudden developmental spurts, or comorbid conditions that influence the progression of therapy.

Phases in the Treatment of Childhood Dissociative Disorders

Phase I: Engagement
Assessment
Reassurance and Education
Stabilization
Identification of the Personality System/Team-building

Phase II: The Trauma Work
Develop narrative of the traumatic events
Process traumatic memories on many levels

Phase III: Resolution
Integrate the dissociated parts
Develop age-appropriate coping

This chapter will provide a basic understanding of this sequence of treatment emphasizing Phase I and II with illustrative examples of cases from our clinical practices. (Phase III issues are discussed at length in the following chapter.) Initially we will discuss some underlying assumptions about work with dissociative children, how to prepare the office, and general issues that pervade all phases of treatment. We will discuss the child's alter system and commonalities that we have observed among many patients and provide examples of techniques for processing trauma and reframing alters. This chapter is not intended to be an exhaustive discussion of treatment issues, as much treatment information is contained in other chapters of the book, and successful treatment may involve many modalities of intervention and multidisciplinary input described in other chapters.

Basic Principles

Kluft (1993) has classified 12 pragmatic principles that underlie successful therapy with adult dissociative patients, and the reader is referred to this discussion for a review of basic principles common to work with dissociative patients of all ages. To highlight sensitivity to special concerns of child clinicians, we would like to supplement Kluft's list for work with dissociative children to include developmental issues as well as principles that highlight the therapist's sensitivity to the context in which the child lives. Childhood treatment is not an isolated event within the confines of the therapy office, but the child therapist is more like a manager, sensitive to a variety of factors that may impede the child's progress and development. The therapist must remain constantly alert to issues of ongoing safety, the input of a multidisciplinary team, and sensitivity to developmental norms. The following list will provide minor modifications to some of Kluft's principles and provide additional therapeutic principles to supplement Kluft's comprehensive list.

1. *The importance of respecting therapeutic boundaries with regard to dual relationships is equally applicable with children as with adults.* However, therapists who work with children do occasionally go to children's schools, performances, or graduations, which helps to illustrate for the child that the therapist is one of the caring adults in his/her environment. The model of therapeutic boundaries for children more resembles that of a teacher than the strict "no contact outside of therapy" rule more appropriate for adult patients. Therapists should use their judgment in maintaining the boundaries that they are accustomed to within their normal practice.

2. *As with adults, the maintenance of a therapeutic alliance is essential, but the alliance with the family in which the child resides is equally important and must be nourished and sustained.* Even if the relationship with the child is outstanding, if the relationship with the parent is strained, therapeutic messages will be distorted and the therapist may become an inadvertent pawn in the parent-child power struggle. This will doom the therapy. If the therapist has judged that the family environment is not an appropriate one for the child, the therapist must expend energy on helping to secure a more appropriate environment—foster care or residential placement. The therapist should never knowingly work with the dissociative child within an environment that is judged to be harmful, and then use that as an excuse to refrain from allying with and providing guidance for the family. This sets up the potential for additional fragmentation in the youngster and will likely result in a premature termination of therapy as the parents become increasingly resentful of the therapist's lack of attention to their family's needs.

3. *The therapist must encourage patient responsibility by requiring that the child be responsible for all of his/her behavior.* Kluft's principle of encouraging patient responsibility is an important one with children, and in our experience we find that it is often violated for newly diagnosed child dissociative patients. Therapists, teachers, or parents may be too quick to absolve the child from responsibility for behaviors of alters when the diagnosis has first been confirmed. We find that the "rule of shared responsibility" helps children decrease inappropriate behavior and may help to ultimately increase co-consciousness. We tell the child that "everyone" (child and his or her dissociated parts) is responsible and "everyone" will have to pay the consequences for wrong behavior. From our clinical experience, the children have re-

sponded with decreased inappropriate behavior and less circumventing of responsibility when the children knew that no matter what "alter" did what, the child must face the consequences. This may help increase awareness of the blocked emotions without forcing confrontation. If children continue to deny responsibility for a behavior, we gently help them appreciate the dilemma of being punished for something they perceive they did not do and help them learn techniques to increase responsibility and internal negotiation.

4. *It is important that the child be in a safe and nurturing environment for treatment to be effective.* To ask the child to remove his or her techniques for surviving in an unsafe environment may contribute to the child's increased vulnerability to ongoing abuse and to internal pain. The techniques described here are not appropriate for children in unsafe environments (see Chapter 15 for some discussion of these). The therapist's first job must be to help promote external safety, and this is a job that occurs outside of an individual therapy session through consultation with family, protective services, or other caretakers (see Chapter 13).

5. *The child interacts with many adults within many environments and each must be respected and included in the therapeutic work for real change to occur.* A multidisciplinary team approach encompassing child care providers, protective service workers, foster care workers, teachers and school counselors, residential staff, or the legal system, is required to assist in a child's total recovery. Sgroi (1982) has recommended that a child's therapist should devote one hour to team consultation for every hour of child therapy. Although this requirement for working outside of therapy is challenging, given managed care constraints, it is essential for the therapist to facilitate smooth team coordination for treatment to be effective.

6. *The therapist should always keep in mind what is developmentally appropriate for the child, and therapeutic goals should work towards developmentally appropriate behavior.* The therapist encourages appropriate activities and skills such as sports, creative activities, reading, clubs, and special interests. These developmentally appropriate activities begin to normalize the child's life and serve to bridge internal separateness, especially if "parts" can agree to engage in them together. Some skeptics have been concerned that working directly with a child's dissociative system may serve to develop and reify the dissociation rather than interrupt it. We believe that if the therapist continues to keep in mind reasonable developmental expectations and works towards these goals, the danger of solidifying the dissociative defenses will be avoided. Children developmentally do *not* call themselves "we," so this is discouraged outside of therapy. Children *are* responsible for all of their behavior, so we don't encourage children to evade responsibility by attributing misbehavior to alters.

Keeping this principle in mind will help guide the treatment when people respond to the child with excessive or special treatment. For example, one enthusiastic and zealous teacher described putting out a chair and paper for a child's alters, and a parent suggested building an addition to the house to be used for the child's anger expression. Awareness of what is normal and appropriate for children suggests that excessive interventions such as these are unnecessary and may serve to reinforce the dissociative defenses.

Kluft's other principles of evenhandedness with all alters, encouraging cooperation, mastery and the resolution of trauma, and correcting cognitive and perceptual inaccuracies are all applicable with child and adolescent patients as with adults and will be described later as relevant.

Preparing the Office

It is recommended that therapists have an office well stocked with a variety of supplies. These might include a large assortment of puppets, doll house with furniture, dolls (including anatomically similar dolls), paints, markers ("changeable," "overwriters," and "3-D"), crayons, colored pencils, drawing paper, clay, feeling games, action figures, animal figures, sand tray, tape recorder and tapes, balls, short-playing fun games, and an assortment of knickknacks, fabric scraps, rocks, and seashells.

Puppets are employed extensively in our practice with young children, as it may be easier for traumatized children to talk to the puppets about their abuse rather than directly to the therapist. F. W. presents a puppet with an "inside family," who is one step ahead of the child in treatment to encourage progress with issues of co-consciousness, cooperation, expression of painful feelings, conflicts, resistance, transference, and integration. F. W. has Hermit, the crab puppet[1] that goes into its shell if afraid of being hurt, or threatened, and comes out when he feels safe and trusting of others. F. W.'s marionette puppet, Dudley the duck, has been extremely useful in demonstrating that his "alters" are not working together, by crossing the strings, which prevents the duck from walking.

Slime or clay has been very helpful to symbolically express separateness, the combination of feelings, and eventual blending of aspects of the self.

A sand tray has been useful for symbolically reenacting external events or internal conflicts as described in treating dissociative adults (Kalff, 1980; Sachs, 1993). As children pick characters for the sand tray and demonstrate conflict, symbolic interventions can help the children make sense of and resolve internal conflicts.

Ball equipment can be used imaginatively to help deal with different

---

[1] Folktails. Folkmanis, Inc., Emeryville, Ca. 94608

forms of abuse and feelings associated with the abuse. Bowling pins or nerf balls can represent perpetrators, as feelings are expressed physically (Graham-Costain, Waldschmidt, & Gould, 1992).

Dolls, particularly the anatomically similar dolls, are a tool in helping the child express what happened and allowing discharge of feelings toward the perpetrator doll. Several sexually abused children have demonstrated cunnilingus and fellatio with these dolls, although they had not previously reported those forms of abuse.

Many dissociative children have used tape recorders to tape songs or plays about their "inside family," about their abuse, or about their new families (adoptive parents). Some have taped symbolic letters to their perpetrators which are used therapeutically.

Phase I: Engagement

Assessment

Assessment of the dissociative child should be an in-depth process in which data are collected from multiple sources and informants in the child's life. Assessment techniques including interviewing, questionnaires, psychological testing, and family interviewing have been described in the first section of the book and will not be repeated. The assessment helps to determine the family's capacity for fully engaging in treatment and the child's strengths and weaknesses, which might help predict the pace of treatment. Assessment of the child's cognitive capacities is important to determine how best to explain to the child about the nature of the dissociative processes and how receptive the child might be to metaphorical communications. The availability of external supports for the child and family is assessed. Are there places the child can go for weekend relief from the parents? Do the parents have a network of support—church, family—so that there is some outlet for stress reduction?

Assessment of the child's and family's capacity for trust may be a useful indicator of whether there is potential for long term commitment to the therapeutic process. Establishing trust with children who were severely traumatized in the first 3 to 5 years of life may seem to be a never ending process. It requires that the therapist exercise patience and understanding when provoked to respond negatively to the child. Abused children will often try to recreate abuse scenarios as a learned response to previous abuse and fear of attachment. Trust is an ongoing issue, which may get tested and retested throughout treatment. However, the authors' experience is that the profound level of mistrust seen in adult patients is not as apparent in children with dissociative disorders. Most have not yet lost their youthful hopefulness that there is someone out there who will finally understand them. Parents who have coped with the traumatization of their own child may adopt a paranoid, accusatory, or hostile attitude towards helping professionals, which may also affect the prognosis for a successful engagement in therapy. The therapist should try to understand the parent's protectiveness and suspiciousness and build credibility and trustworthiness over time. As child and parent act out their fears of vulnerability and abandonment, the therapist is challenged to be calm, accepting, and patient with them.

When the therapist senses that preliminary trust has been achieved, the therapist must assess the dissociative system itself to determine the severity and rigidity of the dissociative defenses. Putnam, Hornstein, and Peterson (1996) have presented evidence that there is some developmental progression so that the older the child, the closer his/her symptoms may resemble the adult disorder of DID. Any given dissociative child may present on a continuum of dissociative severity, from severely rigid amnestic barriers with distinct personalities (DID) to fleeting hallucinatory voices that help the child deal with unacceptable anger. The therapist must assess the degree of co-consciousness of the child or adolescent, the distinctiveness and separateness of the dissociated affect states, and the accessibility of the dissociated states to "being known" by the therapist. This assessment is an ongoing process during the early stages of therapy as communication with the other parts, ego states (Watkins & Watkins, 1993), or voices takes place through drawing, playacting, or directly engaging them (see Chapters 3 and 7 for further discussion of early assessment and engagement techniques).

Reassurance and Education

During this early phase, the therapist begins the process of education and reassurance about dissociation. Simple explanations of how dissociative defenses are used by children may help them begin to feel less weird, less alone, and more in control of the unusual post-traumatic experiences that they have had. Children need to understand what flashbacks are, why they hear voices and how the mind has dissociated to deal with trauma. Explanations of these phenomena in language suitable for children are presented in Chapter 7. Children may benefit from simple books about dissociation (see Appendix) that will help them believe in the universality of what they have experienced and further demystify the diagnosis. Education of the parents should occur simultaneously, so that the parents develop a new context for understanding their child's disruptive and provocative behavior.

Both parents and children must be educated about the process of treatment and what to expect. They need to learn about the importance of respecting all aspects of the mind, the important role that even angry parts have played in the child's survival, and how treatment will involve expression of all feelings with internal cooperation. The therapist also needs to explain to the child the danger of continuing to create new alters as a coping mechanism for new stress.

During this educational phase of treatment, metaphors and symbols may be introduced as a way to dramatize to the child what the course of therapy will be and how the parts of the mind might work together. For example, 8-year-old Joan with DID was told that working together inside was like playing soccer successfully, as each position (symbolic of each alter) is equally important in playing the game well, scoring, and having fun. All team players need to watch, listen, and participate in their positions to play the game. As this metaphor developed through the course of therapy, helpful alters were given jobs of "coaches" and "referees" and the importance of fairness was stressed.

Another useful educational metaphor that the therapist can use to set the stage for a cooperative approach is to compare the child's internal system to his or her favorite dessert. For example, the therapist can say that the flour gives a cookie substance, the baking soda helps it rise, the sugar makes it sweet, the butter makes it smooth, the vanilla adds a special richness, and the chocolate chips provide its scrumptious flavor. Then, the therapist can conclude the analogy by stressing that leaving out any ingredient would not make the cookie taste as good as it could, just like leaving out any part of the child would make him or her incomplete and prevent the child from showing his or her true potential.

When the therapist knows what interests and activities the child enjoys, the therapist can creatively use metaphors and symbols that relate to the child's life to encourage understanding of the idea's of team work and cohesiveness. Mills and Crowley (1986) and Davis (1990) provide abundant examples of metaphors and stories that can be used to illustrate the process of treatment and recovery to traumatized children.

Stabilization

During this initial process of assessment, there is a high probability that the child's internal system will become destabilized. This may be due to the interference of alters that are resentful about the child discussing internal secrets, which may activate any suicidal or self-abusive behaviors to maintain the code of secrecy. It is important to remember that these children have received very strong threats about what might happen if they tell, and many consider telling about the dissociated parts as equivalent to telling about abuse secrets. The following are some techniques for stabilizing the child during this early period.

Contracts. The child and the alters need to be continually reminded that each of them will benefit from controlling self-destructive and aggressive tendencies and thereby gaining more privileges. The therapist can contract with the child and alters to agree to the "No Harm Deal," which reads, "No one will get hurt either inside or outside on purpose or accidentally, and nothing gets broken either on purpose or accidentally until we (child and therapist) see each other again." All parts, or an agreed upon spokesperson, must sign and date the agreement, making it effective until seen again for the next therapeutic session. (F. W. states "until I see them again" instead of putting the date of the next appointment, in case the next session is canceled due to sickness.) If need be, the child may have to continue to sign the agreement during followup sessions until the suicidal or homicidal threats have dissipated. If a threatening alter refuses to sign the agreement, then the child is put on a 24-hour watch by the alerted caregivers and hospitalization is considered. Parts of the child that may be nonaggressive and protective are asked to help prevent any dangerous behavior from occurring. Additional sessions may be scheduled during these times.

Code Words. Like traumatized adults, traumatized children may respond to "triggers," external reminders of traumatic incidents that may cause them to dissociate, remember a painful memory, or be destructive. It is wise to prepare in advance for such encounters. Braun (1980) and Kluft (1983) have used cue words with adult DID patients to elicit an agreed alter to come out and assume control when needed. Preestablished code words can be arranged that signify that the child is exhibiting provocative behavior that could lead to aggression or destruction. One innocuous phrase that has been successfully used by parents and teachers is "Get it together." This phrase signifies that the child is not in control, and the child and the alters need to regroup and cooperate with each other. This phrase does not reveal any confidential information, but concisely conveys to the child the need to reintegrate or cooperate with his or her internal system. One 10-year-old DID child agreed to the word "bubbles," which would signal that it was time to resume control if a destructive alter was emerging or if he needed to be reoriented. The therapist can work together with the child and family to develop code words for specific occasions when the parent needs to alert the child or the child to alert the parent of the child's internal dissonance. To minimize a crisis, it is prudent to arrange with the child and the caregivers such code words early in treatment.

Safe Places. Setting up an "internal safe place," a technique utilized for adult patients (Kluft, 1989), may be beneficial for children as well when therapy begins. The therapist can use the child's imagination to help invent a room or refuge to which the child can escape when feelings become overwhelming. The child and therapist can stock the imaginary room with fantasy tools, such as a magic laser with beams to detect danger, or large screens with favorite movies for distraction. The child can practice having these pictures in the mind during stressful times to help deal with intense feelings. Sometimes developing a safe place involves some negotiation, as demonstrated by one 8-year-old DID patient who wanted a "gun shop" as his safe place, so as to scare any enemies away. The author, F. W., was able to negotiate with him to have an "empty Tommy gun" on his internal "well-stocked private yacht," which emphasized comfort rather than threat.

In our work with dissociative children, we have found that deep trance is unnecessary in having children develop "safe places." Children's imaginations are vivid, and they are able to respond well to simple instructions about visualizing, or drawing relaxing and safe images. Prior to leaving for vacation, it may be useful to describe agreed upon "safe places" on audiotape so that the child can have easy access to them during the therapist's absence.

Identification of the Personality System / Team Building

The therapist's main task at this point in treatment is to begin to identify and understand the parts, alters, or ego states that the child has revealed. As the parts are identified, the child is encouraged to develop an awareness of all parts, termed co-consciousness, and to encourage negotiating and conflict resolution among the parts.

As alters are identified, the therapist can collect information about each part in a book or portfolio that becomes the child's special working document about therapy's progress. Throughout the course of therapy ideas, pictures, or memories can be added to the special book. As the child's internal concepts change over the course of therapy, this therapy book can help to document the changes. It may be useful to have a page in the book for each of the dissociated parts and to fill in information about that part each time new information is learned. In exploring the different alters and their roles the therapist can ask the following questions: What feelings does each of the child's parts/alters/ego states have most predominantly? How are these feelings similar or different? What were the roles or purposes that each part held in containing the feelings? What conflicts exist among the parts? What identification did the parts assume? Each part may contain similar or contradictory feelings toward abuser, non-perpetrating parent, the abuse itself, and one another. How old was the child when that part developed and how old does that part see itself now? The answers to these questions and associated drawings can be tracked in the child's special therapy book (see Figure 1).

Our clinical cases, as well as other reported cases (Fagan & McMahon, 1984; Hornstein & Tyson, 1991; Kluft, 1985), suggest that for most dissociative children the boundaries within the child's personality system ap-

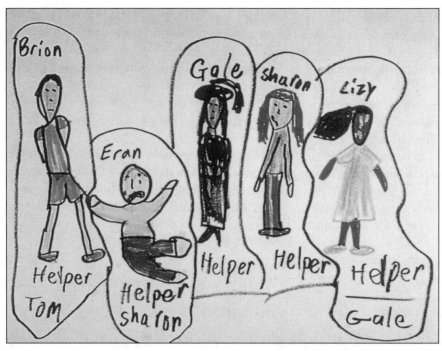

Figure 1. This picture shows a page from a child's therapy book in which she is organizing her parts by their functions.

pear more fluid and flexible than adult DID internal boundaries, and co-consciousness seems to be attained more readily. The simple suggestion for all parts to "watch and listen" during therapy may be enough to encourage more full awareness. One might ask the child, "Did Big Albert hear that? Please tell him to listen," particularly at an important therapeutic moment. One 11-year-old with DID reported that she imagined an internal TV set with a VCR with play and rewind buttons, tapes, and speakers. She could keep the internal communication system "on" at all times, but if she missed something, she would rewind the tape to learn what happened. For some children, it is useful to ask them to close their eyes and listen carefully in their mind to find out what another part feels about an issue being discussed. Children are frequently surprised that they can "hear" answers directly from parts that they had not previously known about. As internal awareness and communication increases at this early stage, the child is encouraged to show appreciation, acceptance, and respect for all parts of the mind, which is modelled by the therapist's accepting and nonjudgmental attitude. It is often a shocking realization to the child that it is possible to show respect and appreciation for an "angry part," as frequently the child has learned that anger and negative affect are unacceptable; this attitude may have resulted from environmental pressure that led to the dissociation in the first place. The realization that acceptance is possible for the dissociated negative affect is often relieving to the child. One 6-year-old DDNOS patient stated to J. S., "I always knew that my 'Devil' had a nice side of him, but I was afraid to be nice back." At this point, the therapist suggested changing the "Devil's" name to "Mr. Mad but Nice." Audiotaped or written plays in which the parts talk and express understanding for one another, as well as "thank you cards," "get well cards," and other polite gestures can be useful at this stage.

In cases of strong amnestic barriers between the parts when the child denies being able to understand the feelings or behaviors of other alters, it may be useful to have the child "role-play" what it might feel like to have done the behavior in question. The author, J. S., used this technique with a 9-year-old boy with DDNOS, Tom, who denied that he had strangled his pet rabbit. The therapist and child together alternately role-played the feelings of the rabbit and then the feelings of the rabbit's "unknown" attacker. As the child role-played the rabbit about to be strangled, he got in touch with his own feelings of fear and vulnerability. As he role-played the attacker, he experienced the feelings of fear of vulnerability and trust. After several successive role plays of this event, Tom quietly admitted, "I strangled the rabbit." By encouraging the expression of feelings without confrontation, the therapist allowed Tom the opportunity to overcome the dissociative barrier between feelings of victimizer and victim and to understand his destructive behavior.

Another technique for dissolving amnestic barriers, is to ask the child to imagine an alter as a perfect mask of the face which is overlaid on the child's own face. The child is asked to imagine that the mask has eyeholes and earholes so both child and alter can see and hear simultaneously. Children are very receptive to simple suggestions and visualization techniques such as this.

Once there is some ability of the parts to communicate with one another, the therapist may use the term "inside family" to describe the child's internal system. This promotes a sense of cohesiveness, particularly since many of the children have come from disruptive families and long for a caring family. Understanding that the inside parts are like a family helps to emphasize for the child that the parts must get along and must learn the negotiation and mediation that families use to solve problems. Many teenagers have had experience with family therapy, and explaining to them that the work they need to do is like family therapy appears to be a helpful metaphor.

As alters are identified, it is important to explore the names of the alters, which frequently relate to their roles in the trauma. Their initial roles may have remained the same or become redefined as the child ages. Several of our DID children have taken on alter names of hero figures or cartoon characters such as Mr. HeMan or Raphael the Ninja Turtle, as did cases described by Kluft (1985). Other names will pertain to significant others in the child's environment, like special best friends, understanding teachers, or perpetrators. Other alters may have names of stuffed animals, imaginary friends, or pets. Many children use feeling names to identify their parts, such as "Sad Adam and Mad Adam" or "Laffy and Crybaby." Questioning the child about how the name was chosen can be an initial step in getting to know that dissociated part. Some children do not have names for their dissociated states. In this case, providing the child with temporary names that are descriptive of the feeling states can be helpful—"Debby when she feels lonely" or "Debby when she's real mad." However, the therapists should avoid helping the child elaborate on undeveloped fantasy projections that the child has not already envisioned and created. If the therapist is unsure if the patient seems to be "making it up as he/she goes along," the therapist might stop discussions about the alters temporarily, and then listen for what the child spontaneously describes next time the topic is mentioned. The therapist should look for clues that the dissociated descriptions have stable qualities over time, which is different from the fluidity of a normal child's spontaneous fantasy creations.

There may be many classifications within a child's personality of alters that assume varied roles. We have found surprising commonality in our caseloads. Below is a brief categorization and description of some of the more common alters we have encountered and therapeutic approaches to them.

Perpetrating/aggressive/self-abusive Alters. Internal perpetrating alters may have experienced the severest forms of abuse and consequently identified with the external abusers by assuming their names and/or temperamental behaviors. It is advisable to establish an alliance early in treatment with abusive alters to gain their respect and cooperation, as suggested in the adult literature (Kluft, 1993; Putnam, 1989). These alters may be responsible when the child engages in self-abusive behavior. Through careful inquiry, the therapist can learn from the child what was the meaning or purpose of cutting his or her wrist or attempting to stab himself or herself, and what part/alter was involved. An abusing alter may be hurting the host personality because he or she is telling about the abuse, which violates the code of secrecy. An abusive alter may be hoping to stop the pain by ending the child's life. Strategies that encourage empathy and gratefulness to the perpetrating alters for their original role in coping with the trauma are useful.

The following therapeutic approaches may be recommended with the abusive alters:

1. Inquire about their motivation to harm.
2. Help them to process the painful feelings and thoughts associated with trauma.
3. Cognitively process with them the reality of their current environment with adults available to support them.

4. Point out to them that their strength and power, which were required to survive the assaults, were courageous and admirable.
5. Discuss with them how their strength and power can be utilized in other ways now to help the child adjust and recover; process with them how their strength can be constructively employed.
6. Discuss with the abusive alters the idea of degrees of strength needed in various situations. (This is critical because minor conflicts can be met with an exaggerated response by the child.)

One common problem that dissociative children encounter from peers is teasing due to perceived oddness, spaciness, destructiveness or other behavioral symptoms that isolate the child. This may set up a cycle of further rejection, as the aggressive alter may seriously attack another child for name-calling. Role-playing with the aggressive alter (while the other alters watch and listens) peer conflicts with different nonviolent solutions can help the aggressive alter learn to judge what is an appropriate response.

In addition, setting up safe ways to discharge angry feelings at home is helpful. Ten-year-old John was physically abused by his father from infancy until he was approximately 3 years old. He reported a violent "voice/part" of him who would explode at home and at school with little provocation. John was amnestic to these explosive incidents. John and his "angry part" signed the No Harm Deal, and the angry part of him agreed to contain and release appropriately his rageful feelings through exercise. The agreement indicated that John would earn 10 minutes on the video game system if he spent 10 minutes on the step exercise machine to release his anger. If he worked out on the exercise machine on his own initiative before he began losing control, he would earn an additional 10 minutes of time playing video games. This behavioral contract tempered his rageful behaviors at home while F. W. worked with John in therapy to process his feelings toward his father. To help John at school, with his mother's permission, F. W. met with his teacher to explain his dissociation and his vulnerabilities to peer teasing. The parent, teacher, and therapist agreed on several approaches, one of which was the use of the verbal cue, "Get it together," which triggered John to take a deep breath, count to 10, and ask for help inside to control his temper. John's outbursts decreased at school and at home in frequency and intensity.

Sexually Obsessive Alters. Dissociative children who have been sexually abused may have an alter or unconscious part that influences them to have sexually obsessive thoughts and compulsive sexual behaviors. Sexually abused children may engage in excessive masturbation that physically hurts themselves, or they may sexually perpetrate on other children (Briere, 1992). These children appear extremely remorseful and guilty but seem to have little control over such thoughts and behaviors.

Until the dissociated, influencing part is accessed, the child may continue to be at high risk for sexually abusing other children.

F. W.'s case of "Sam," a 7-year-old sexually compulsive DDNOS child, illustrates this process. Sam had been sexually abusing his 2-year-old half brother and had identified perpetrating parts who had assumed the same names as the teenage perpetrators who sexually abused him. After Sam learned that the internal perpetrators had experienced his sexual abuse, his ability to control his impulses increased. The process of co-consciousness and cooperation developed. Several techniques were useful in helping him gain control. He was a visually oriented child who liked to draw pictures, and he was encouraged to draw in therapy sessions and at home whenever he felt as though he was going to touch his brother. He would draw himself with large, out of proportion hands, which appeared to signify the power the hands had over him (see Figure 2). During one therapy session, F. W. requested him to draw a picture of something that could help him control the overwhelming feelings and thoughts about sexually touching his younger brother. He drew a picture of his head containing an internal laser machine that would be activated when he had feelings or thoughts of touching his brother. The alarm system would alert him to tell his parents, to get away from his younger brother, or find something to divert his attention. This was an effective tool in containing his impulses as therapy progressed towards uncovering more details of his sexual abuse history. Additionally, parents were alerted to maintain close supervision and clear boundaries between Sam and younger children. Sam expressed shame, guilt, and regret for abusing his younger brother and apologized to him.

The therapeutic goals with sexually obsessive alters are listed below.

1. Explore their original role in the sexual abuse and encourage expression of the feelings associated with this abuse (generally in Phase II).
2. Learn empowerment techniques through internal and external control strategies.
3. Alert caregivers to closely monitor and structure the child's environment to protect other children.
4. Help the children to learn empathy towards their victims and self-forgiveness.

Maternal Alters. Traumatized children may have formed "maternal" alters to compensate for the lack of protection when abused. The therapist may have to simultaneously work through internal and external conflicts with a child's maternal alter. A mother alter, who has been the protector and comforter of the repeatedly traumatized child, may be very jealous or resentful of mother figures in the child's life and may be the source of oppositional and defiant behavior. Many adoptive mothers of dissociative

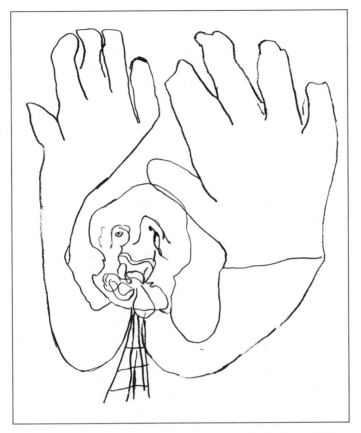

Figure 2. A child with a sexual compulsion illustrates the feeling of his "out-of-control" hands.

children have reported angry scenes with the pseudo-mature internal mother vying for control over a situation.

In this case, the therapeutic strategies are:

1. Help the maternal alter deal with the pain, anger, sadness, and burden that she felt while protecting the child.
2. Help the maternal alter to accept and trust the parent figures in the child's life so she can release that responsibility. Getting the parents involved in the treatment is an essential part of the conflict resolution with the maternal alter.
3. Help the maternal alter to redefine her role so that it is compatible with the child's age and development.

The following case exemplifies this treatment process.

"Susan" was the name of a maternal alter of Darla, a 12-year-old with a long history of sexual abuse. "Susan" had comforted Darla when she was being sexually abused. Initially "Susan" was resistant to giving up this role until she was acknowledged and praised for her fine work of comforting Darla. She shared with Darla details about her history and together they did a number of therapeutic exercises to work through their rage at the biological perpetrating parents. "Susan" was encouraged not to carry this burden anymore, since Darla was in a safe adoptive home and had a mother wanting to support and protect her. The next crucial step in giving up Susan's role as internal mother was a formal meeting with Darla's adoptive mother and an agreement for Susan to "adopt" her as well. At a family therapy session, the two who had been previously acquainted through arguments formally met, and discussion occurred about what Susan had done for Darla. The adoptive mother praised Susan for helping Darla, and Susan agreed to let go of her earlier role and accept the adoptive mother as being in charge of caring for Darla. In time, Susan became the same age as Darla and integrated with her (see Chapters 9 and 13).

Bereaving Alters. When treating dissociative children, it is important to explore with them and their alters what their feelings are toward their birth parents who abused and neglected them. In spite of how horrendous the abuse was, the therapist needs to be understanding of the infant/parent bond formation (Ainsworth, 1979; Bowlby, 1969), and to be careful not to appear critical of the abusive parent; this could inhibit the child from expressing and resolving his or her attachment and separation issues with these parents. The intensity of these trauma-based attachments have been described by James (1994). Dissociative children frequently have unconscious parts that retain these strong attachments to the birth parents. The bereaving alter may have spent positive time with the abusive parent or received special attention from his/her parent, even though significant abuse was incurred as well. The bereaving alter must deal with the traumatic aspects of the relationship to the primary parent as well as grieve the loss of the positive aspects of the primary relationship. Healthy attachment to a new parental figure can occur only after this process has been completed. Children who remain in their family of origin also need to grieve the loss of a nurturing and protective parent in order to forgive, accept, and resolve their ambivalent attactment toward the parent.

The therapist needs to explore with the child and his/her dissociative system what each of them feels toward their abusive parents and to facilitate the child's mourning over the loss of his or her parents. Mourning can be done through writing letters or making tapes to the parent, even though these are not sent. One adopted child treated by J. S., whose father was imprisoned for murdering her mother in front of her, was helped to write a play with roles for her abusive parents expressing regret and apology for their behavior. This play was then put on audiotape (with appropriate voice changes) for the adoptive parents and other important people and it provided a sense of healing and resolution. The processing of these issues of loss of parents may prevent these feelings from being acted out in severe conduct problems in later years (Greenberg & Speltz, 1988).

This therapeutic mourning process will enable children to appropriately release painful feelings and thus pave the way to accept adoptive parents or to resolve feelings of rejection, abandonment, and hurt toward biological parents who have ceased their abuse and are providing a safe environment.

Therapeutic goals in dealing with bereaving alters of adopted children are:

1. Mourn the loss of their biological parents and their idealized early childhood.
2. Express sadness to their adoptive parents and accept their comfort about their early childhood trauma inflicted by biological parents.
3. Develop symbolic adoption rituals to encourage attachment with adoptive parents.

With children who remain in their biological home, it is imperative that their environment remain safe for the child's bereaving alters to mourn. Therapists need to help parents to work through their guilt and shame about the pain they administered to their child and learn to comfort their child as they acknowledge full responsibility.

Ego Ideal or Helper Alters. All dissociative children whom we have worked with have had alters that represent the positive attributes of their personality and their capacity for coping and survival. Frequently these alters have facilitated reporting about the abuse and thereby have obtained safe environments. Accessing these alters is important, as they can assist the child in controlling destructive impulses and self-destructive behavior. However, it is important for the therapist not to show undue favoritism to these alters, or the other parts may feel jealous or resentful, and sabotage the therapy. These helper alters can help to set the tone for fairness, cooperation, and team-building.

Gregory was a 6-year-old boy with DDNOS who told author J. S. that he had a "pink hamster" living in his brain that told him to "calm down" and to accept living in his new foster home. This "pink hamster" had many ideas about how to help Gregory in treatment but was not willing to let Gregory express positive memories about his birth parents. After the therapist negotiated with the "pink hamster" and provided reassurances that contact with his birth parents would not resume, the "pink hamster" was helped to accept the reality of Gregory's attachment to his birth parents.

Therapeutic strategies for working with "ego ideal alters" include engaging to assist with positive therapeutic change and resisting favoritism, while encouraging a cooperative attitude.

Other Classifications of Alters. Other alters that we have encountered include "laughing alters" ("Giggles," "Laffy," "Jokester") whose job it is to deny painful feelings, baby or younger age alters that may contain intense needs for nurturing, and depressed alters that may be responsible for suicidal behaviors. In young children, we have often observed "animal" alters including dogs, cats, horses, and birds, which may have varying roles. One 9-year-old DID boy had incorporated several dog alters as a result of witnessing his parent kill his pet dogs. In each case, the therapist must elucidate the alter's needs and feelings and assist with expression, positive reframing, and growth. As work with the dominant alters progresses, many of the less important ones may spontaneously merge with others or fade. This process is discussed in the following chapter.

Retracting or Disappearing Alters. On several occasions in our own cases or in consultation with other clinicians, we have come across patients who come to a therapy session and state "I made it all up. I don't really have those voices (parts, inside friends)." When this happens, it may represent a child's attempt to divert the treatment process to avoid painful issues or to regain control in the therapy setting. Somehow the child may feel that the therapist has become overly invested in hearing about the parts, or that someone outside of therapy is pressuring them in an uncomfortable way about talking about this. The recommended stance in this case is to ally with the child's current perception. One might say something like "You made these up. Sometimes things that we make up can seem more real than we expect. A lot of children find it helpful to deal with scary things by doing that. It's okay if that's not the best way for you to talk about these problems right now. If it is useful for you to think about it in this way again, we can talk about it again. This is your therapy and you know best what it feels like to be you." The therapist should try to avoid getting into a power struggle with the child about whether he or she does or does not have "parts." Since we understand that personality "parts" are internal representations formed from traumatic episodes, reference to "parts" is a useful metaphor for later discussion when the child is more comfortable. Therefore, if this is handled in a matter of fact way, without the child sensing that the therapist is experiencing a narcissistic loss, the child may again bring up the "parts" at a time when he/she is feeling more in charge or when his/her ego feels stronger to manage the disturbing memories contained by the "parts." However, it is important to assess, if this retracting of "parts" occurs, whether the child has become exposed to some current danger which is making it unsafe to tamper with the dissociative protections.

If talk about the parts does not reemerge spontaneously and the child's symptomatic behaviors lessen, the therapist may move on to other developmentally normative topics and assume that the child has experienced spontaneous fusions or that the previous self-description is no longer needed. True dissociative parts that remain a significant influence on the child's behavior will present themselves again for therapeutic intervention as the child continues to display disruptive symptoms.

This "retraction" is to be distinguished from the "retraction of abuse" which is a frequent characteristic of abused children in general as part of the "child abuse accommodation syndrome" (Summit, 1983), which will be alluded to in the following section.

Once the therapist has stabilized the child, become acquainted with the alter system, and encouraged co-consciousness and team work, work on the second phase of treatment may begin.

Phase II: The Trauma Work

At conferences participants frequently ask the authors how important it really is to deal directly with traumatic material. This question is motivated by the concern that the material may be re-traumatizing, and the instinct is to protect the child from further harm. The consensus of most trauma therapist is that this work is essential (Friedrich, 1990; Gil, 1991; James, 1994; Jones, 1986). The retelling of the trauma story helps to validate children's feelings, empower the children through constructive techniques, and help them learn to accept what happened before storing it in their memory (James, 1994). However, James wisely points out that "forcing children to face their terror" is dangerous. Sensitive pacing of traumatic material is essential to avoid overwhelming or destabilizing the child.

There is a delicate balance between pursuing the traumatic memories, waiting for them to unravel, and respecting the child's need to stay defended. For many children with trauma histories the material is close to the surface, and simply providing unstructured materials and a safe environment may stimulate their disclosures and play about traumatic themes. Some children, however, are guarded, well-defended, and avoidant. We recommend providing an environment in which the child knows that disclosure is safe and expected and in which other children have successfully disclosed. The therapist presents himself/herself as someone who is an expert on children who have "had really bad things happen to them," is not afraid of the material, and is willing to listen empathically without being horrified. The therapist reassures the child that the office is a safe place to talk and together they will work on alleviating painful feelings. For some children for whom the traumatic events are overwhelming and whose defenses are weak, it may be appropriate to wait until another developmental stage to deal with traumatic memories. This is particularly true of patients who enter treatment during adolescence, whose treatment must emphasize coping with the numerous developmental tasks of their teen years. As long as they remain stable, it may be possible to avoid direct work on the trauma, which could stimulate regression and impede their teenage life experiences.

Developing a narrative

The first goal in the processing of traumatic material is having the child tell the story of what happened. This story is usually told in bits and pieces over time, and is rarely a completely coherent, sequential narrative (Coulborn Faller, 1988; Sgroi, 1982). The child's "telling" can be done through drawing pictures, making clay figures, puppet or doll play, or dramatic role play. During the telling phase, assisting the child to describe specific physiological sensations, emotions, and thoughts encourages the child to connect and integrate many domains of experience. As described by Braun (1988), the reconnecting of behavior, affect, sensation, and knowledge helps to overcome learned dissociative barriers. Through the telling and retelling, the child's cognitive task is to attribute responsibility appropriately and avoid self-blame. When reenacting abusive events it may be useful to help the child come up with alternative endings that reinforce empowerment and strength: "Let's pretend you got to the telephone and called the police; what would you say?"; "Let's pretend the door wasn't locked; how would you get away?" (As a note of caution, this technique would not be advisable to employ if the child was preparing to testify in court regarding the abuse and needed to maintain accurate details in his or her memory.)

During the telling process, abused children go through periods of time when they will deny what they reported. This is particularly true immediately preceding court hearings, protective service visits, or contact with birth parents from whom they had been removed. Usually these are short-lived and represent the internal struggle to reconcile the competing memories that they hold of their abusive but sometimes loving parents. Sometimes retraction is due to the family's attempt to supress honest disclosure. Our approach in these cases is to be tolerant, patient, and nonconfrontational.

Summit (1983) described retraction as one of the key features of the "child abuse accommodation syndrome," which also includes delayed, conflicted, and unconvincing disclosures. Summit writes, "Beneath the anger of impulsive disclosure remains the ambivalence of guilt and the martyred obligation to preserve the family" (Summit, 1983, p. 188). Retraction of stories of abuse among adult patients has received attention in the popular press; this may make nonprofessionals overreact to retractions by children. Although attributing retraction to this syndrome cannot be used in court proceedings against alleged perpetrators (Myers, 1996), professionals are becoming increasingly skilled at making the determination between "true" and "false" retractions (Whitfield, 1995). Characteristics of truly abused patients who retract their story include presence of flashbacks, serious psychopathology, and fear or knowledge of the perpetrator's response to their disclosure (Whitfield, 1995). Many of the sensationalized media presentations of adults who recant abuse have little bearing on childhood cases in which physical abuse evidence is often blatant, protective services investigations have been thorough and repeated, accused perpetrators have harmed more than one child victim, and the children corroborate one another's report.

Processing Trauma

There are many types of exercises for working with traumatic material. As discussed by Gil (1991), the therapist must try to take an active role to help move the child past traumatic reenactment (Terr, 1990), in which the same scenario is continually replayed, as if the child is "stuck" in a traumatic moment. The play is modified through therapeutic intervention to encourage mastery of experiences, express feelings that were unexpressed at the time of the abuse, or play the scene out differently with a wished-for fantasy conclusion. Techniques for processing trauma are limited only by the imagination and creativity of the therapist and the child, and many have been described in other sources (Friedrich, 1990; Gil, 1991; James, 1994; Jones, 1986).

We believe that the standard trauma techniques should be modified with dissociative children to include the whole host of internal characters that will participate, overtly or covertly. The involvement of the other "parts" should be made explicit before the trauma exercise. As in group work, all "members" of the group will influence the process and outcome of the group. It is useful to inform the child before beginning the exercise that the child will be able to choose an activity after the trauma work and the child can negotiate with the alters about a fun activity that will follow. Inquire which ones, voices, parts, alters were involved in a particular abuse or trauma, and ask them to participate in the exercise together as a team. Others not involved will be encouraged, if feasible and appropriate without traumatizing or overwhelming them, to watch, listen, and learn from techniques that may later assist them in appropriate expression of their feelings. They will be asked to support, comfort, and cheer those "parts" doing the trauma intervention. The therapist can draw on examples of cheerleaders or spectators of sports events to emphasize the importance of building team spirit, endurance, and strength in their successful recovery. Alters who are too young or unable to handle the intensity of the expression can be kept in an established internal "safe place" with stuffed animals and an internal "parent" nurturing them. It is important to cover all bases and to include others that may not have been identified but may be helpful to the team by saying to the child, "If there are others that I (therapist) have not met, ask them to watch and listen or participate in a way that will be helpful." This statement addresses itself to possible fragments of the personality that may have been involved directly or indirectly in the original abuse.

To avoid sabotage of the activity by aggressive "parts" it is important to set structure and clear limits. The "No Harm Deal" may need to be reiterated and specific guidance given about how to carry out an activity that involves the expression of physical rage. For example, in a ball activity in which a child puts a drawing of the perpetrator on the wall, the child is instructed to throw the nerf ball on the specified wall and nowhere else.

When children are recounting trauma memories, affects can become intense. Children can be helped to store "bad feelings" in magical vaults, trash bags, or specially marked "bad memory" boxes (James, 1989). For some children, there seems to be a sequence of feeling expressions which move from fear, helplessness, and guilt, to rage, and then to grief and depression. There may be some sex differences in this sequence, as boys appear to be more in touch with their rage initially (see Chapter 4). Children may graph the progress of feelings using colorful graphs in which each marker color represents another feeling or alter state. Therapists can create large pictures of the child which can be segmented and then joined together as common feelings are expressed and shared. Angry feelings can be expressed with physical activities of pounding clay, coloring over pictures of perpetrators, tearing pictures, or throwing balls.

Trauma to the body may leave emotional scars which can become fixated in the traumatized part of the body. Children may experience severe psychosomatic complaints, such as headaches, intense olfactory sensations—"bad smells"—or pain at the site of a known physical trauma. Anita was a 7-year-old patient with DID who experienced intense pain at the site of a healed cigarette burn inflicted by her father. The therapist and child created a pretend magical secret lotion that the therapist and foster mother rubbed on the child's leg to alleviate the pain. During the course of the session, the foster mother was instructed to repeat, "I can love you enough to make all the pain go away." Symptoms diminished after this exercise. F. W. treated a 10-year-old child, John, who had no memory of being placed in a freezer as an infant, a memory reported to the therapist by an older sibling. John experienced an acute "icy sensation" on his back. F. W. instructed him to draw something that might remove the "icy spot," and he drew his adoptive mother breaking up the ice with an "ice cube muncher" (see Figure 3). John indicated that the icy sensation disappeared. His adoptive mother reported that after this session, he

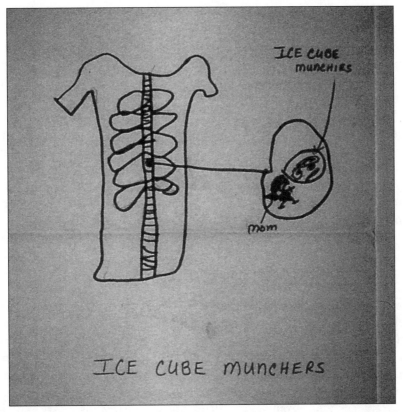

Figure 3. An "ice-cube muncher" drawn by a child with a somatic memory of being placed in a freezer.

was able to play outside in the snow, an activity he had previously avoided.

A traumatic history affects all aspects of the child's functioning—cognitive, emotional, interpersonal, physical, and spiritual. These aspects of functioning and how they are impacted by trauma have been reviewed in the previous chapter. The most effective techniques utilize many modalities of experience simultaneously. For example, children who are expressing rage at a past abuser by physically pounding a clay figure representative of abusers can be encouraged to make statements about the abuse—"You had no right to treat me that way"—and to work on cognitively modifying their perceptions about the events. They are concurrently encouraged to discuss how their body may have been affected, how their relationships to their family and others were influenced, and how their belief system helped them to survive. Another technique for simultaneous processing is to request that the child use cartoon balloons to describe emotions of anger, fear, hopelessness, loss, and guilt while drawing cartoon pictures depicting abuse events (Doyle & Stoope, 1991). While the child draws these pictures, the therapist helps the child to cognitively process the events and to develop a sense of hope. Therapists are encouraged to use their creativity to develop techniques such as these which promote positive parental bonding, expression of feelings, and imagination for positive coping.

An essential factor in successfully processing traumatic events with dissociative children is including the appropriately involved parts or alters. Unless their feelings and thoughts are considered in the therapeutic techniques, a complete and successful recovery may be inhibited. Engaging the child's milieu—the family, school, and significant others—is recommended, as in other child-oriented treatment, so that new skills learned generalize across many facets of the child's life.

Treatment Considerations Regarding Teens

Teenage years can be turbulent even for non-abused children, but for dissociative teens who have experienced early and repetitive abuse, adolescence can be extremely chaotic. The treatment of dissociative teens is challenging (Kluft & Schultz, 1993), particularly if they have not been diagnosed prior to the intense activation of the issues of separation, individuation, and trust typical of adolescence. Symptoms in sexually abused children, such as promiscuity, drug abuse, eating disorders, suicidal thoughts/attempts, depression, and anxiety tend to be magnified during the teenage years. Frequently in adolescents these maladaptive behaviors are isolated within different alters—an alcoholic alter, a promiscuous one, one with an eating disorder. Assessing what part or alter is exhibiting such symptoms is the pathway toward alleviating the symptoms. Many dissociative teens demonstrate borderline characteristics as a defense mechanism to their fear of trusting, getting close, and feeling vulnerable. Frequently this causes others to see them as manipulative and deceitful, and the trauma basis of their dysfunction is not appreciated. Feelings of fear, pain, sadness, loss, and vulnerability are difficult for dissociative teens as their defenses are becoming more rigid. The therapist needs to be aware of transference and countertransference issues, in order to avoid power struggles which are easily aroused as the teenager tests the trustworthiness of the relationship. F. W. treated Tammy, a DID teen who was severely traumatized repeatedly from infancy until she was 8 years old, when she was removed from her biological home and adopted. Tammy would project the anger she held for her abusive parents onto her adoptive parents and therapist, particularly when she was being confronted for inappropriate behavior. In spite of the commitment to her and intensive therapy with her on rage and distrust, she continued to struggle with issues of trust. She ran away from home several times and was placed in a residential treatment center and later a foster home. Tammy reported in therapy that the dissociated parts had integrated, but still she could not make peace with her adoptive parents. With some severely abused dissociative teens, it may be too much to expect them to completely resolve trust and attachment issues during these turbulent years. Keeping goals limited to basic survival needs, such as maintaining physical safety, a drug and disease free lifestyle, and avoiding pregnancy, may be seen as successful therapy in some cases, until a more stable developmental period allows more work on trauma and attachment issues.

Expressive arts and journaling are very useful for teens who may have difficulty with straight verbal therapy. It can be a therapeutic outlet for a teen and his or her alters to journal throughout the process of treatment on traumatic issues as well as developmental issues (dating, peer pressure, etc.). Some teens who have been abused are exquisitely sensitive to their effect on others and may experience minor peer rejections as a further traumatizing event. The author J. S. worked with a 15-year-old DID girl who struggled with profound feelings of rejection from peers. In this case, the treatment technique involved letter writing between alters about how to manage feelings of rejection without resorting to suicidal behavior (see Figure 4). Creative activities are also encouraged for teenagers who may portray their alters, their inner life, and their integration in poetry, songs, short stories, and paintings.

One creative DID teen, "E.," used poetry to describe her inside family. She wrote the following:

MY INSIDE FAMILY
The darkness surrounds me
But the light still shines
Down.
The far seems farther away.
But there they are.
My friends, My family,
Held together. We, the moon
in the sky.
Though something connects
Our hearts,
It's something that can't
Be explained.

As teenagers are beginning to think abstractly, it is very important to include the spiritual domain in the therapy. They are beginning to wonder about life's meaning, their own purpose, the unfairness of their life experience, and if there is a God. Therapeutic exercises which highlight hope and future potential are important. One 14-year-old DDNOS teen drew a symbolic picture of how she felt toward her alcoholic, neglectful,

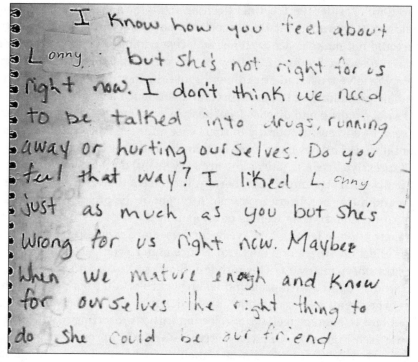

Figure 4. A teenager communicates with an alter through a letter to deal with issues of peer rejection.

and abusive parents. She drew a picture of palm trees being struck by a hurricane, representative of her rage toward them. At the end of therapy, she drew the palm trees again, this time with a bright sun covering the page, and herself smiling in the center, suggesting her hopeful outlook towards the future.

Integrated teens or teens who have made significant gains in the trauma phase can benefit from a teen group for sexually abused girls to receive peer support. Other beneficial groups may focus on conflict resolution or communication skills (see Chapter 11).

Summary

Treating dissociative children and adolescents is challenging and yet rewarding as the therapist moves the child forward from living with the pain and horror of past abuse into a sense of hopefulness about the future. To successfully treat such children, the therapist needs to understand child development, how developmental processes are thwarted when trauma occurs, and the dynamics of dissociation. Therapists must show sensitivity to the underlying dissociative parts, with an emphasis on negotiating and conflict resolution before engaging in trauma-specific techniques. Many play therapy techniques can be adapted to work with dissociative children, and techniques should attempt to involve the whole child ("alters," "parts," or "voices") on many levels of experience—cognitive, affective, physical, interpersonal, and spiritual. Involving appropriate parental figures in the therapy will assis the child to resolve issues of rejection, abandonment, grieving, and trust and facilitate the child's development of healthy attachments to adults.

This chapter serves as an introduction to approaching therapy with dissociative children, who must learn to understand and communicate with all split-off internal parts, cooperate, and express feelings related to the trauma history. When this work is complete, the child is ready for the third treatment phase—integration—covered in the next chapter.

References

Ainsworth, M. D. S. (1979). Infant-mother attachment. *American Psychologist, 34,* 932–937.

Benjamin, L. R., & Benjamin, R. (1993). Interventions with children in dissociative families: A family treatment model. *Dissociation, 7,* 47–53.

Bowen, M. (1978). *Family therapy in clinical practice* New York: Jason Aronson.

Bowlby, J. (1969). *Attachment and loss: Vol. 1.* New York: Basic Books.

Braun, B. G. (1980). Hypnosis for multiple personalities. In H. Wain (Ed.), *Clinical hypnosis in medicine.* Chicago: Year Book Medical.

Braun, B. G. (1988). The BASK model of dissociation. *Dissociation, 1,* 4–23.

Briere, J. N. (1992). *Child Abuse Trauma.* Newbury Park, CA: Sage Publications.

Coulborn Faller, K. (1988). *Child sexual abuse: An interdisciplinary manual for diagnosis, case management and treatment.* New York: Columbia University Press.

Davis , N. (1990). *Once upon a time . . . Therapeutic stories.* Oxon Hill, MD: Psychological Associates of Oxon Hill.

Doyle, J. S., & Stoop, D. (1991). Witness and victim of multiple abuses. In N. Webb, *Play therapy with children in crisis.* New York: Guilford Press.

Fagan, J., & McMahon, P. P. (1984) Incipient multiple personality in children. *Journal of Nervous and Mental Disease, 172,* 26–36.

Friedrich, W. N. (1990). *Psychotherapy of sexually abused children and their families.* New York: Norton.

Gil, E. (1991). *The healing power of play.* New York: Guilford Press.

Graham-Constain, V., Waldschmidt, C., & Gould, C. (1992). Creating play interventions for use in therapy of children and adults with dissociative disorders. Paper presented at the meeting of the Ninth International Conference on Multiple Personality/Dissociative States, Chicago, IL.

Greenberg, M. T., & Speltz, M. L. (1988). Attachment and the ontogeny of conduct problems. In J. Belsky & T. Nezworski (Eds.), *Clinical implications of attachment* (pp. 177–218). Hillsdale, NJ: Lawrence Erlbaum & Associates.

Herman, J. L. (1992). *Trauma and Recovery.* New York: Basic Books.

Hornstein N. L., & Tyson, S. (1991). Inpatient treatment of children with multiple personality/dissociative disorders and their families. *Psychiatric Clinics of North America 14,* 631–647.

James, B. (1989). *Treating traumatized children: New insights and creative interventions.* Lexington, MA: Lexington Books.

James, B. (1994). *Handbook for treatment of attachment-trauma problems in children.* New York: Lexington Books.

Jones, D. P. H. (1986). Individual psychotherapy for the sexually abused child. *Child Abuse and Neglect, 10,* 377–385.

Kalff, D. M. (1980). *Sandplay: A psychotherapeutic approach to the psyche.* Boston: Sigo Press.

Karpel, M. A., & Strauss, E. S. (1983). *Family evaluation.* New York: Gardner Press.

Kluft, R. P. (1983). Hypnotherapeutic crisis intervention in multiple personality. *American Journal of Clinical Hypnosis, 26,* 73–83.

Kluft, R. P. (1984). The treatment of multiple personality disorder: Results in 33 cases. *Psychiatric Clinics of North America, 7,* 9–29.

Kluft, R. P. (1985). Hypnotherapy of childhood multiple personality disorder. *American Journal of Clinical Hypnosis, 27,* 201–210.

Kluft, R. P. (1986). Treating children who have multiple personality disorder. In B. C. Braun (Ed.), *Treatment of multiple personality disorder* (pp.79–105). Washington, DC: American Psychiatric Press.

Kluft, R. P. (1989). Playing for time: Temporizing techniques in the treatment of multiple personality disorder. *American Journal of Clinical Hypnosis, 32,* 90–98.

Kluft, R. P. (1993). Basic principles in conducting the psychotherapy of multiple personality disorder. In R. P. Kluft & C. G. Fine (Eds.), *Clinical perspectives on multiple personality disorder* (pp. 19–49). Washington, DC: American Psychiatric Press.

Kluft, R. P., & Schultz, R. (1993). Multiple personality disorder in adolescence. In S. C. Feinstein & R. C. Marohn (Eds.), *Adolescent Psychiatry, 19* (pp. 259–279). Chicago: University of Chicago Press.

McMahon, P. P., & Fagan, J. (1993). Play therapy with children with multiple personality disorder. In R. P. Kluft & C. G. Fine (Eds.), *Clinical perspectives on multiple personality disorder* (pp. 253–276). Washington, DC: American Psychiatric Press.

Myers, J. E. B. (1996). Expert testimony. In J. Briere, L. Berliner, J. A. Bulkey, C. Jenny, & T. Reid (Eds.), *The APSAC handbook on child maltreatment* (pp. 319–339). Thousand Oaks, CA: Sage Publications.

Mills, J., & Crowley, R. (1986). *Therapeutic metaphors for children and the child within.* New York: Brunner/Mazel.

Peterson, G. (1996) Early onset. In J. L. Spira (Ed.), *Treating dissociative identity disorder.* (pp. 135–173). San Francisco: Jossey-Bass.

Putnam, F. W. (1989). *Diagnosis and treatment of multiple personality disorder.* New York: Guilford Press.

Putnam, F. W., Hornstein, N., & Peterson, G. (1996). Clinical phenomenology of child and adolescent dissociative disorders: Gender and age effects. *Dissociative disorders: Child and Adolescent Psychiatry Clinics of North America, 5,* 351–360.

Sachs, R. G. (1993). Use of sand trays in the beginning treatment of a patient with dissociative disorder. In R. P. Kluft & C. G. Fine (Eds.), *Clinical perspectives on multiple personality disorder* (pp. 301–310). Washington, DC: American Psychiatric Press.

Schaeffer, C. E. (1979). *Therapeutic uses of child's play.* New York: Jason Aronson.

Sgroi, S. M. (1982). *Handbook of clinical interventions in child sexual abuse.* Lexington, MA: Lexington Books.

Shirar, L. (1996). *Dissociative children: Bridging the inner and outer worlds.* New York: W. W. Norton.

Summit, R. C. (1983). The child sexual abuse accommodation syndrome. *Child Abuse & Neglect, 7,* 177–193.

Terr, L. (1990). *Too scared to cry.* New York: Basic Books.

Watkins, H. H., & Watkins, J. G. (1993). Ego-state therapy in the treatment of dissociative disorders. In R. P. Kluft & C. G. Fine (Eds.), *Clinical perspectives on multiple personality disorder* (pp. 277–299). Washington, DC: American Psychiatric Press.

Whitfield, C. L. (1995). *Memory and abuse.* Deerfield Beach, FL: Health Communications.

Promoting Integration in Dissociative Children

Frances S. Waters and
Joyanna L. Silberg

Integration has been defined as a "pervasive and thorough psychic re-structuring" (Kluft, 1984). It is viewed by adult dissociative therapists (Kluft, 1984; Putnam 1989) as an ongoing process in the latter stages of treatment wherein the barriers between the separated self-states slowly erode and new, blended configurations of self-representation emerge. Integration, which is an ongoing process, is distinguished from "fusion," which is the specific "compacting" process (Kluft, 1984) at a given point in treatment wherein the blending of two or more states occurs. These definitions and distinctions may not be as appropriate for the understanding of the final stages of child and adolescent dissociative treatment, as the "psychic structuring" of younger patients is not as rigid or well-developed, and the moments of "fusion" are less specific during the ongoing integration process.

In fact, many therapists who have described childhood integration view the process as more simple, natural, and developmentally driven than adult integration. Albini & Pease (1989), in discussion of treatment of young latency children, suggest that it is preferable to "allow the natural, more gradual establishment of cohesion to unfold" (p. 149) rather than using hypnotic or other intrusive techniques. Peterson (Chapter 1, this volume) as well as Silberg (Chapter 3, this volume) have described that dissociative children's "voices" will often spontaneously disappear even after an initial interview. LaPorta (1992) describes a case of a child who spontaneously reports "We are now one" from under a blanket in a play therapy session.

Other therapists report more focussed fusion rituals to promote childhood integration, but these are reported to be easier, quicker, and less complex than with adult dissociative treatment. Fagan & McMahon (1984) describe an imagery-building technique in which the child is asked to imagine the personality states "hugging" until they are joined. Initial followup after integration of these cases of "incipient multiple personality disorder" suggested that the integrations held, and there was impressive symptom reduction. Kluft (1985) described the use of hypnotherapy techniques to promote fusion, utilizing images crafted from the child's interest or experiences (e.g. "star trek images") and determined that the children achieved integration rapidly, and that dissociated parts at times requested to "join" the others. Followup on some of these cases suggested that these fusions held (Kluft, 1985; 1990).

In addition to the shortened time involved to achieve fusion of personalities and eventual integration, integration-focussed therapy for dissociative children has other differences from the therapeutic approach with adults. Play therapy with dissociative children relies on many concrete ways of demonstrating the ideas of integration and unification, and this fantasy play is a primary vehicle for experiencing integration. Concrete play rituals to promote the process of integration have also been described by McMahon and Fagan (1993) and Shirar (1996).

This chapter describes specific fusion rituals and techniques that promote integration that the authors have found useful in treating over 50 dissociative children and adolescents. Techniques for working with DDNOS and DID will not be distinguished, as the process is similar whether the parts are more differentiated and autonomous as in DID, or more passively experienced as in DDNOS. The authors' experience suggests that unification of the personality is often a natural development at the latter stages of treatment, but that some children may report spontaneous fusions throughout the course of treatment. Length of time to achieve full unification will vary depending on the severity of the initial trauma, the consistency and availability of appropriate parenting, and the child's cognitive and emotional strengths. The authors acknowledge the creative input of other authors (Fagan & McMahon, 1984; Kluft, 1985; McMahon & Fagan, 1993; Shirar, 1996) but seek to expand the developing literature on childhood integration by describing some new techniques, by emphasizing a variety of modalities for promoting integration experiences, and by highlighting the use of the family to enhance the integration process.

The Importance of Integration

The authors believe that the fusion and eventual integration of all of the dissociative child's split-off parts is crucial to assisting the child to learn in school, to engage in appropriate behaviors, to develop his/her capabilities, and to form meaningful and lasting relationships. As long as fragmentation exists, the dissociative patient relies more on his or her disso-ciative defenses, and this coping style becomes increasingly more in-grained. As the literature on adult dissociative disorders expands, the overwhelming morbidity of this disorder in adulthood becomes clearer, making even stronger the imperative to strive for total integration in childhood cases.

In our experience, most children do not resist the concept of eventual unity of the personality, especially if the concept of "togetherness" has been emphasized throughout the therapy. This is consistent with the ob-servations of other therapists (Kluft, 1984; Laporta, 1992; Shirar, 1996) who report that children have an almost instinctive awareness of what the natural course of therapy will be. Before adolescence, children appear to have less investment in the separateness of the parts. The following essay written by a 10-year-old describes her perception of the positive po-tential of integration.

> A inside part is like a friend. They are helpful sometimes. Sometimes they distract you or do wrong things. Sometimes in life they join into one, but they will always be here. There can be little ones and big ones. They come in all different ages. Some are playful, some are not. It's very surprising to know you have an inside part, but it's perfectly fine to have an inside part. When you get hurt, they will make you feel better. Some are very creative. Some are humorous. Inside parts have feelings too. They are all good at different things. They have different preferences. I was very startled when I found out I had inside parts. There is a so-called MPD. If you go to a therapist it won't be so seri-ous. One day they will all come together and they won't be separated.
> —Melissa, age 10

Most children who have been diagnosed with a dissociative disorder and educated about it will readily accept the idea that "all parts" will one day be so "close that it will be difficult to tell them apart." In early stages of treatment, children are not required to understand clearly how this might be so, and lengthy discussions about it may serve to frighten the child or other alter states. If children seem to express a high degree of anxiety about this potential process, the therapeutic stance is a "let's wait and see" approach (Kluft, 1993) assuring them that the therapist will never impose anything on them which is against their will or the will of the other parts. (Although forced integrations have been described for adults [Putnam, 1989], they are clearly not advocated for children.)

With adolescents, the idea of eventual integration may be much more frightening. Dell and Eisenhower (1990) and Kluft and Schultz (1993) have expressed similar observations about adolescent patients who may have become more invested in the separateness of the personalities and more reliant on this defensive style. Our adolescent patients have expressed fear of "being lonely" without the accustomed friendly chatter in their mind or fearing that integration may be a kind of "death. " With adolescents, the emphasis is always on the patient's own potential for decision-making about this and on respect for the patient's pace and choice in the process. As adolescents may never be completely open about their internal experience, the therapist really has no choice but to be a "coach on the sidelines" respecting the adolescent's own decision-making about how and when integration may occur.

Other adolescents may have unrealistic notions that integration may produce magical alleviation of symptoms, reduction in learning disabilities, or an improved social life. These notions need to be dispelled, so that the teenager does not try to prematurely squelch the legitimate expression of all of his/her dissociated self-aspects.

Integration is equally important for the child with dissociative disorder not otherwise specified (DDNOS) who may have internal personality fragments or ego states. Our observation is that these children do not make continued and consistent progress in symptom reduction until their fragmented personalities or ego states have become integrated into the child's personality. Regardless of the severity of the dissociation and the degree of splitting of the child's personality, eventual integration is required.

When is the Patient Ready for Integration?

Integration is not a discrete point in time but a gradual process, even more so with children than with adults. Work on integration actually begins at the early stages of treatment when alters are identified and respected, and when the importance of the role of each internal part has been recognized. Throughout the therapeutic process, metaphors about unity, team cooperation, and joint ventures are stressed in play activities and therapeutic conversations which continue to build momentum towards the goal of final integration. Kluft (1993) has identified several "pathways" to integration in adults—some fostered by therapist intervention (fusion rituals, blending interventions) and some initiated by the patients spontaneously after processing traumatic memories or other internal reconfigurations. The integration pathways for children are similar but may more often be initiated by the child naturally as the child develops in therapy. Although some children may be receptive to planned fusion rituals, particularly if they have heard about these experiences from a dissociative parent, many report more spontaneous blendings and fusions which occur outside of therapy. Sometimes dramatic spontaneous fusions have occurred with DDNOS and DID children during early sessions, just through recognizing and reframing alter presences, as has been reported by Kluft (1985).

Formal fusion ceremonies are most appropriate during the latter stages of treatment when the traumatic materials contained by the alters have been adequately processed, the alters' original purpose is no longer needed, and their roles have been redefined and focussed towards joint problem solving. However, Shirar (1996) reported that she agreed to conduct a fusion ritual early in the treatment for a young adolescent boy and then deal with the continuing emotional conflict in treatment after integration. Kluft (1993) also reports some variations in timing among different patients who may prefer to have fusions facilitated earlier, while continuing to work on the overall personality integration in the course of treatment.

If a formal fusion ritual is tried, and there is a failure in a dissociative child's attempt to unify the personalities, the therapist needs to explore with the child several possibilities that may be impeding integration. Is the child currently being abused? Are there stresses in the child's environment for which the child continues to rely on his/her dissociative defense mechanisms (e.g. testifying in court, placement changes, school transfers, or new memories)? Is there a hidden alter who is causing a sudden change in behavior resulting in serious, destructive actions? These issues will be detailed under the heading "Relapse" later in this chapter.

Integration Techniques: From the Abstract to the Concrete

Metaphors and Imagery

Initially, ideas about integration and what it may mean are illustrated to the child through metaphors that relate to his/her own experience. Selecting a metaphor or a symbol that pertains to the child's interests will increase the likelihood of the child understanding the significance and meaning of integration.

There are many everyday activities and experiences with which children are familiar that can be used to explain to a child the relationship of parts to a whole. Sport teams supply an excellent metaphor for "parts working together" to accomplish a goal. One DID child, Donna, who loved soccer, displayed a temporary regression when a younger alter wanted to do Donna's homework on her own, resulting in many mistakes. Donna was told that this was like letting her younger sister play soccer for her. Through this analogy, Donna's younger alter understood that she needed to allow Donna to do her homework, but she could learn about school work by internally watching and listening. When Donna was in the stage of unification, she drew a beautiful, full-size picture of herself playing soccer on the field and successfully hitting the soccer ball, symbolizing her integration (see Figure 1).

One child who had an obsession with television news shows was told that his dissociative system was like Channel 7—someone does the re-

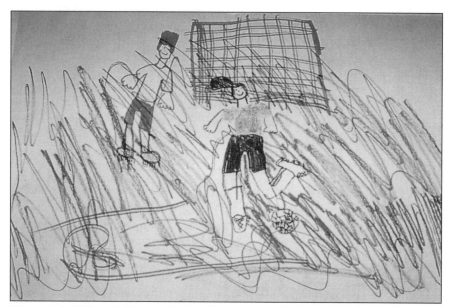

Figure 1. A child symbolizes her feeling of integration with the metaphor of playing soccer successfully.

search, someone edits, and someone presents the news on camera. All members of the news room are required for a successful news program, even though we don't see all of them on camera. This gave the alters who were not "out" a feeling of confidence and importance and helped them appreciate their input even when it was more covert. For this patient a metaphor for moments of integration was "being on the air." The part-to-whole relationships in desserts, where various ingredients come together to make a final whole, is a particularly powerful way to describe the concept of personality integration. Children are well aware that the final product—a delicious cookie or cake—is much better than each part alone, and this point is stressed when discussing integration. This metaphor was used with a patient who picked pumpkin pie as her favorite dessert. References were made frequently to her and her inside family coming together as "one delicious pumpkin pie." After one particularly resistant but significant alter, Lucy, decided to join with the others, the child reported enthusiastically that "Lucy was the pumpkin added to the pie, and the pumpkin pie tasted scrumptious!"

Shirar (1996) describes a child's poignant analogy that her traumatic splitting was like a "tree stump," in which all of its branches have been cut off. As healing progressed, this patient was able to visualize the tree being "grafted" back together.

As demonstrated by the above examples, once the child has become familiar with a metaphor used throughout therapy, that metaphor can be utilized in visualization exercises that symbolically represent a "coming together. " Exercises involving the visualization of images associated with unity are standard work with adults (Kluft, 1993) and are also useful with children. Shirar (1996) describes having the child pick an imaginary place, such as a beach or meadow, for two parts to fuse together, and then describes the parts joining "from the feet up to the head and from the tummy all the way to the backbone."

Kluft (1985) describes the use of imagery for childhood fusion rituals taken from television science fiction: "beaming up" as seen on *Star Trek* helped several children visualize the internal experience of alters coming together. Images of two parts "dancing together" or "hugging" have also been described by Fagan and McMahon (1984).

In our visualization work with children, we have generally not found it necessary to use formal hypnosis. Children often enter spontaneous trance, and play itself has been seen as a form of trance (Donovan & McIntyre, 1990). Children's visual imagination is often superior to that of adults and they seem not to require the formal elements of trance induction in order to visualize successfully. In addition, the issue of informed consent is trickier with children, as it is not clear that they have a complete understanding of what they are consenting to. Children may have distorted ideas about what hypnosis is and fear a loss of control. Similarly, parents who have heard news media reports about "false memories" may have undue fears of formal hypnosis and it may add an unnecessary element of confusion into the therapist-parent alliance. In addition, children may be asked to testify in court regarding abuse, and some state guidelines prevent information obtained after hypnosis to be used in court testimony. These cautions aside, hypnosis can be a powerful technique for fusion rituals with children as described by Kluft (1986), as long as therapists are aware of the risks and legal consequences in each particular case. If hypnosis is employed, the therapist needs to explain the purpose of hypnosis and dispel any myths the patient or parents may believe. An informed consent signed by the parent or legal guardian is recommended.

However, hypnosis, formal visualization exercises, and metaphors are only part of the necessary tools to facilitate personality integration for childhood dissociative disorders. In our work with dissociative children and adolescents we have found it most useful to incorporate a variety of techniques that provide concrete dramatization of the concepts of integration along with formalized play rituals to encourage specific fusions. These concrete activities are helpful for many reasons. Children are often not capable of the abstract thinking which would allow them to conceptualize what integration may be from verbal conversations and explanations alone. Learning specialists know that children's learning is enhanced though multisensory experience (see Chapter 15) and concretized integration techniques facilitate this multisensory learning by providing visual, verbal, motor, sensory, proprioceptive, or even olfactory and gustatory input. In addition, as Donovan & McIntyre (1990) have pointed out, children believe in "magic," that is, the powerful effect that concrete rituals can have in changing their experience of the world. Thus, children may readily buy into the "magical" ritual elements in a fusion intervention. Finally, these concrete experiences are fun for children and may be perceived as a form of constructive play in which important new challenges are mastered. As Piaget (1951) has pointed out, "play" is in fact the "work" of childhood, and thus it is often in play that new, important, growth-enhancing experiences take place. We will explore various sensory modalities to describe how concrete activities involving sensory experiences can be structured to enhance feelings of unity and cohesion in dissociative children.

Sensory Modalities

Visual Art. Art is a powerful modality for children and, as stated by Sobol, "Images developed and changed through art-making may alter or amend internal imagery" (see Chapter 10). A picture, diorama, or collage made by the child can be used to depict the ongoing process of integration or can be incorporated into a fusion ritual. It is important that the child and alters equally participate, negotiate, and agree on the symbols, colors, designs, etc. to be used in the visual art. A session can be devoted to talking about symbols with the child and his/her alters, and their significance to the child's healing and integration. What the child says about the visual art can then be used in an integration story: "This is a picture of how you look when you are whole. The buttons are for eyes that let all of you see the good in the world, the cotton, for the soft feeling of love all of you share . . . etc." The creation of the art may be trance-inducing, and the therapist's storytelling tone similarly helps the patient achieve a feeling of concentrated relaxation and focus that heightens the experience. The concrete experience of creating the picture imbues the fusion ritual with a kind of "magic" which allows the child to believe that he/she can construct an "inner whole self" as well as the external art creation.

Jane, an 8-year-old DID girl, used a picture she created of "the love lines" connecting her and her alters to finalize a fusion with her alters. While she drew this picture, a discussion occurred about Jane's and her alters' individual strengths being combined, reinforced, and connected through the "love line. " It was stressed that the "love line" will help them come together as one, experiencing life simultaneously, playing, learning, and loving her adopted family.

Pam, a DDNOS teenager with three ego states, drew a picture of a kite to represent her growth and integration. Each ego state picked a favorite color and design to put on the kite. One of her ego states, Lisa, had pulled off the petals of daisies and played the game of "He loves me, he loves me

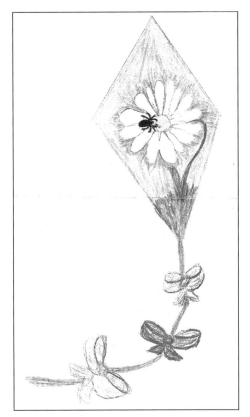

Figure 2. This picture of a kite was drawn by a teenager with DDNOS to symbolize integration.

not," when questioning the love of her father who abused her. Pam drew a large daisy with all of the petals intact on the center of the kite, symbolizing the resolution of that conflict, with a spider symbolizing the ongoing need for protection. Integration occurred as Pam looked at her picture, while F. W. told an integration story about Pam and her parts joining together and soaring high, like the kite, free of abuse and fear (see Figure 2).

Several patients have chosen the image of a rainbow to represent integration experiences and have drawn rainbows with their alters' favorite colors. As children experiment with mixing paint colors during play therapy, the idea of colors blending together can be used to describe how parts are not lost but transformed by the process of integration. A ceremonious mixing of paint colors can then be used in a fusion ritual (Marcia Waterbury, personal communication).

Another interesting visual tool developed by F. W. is creation of a crossword puzzle with the names of the child and the alters connected. The child can add the alter's qualities to the puzzle or put the qualities in a separate crossword puzzle. These qualities, such as strong, kind, musical, artistic, are included in a mutual storytelling by the therapist and child after the crossword puzzle is created, to describe how they will feel when interconnected into one like the crossword puzzle.

Dr. Priscilla Cogan, a therapist in Maryland, has described her use of a picture puzzle to help explain, encourage, and symbolize integration (personal communication). She sent a photograph of a patient to a company that will make a puzzle with the child's face on it. As the therapist and patient worked together in therapy, the pieces of the picture puzzle of the child's face were slowly pieced together. The author J. S. has used makeshift puzzles, paper drawings with pictures of the child on them, that have been cut apart. As new feelings, or memories are shared, the child ceremoniously begins to tape the pieces of paper back together.

Tactile Experience. Clay and sand tray provide tactile experiences for a child in which the child can touch, create, or form objects with his/her hands to symbolize the blending of feelings or attainment of wholeness. The child and the alters might be asked to each pick their favorite color of clay which has special meaning for each of them and to form it into a ball symbolic of unification. This can be done in the early part of therapy to help symbolize what might be accomplished as therapy progresses. Later, if a fusion ritual is needed to help cement the integration process, the child can be asked to mix the clay more thoroughly, while the therapist discusses the strengths of the various parts of the self contributing to the whole child. The child is permitted to take the ball home to keep as a reminder of the personality unification.

If the sand tray has been used in the early stages of treatment, as explained by Sachs (1993), then it will feel natural to use the sand tray to demonstrate continuing integration as well. The child can arrange objects and figures depicting his/her personality system coming together and move them ceremoniously closer in the sand tray from week to week in therapy. To turn this technique into a more formalized fusion ritual, the child and therapist can tell a story together about the significance of each character and its role in promoting the total well-being of the whole child.

Auditory and Language Techniques. Children are fascinated and intrigued by the sound of their own voice on tape. For dissociative children whose identity is fragmented and confused, it is as if this concrete auditory feedback provides external confirmation of their identity. The tape recorder can be used in many ways to facilitate the child's ongoing appreciation of the integrating aspects of the self. The author J. S. will frequently have children write play scripts, recounting past events, reflecting internal dialogue between the parts, or depicting wished-for reconciliations between parents or siblings from whom they are separated. As the play scripts develop, the therapist can move the play in the direction of personality unity and recovery, so that the play has a healing effect. These plays can then be recorded on a tape recorder, with different voices if desired, and the final tape of this play can become an important object symbolizing the completion of therapeutic work. For one child, a play about the aftermath of her father's murder of her mother (which she had witnessed) eventually contained themes of anger resolution, forgiveness, and faith. Listening to this tape allowed her to deal with the conflicting emotions of this tragedy and provide some soothing. Therapists and patients can develop stories together which can be taped and then played at home for the child to facilitate work on continuing integration. Sometimes spontaneous fusion is reported after children have listened to these tapes.

Some dissociative children are particularly gifted in music or poetry and have created songs or poems about the process of integration which can be utilized as part of a fusion ritual. The following poem was written by a teenage patient during a fusion ritual when a particularly religious alter fused with other personalities.

> You have a bright light of God within you.
> I will be there with you in your prayers.
> Love, H.

Other sensory modalities. Children love the sensation of passive movement, on rides, bicycles, or playground equipment, which seems to have trance-inducing qualities. Author J. S. utilized a child's proprioceptive sensory awareness to enhance integration during outdoor play. While the child was on the inpatient hospital's playground merry-go-round and asking to be spun "faster and faster," integrating messages were conveyed: "As you spin, the walls between the feelings will melt away and get blended more and more together." As work progressed, repeated playground excursions to the merry-go round were used to help cement therapeutic gains and reinforce the messages about unity.

The experience of eating a delicious dessert, shared with special family members and the therapist at an "integration party," can serve as a unifying fusion experience, especially if the metaphor of a delicious dessert, as presented earlier, has been used to illustrate unification throughout the therapy. In this case even gustatory and olfactory sensation can be utilized to heighten the sensory experiences which symbolize personality integration.

Creative Play and Toy Symbols

The play therapy itself in which dolls, puppets, or other toys are utilized in therapeutic creative play can serve as the medium for integration work. Techniques that use concrete doll symbols to represent split off parts during play therapy have been described by Gil (1991), McMahon and Fagan (1993), and Shirar (1996). McMahon and Fagan (1993) describe using a doll to represent the "new" child; the different elements of the child can give symbolic gifts to represent their continuing characteristics. The therapist can have the child enact joining the elements into each other with a play hugging of the dolls.

Throughout the various stages of treatment puppets can be employed to demonstrate "inside families" and trauma issues. The puppets can be one step ahead of the child in order to guide the child through the treatment process. In the integration phase, the puppet will tell the child his/her feelings and thoughts about unification and improvement as integration has progressed. When the child is ready for personality unification, the child's favorite puppet can talk and cheer them during and after a fusion ritual. One particularly useful marionette puppet, Dudley, frequently struggles with tangled strings, a useful metaphor for the child of "parts not working well together."

Toy symbols can be helpful to children in understanding cooperation, co-consciousness, and eventual integration. One particularly useful toy is a wind up caterpillar that sits on author F. W.'s desk. This caterpillar's body has joints connecting the four separate body parts with wheels that move it (see Figure 3). The caterpillar's parts are compared to the child's alters, fragments, or feeling states. When the child is having conflicts with the alters, one or more of the body joints of the caterpillar will be turned upside down, which inhibits it from moving. The immobilized caterpillar is compared to the impaired child who is experiencing internal conflicts with alters or external conflicts with family. It is explained to the child that when a caterpillar grows, it becomes a beautiful butterfly, just as when the child grows and the personality integrates, he/she will become a healthy man or woman who will be able to utilize all of his/her strengths and skills. The child may be given one of the caterpillars to safeguard and protect, and a fusion ritual may involve creation of a butterfly.

Sometimes toy symbols can be created by the child with clay or other medium. These toy symbols, when combined with creative play experiences, may be particularly powerful in encouraging integration episodes. F. W. has used clay figurines created by the child to help age progress and eventually facilitate the integration of split-off "baby parts" in several adopted children. These children, who were between the ages of 3 and 9 years old, had documented abuse histories predating their adoption and exhibited many infantile symptoms, such as sucking their thumb, baby talk, spitting food, walking on toes, and wetting. It was surmised that their problematic, regressed behaviors were associated with preverbal trauma which impaired their ability to attach to their adoptive parents.

Each child was asked to make the "baby part" of herself out of clay while the therapist made a rocking chair and "a mom" out of clay. The

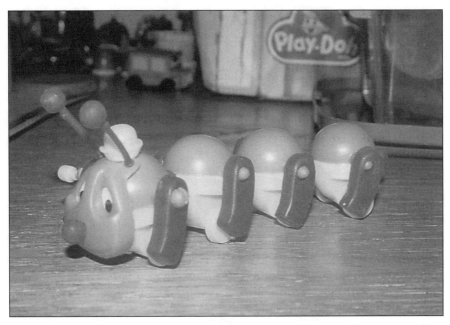

Figure 3. A therapist can utilize toys such as this caterpillar to symbolize parts working together.

child was asked to identify the clay mom as either her biological mother, adoptive mother, or simply a mom. In this first stage, each of the adopted children identified the clay mom as her biological mother. Then, the child was instructed to place the clay baby figure in the arms of the clay mom figure which was sitting in the clay rocking chair, and rock the sculpture in her hand as she sat in the office rocking chair (see Figure 4). It was explained how, when she was a baby, she had been hurt and was unable to be comforted by her mom, who was perhaps unaware of the abuse, or abused herself and prevented from protecting her daughter. The child was asked to pretend that the clay mother was providing the comfort that the baby needed through rocking. The child was asked to count slowly from the "baby" age to the child's age as the baby part was rocked so that it could grow up to the child's current age. The therapist participated in counting as the child rocked the sculpture in her hand. The child was instructed to carefully take the clay sculpture home and rock it daily to continue to help the "baby part" grow through this comforting process.

In the subsequent sessions in which the instructions were repeated, each of the children reported that the infant part had age progressed to an older age and then to the child's current age. After the initial session in which the children were able to process their grief and loss over their biological mothers, the adoptive children consistently chose their adoptive mother to be represented by the clay mother. This reinforces Bowlby

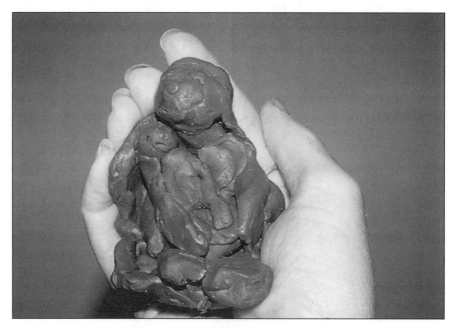

Figure 4. Clay figurines are used in an age progression technique.

(1980) and James (1994), who describe children who have been separated from their primary caregivers and need to resolve feelings of loss, abandonment, and grief. Once these children in treatment were given an opportunity to process the loss and grief regarding their biological mothers, they were ready to attach to their adoptive parents.

In the final steps, the clay technique was used in a formal fusion ritual as the therapist suggested that through rocking and loving the symbolic clay sculpture, the age-appropriate part could become one with the child and their good qualities would be shared.

This symbolic clay technique highlights several important implications for working with children who may have had early abuse, a dissociated infant, separation/loss issues with primary parents, and attachment problems with adoptive parents. Significantly, after the initial session of rocking the infant part, the infantile symptoms ceased without the need to retrieve the specific early memories. When the infant part resolved the loss of her biological mother, that part was able to age progress, which paved the way for the child to integrate and attach to her adoptive parents. Because the children took their clay sculptures home, parents and siblings became involved in the healing process by enthusiastically participating in rocking the sculpture. This technique highlights the importance of family involvement in integration techniques which will be emphasized in the next section.

Family Involvement in Integration and Fusion Rituals

As illuminated above, in many of the techniques, we view family involvement in the therapeutic process as a key to solidifying integration with
children. One of the primary ways in which working with dissociative
children differs from work with adults is the opportunity to resolve and
intervene in promoting appropriate attachment experiences. Although
the therapist for an adult patient is an important attachment figure, the
therapist can never truly re-parent or make up for the profound loss of
consistent nurturing of which these children were deprived. However,
with dissociative children, the optimum goal is to help them develop an
appropriate attachment to a consistent, caring parental figure in their life
who can accept and attach to all of the split-off aspects of the child. Many
child DID patients initially come into therapy reporting that one or more
of their alters do not have a mother, or have a different mother than the
identified caregiver. Although the child may be able to cooperate and
share feelings among the parts, successful personality integration will be
impeded unless all of the parts recognize and accept the same parental
attachment figure. Both authors have used adoption ceremonies for alters
as an important fusion ritual.

One DDNOS child, Nikki, had been adopted at age 6 by an aunt from
another city whom she had rarely seen before the adoption. Her birth parents, both substance abusers, had abandoned Nikki at a homeless shelter
at age 5. On occasion, 10-year-old Nikki would spend therapy sessions
looking through the phone book to try to locate her birth parents, with
whom her aunt had lost contact. This behavior was in marked contrast to
her playful engagement and positive attachment to her aunt at other
times. We identified this obsessive phone book reader as a part of Nikki
whom we named "the Nikki not attached" to Aunt Rose, and planned an
adoption ceremony for her. A chair was prepared for "the Nikki not attached" and a doll was chosen to represent this aspect of Nikki. Aunt Rose
ceremoniously talked to the symbolic doll and described how she had first
heard about Nikki's birth, the occasions when she had seen her as a baby,
and how she had made preparations to adopt her. After this session was
over, Nikki stated "The Great Wall of China just fell down," and the obsessive reading of phone books stopped. "The Nikki not attached" had integrated and attached to her aunt.

In another dramatic fusion ritual involving a parent, an aggressive alter who had denied that the patient's mother was her own asked to be
joined with the host personality during a family therapy session. The
mother had used the session for a tearful apology about not knowing
about the "bad people" in the neighbor's house where the child had been
abused. This apology allowed the alter to feel forgiveness and sympathy
and she stated, "I am not needed now. " A visualization involving the

metaphor of water flowing together was used with this older adolescent while her mother held her hands.

Even when not directly included in the therapy sessions during fusion rituals, parents can be involved in celebrating integration by listening with the child to taped stories or poems about the integration. Preceding fusion rituals, parents can be involved in writing letters to the child and the alters about their recovery, or giving special "thank you cards" to "adult" parts that helped the child during traumatic times. Shirar (1996) describes allowing the parent to have a session for a final goodbye to an alter before integration. Parents can be instructed to celebrate unification with the child by baking together, especially desserts, which have been used as metaphors for integration, or working together on special craft projects that have been linked to the child's attainment of unification. Families may work together on special picture albums or scrapbooks that help unify the child's memory into a coherent narrative and provide a unifying record of the child's complete history. All of these family techniques help to provide some insurance against re-fragmentation as the child has the opportunity to process important feelings towards the primary attachment figures and attach to them in their new reconfigured state.

The Assessment of Integration in Dissociative Children

The assessment of whether successful fusions have occurred may be tricky in children who falsely report that spontaneous fusion of personalitites has occurred to please the therapist, to interrupt the treatment process, or to have time to engage in activities that are more "fun." Children may go through periods of distrust of the therapist and transference issues can arise, particularly when the child is confronted with his/her aggressive or destructive behaviors. Children may blame therapist, parents, or others, or minimize the seriousness of such behavior, and contend that "everyone was out and together as one," hoping that the therapy will end soon. These are tedious sessions for the therapist who does not want to become enmeshed in the power struggle or allow countertransference issues to interfere in processing conflicting issues with the child. During these times, it is best not to argue with the child as to whether personality integration has occurred successfully, but to provide support and understanding about the time and pain involved in recovery. Shifting the focus of discussion temporarily from the aggressive episode to a time when the child responded appropriately may encourage the child to be reengaged in the therapeutic process.

Kluft (1993) has presented six research-based characteristics of adult patients with stable fusions, which include memory continuity, no behavioral signs of MPD, the report of subjective unity, an absence of alters, modifications of transference, and clinical evidence of unity. Although no research on the characteristics of children in the post-unification phase is available, our experience suggests that Kluft's list of characteristics may be equally applicable to children. However, the assessment of these characteristics differs in children, as these assessments are more reliant on multiple adult observations and give less credence to subjective expressions of the child unless particularly clear and striking. Hypnosis to elicit alters is not generally used to test for continued alter presences in our work with children. Instead the therapist may ask for alters directly. The child who has achieved a successful fusion will seem perplexed by this and may reiterate that they are all "one" with her. Sometimes, the alter will seem to reappear and state that she is the spokesperson, but "we are all together." In this case, the "alter" appearance will not be accompanied by noticeable changes in voice, facial expression, or body language.

The following list of methods to assess whether stable fusions and ongoing integration have occurred in children and adolescents may provide a structured guide for families and therapists. It is hoped that future research can assess whether these preliminary guidelines continue to be useful as clinicians from various settings gain increased experience with children in the post-unification phase of treatment. These guidelines might also be useful for determining the efficacy of treatment, the continued maintenance of unification, and the child's adjustment after post-unification therapy has been provided. Many of the manifestations of integration listed below would not necessarily be achieved at the moment after a fusion experience, but during the post-unification phase when continued therapy has been provided to teach coping skills and ongoing resolution of developmental issues.

Guidelines for Assessing Childhood Integration

1. *The child's subjective report of a unified self, and accompanied sensory changes.* Adult reports of subjective unification may be much more reliable than children's reports. Children may engage in many playful tactics to fool the therapist if they are tired of therapy or want to avoid responsibility for inappropriate behavior. Nevertheless, self-report of unity by the child is one assessment criterion, particularly if the child is articulate and specific about the changes he/she has experienced. Children have described sensory changes after final fusions in which their hearing, sight, touch, taste, and smell are clearer and more distinct, much like what has been reported in the adult literature (Kluft, 1988). Children may say that colors are more distinct and vision is clearer. One integrated 9-year-old DID girl articulately described how much easier it was for her to ride her horse, as she sensed that the horse felt less confused by mixed messages and was more responsive to her direction. This girl described the sensory

changes in her inner world when she had finally integrated as follows:

> "I don't blank out a lot because I don't need to do that anymore. I have a new home . . . It's like you're in a new world. I used to be all black. My eyes would be cloudy. My mom and dad would sense that something's wrong. But now it's like you're in a new world and you aren't cloudy. You're really happy and you laugh and play a lot. It's like you're in a new world!"

2. *Observed changes in physical characteristics.* Author F. W. has observed dramatic physical changes in children following fusion including facial, body posture, and gait changes. The face may appear more relaxed, and most notably, the eyes appear brighter, softer, and more open. Circles under the eyes may not be as dark or may disappear. The child's complexion may have more color and the forehead may appear smooth without lines between the brows. The body posture may be more erect and the head is held straighter. The child may have a spring in his/her gait. The child's voice may develop a more musical lilt. These physical changes of voice, facial appearance, and body movement remain without the variations noted prior to the fusion.

3. *Observed affective changes.* The parents may notice a more cheerful disposition and see that the child smiles more readily and easily and can demonstrate humor. When conflicts or obstacles occur the child has a more optimistic approach to solving them. The child shows more resiliency and can return to a playful state soon after the conflict. There are unhappy feelings, but they do not seem to dominate the child's entire day or have the intensity that they had before. Moods are more constant, consistent, and predictable. There seems to be a significant shift from a sense of hopelessness and despair to a sense of hope for the future. The child anticipates activities, discusses future plans, and conveys optimism.

4. *Observed and measured cognitive changes.* McMahon and Fagan (1984) reported a 14-point improvement in IQ for one child following fusion. Similarly, we have observed the child's cognitive processes have become more organized, clearer, and logical. Cognitive deficits to some degree may continue as the child struggles with processing current events, relationship issues, and situational conflicts. However, the presence of the victim/persecutor attitude which previously dominated many of the children's thinking about life situations, relationships, and their future is less pervasive.

    Most notably, the child's attention span increases, improving the child's responsiveness to the teacher and leading to more appropriate behavior in the classroom. The child may not be as easily frustrated when he/she cannot accomplish an assignment and may show more consistency in learning, completing homework, and on test performance.

5. *Observed changes in family relationships.* The trust and attachment issues continue to be difficult for the child, but there are positive signs that the child is forming more meaningful family relationships, particularly in adoptive homes, with less frequent episodes of testing. The child may be more willing to participate in family activities and may be more willing and able to complete chores.

6. *Observed improved peer relationships.* The child is able to form meaningful relationships and maintain them for 6 months or longer. He/she may begin to receive invitations from school friends to attend birthday parties. He/she may be included in playground activities, be better able to share with peers, negotiate over activities, and not bully or intimidate if he/she does not get his/her way.

7. *Behavioral improvement in a wide variety of settings.* The child's impulse control appears to improve across a variety of settings. The parents feel more comfortable about exposing the child to new unfamiliar people and places. The child may display more sensitivity to others and respect for property.

8. *Increased interest in hobbies, special projects, age-appropriate pursuits.* The child may show an interest in extracurricular activities offered through the school or community, and begins to participate in sports, learning a musical instrument, drama, dance, skating, hiking, etc. Friendships are made through these activities, and anticipation and enthusiasm are expressed.

9. *Observed decrease in memory lapses and fluctuating behavior.* The child who has achieved a state of personality integration no longer appears perplexed about events that family and friends recall. Preference in clothing, food, activities, music, etc. , may change with the child's development, but do not change from moment to moment.

10. *Observed changes in therapeutic transference.* The child no longer appears to fluctuate dramatically in relationship to the therapist. There is less testing, sporadic aggressiveness, and resistance.

Many of these guidelines do not reflect a qualitative level of change, as assessment must include sensitivity to gradations in improvement during the ongoing process of integration. The child's continued improvement after the final fusions may involve sporadic variations in functioning, as temporary splitting during new life crises may occur in the post-unification phase. However, the variations are relatively mild and brief in duration and not so intense as to impair the child's overall adjustment at school, home, or in the community. If the child temporarily "splits off," he/she is able to reunite within a short period of time. This transient splitting after integration is generally not rooted in unresolved past trauma issues but due to a current environmental stressor or activity, such as going to a school function or extracurricular activity. One integrated 8-year-old girl had momentarily dissociated when her younger alter wanted to be the only one out to skate at a recital. The parent indicated that this younger alter separated for part of the performance and then rejoined the child. The subtle manifestations of this temporary occurrence were noticeable only to the parents and later confirmed by the child's report.

Post-fusion Relapses

Relapses differ from the transient and momentary appearance of alters described above. When the child "splits off" and an alter personality appears for hours or days at a time, resulting in developmentally inappropriate behavior, embarrassment, and confusion, it may be considered a relapse. Kluft (1988, 1984, 1986) indicates that the majority of unified patients will experience one or more relapses, and a certain percentage of patients will continue to have such events over time until the full domain of their multiplicity has been explored and resolved.

Significant relapses have occurred with F. W. 's dissociative children when the following conditions occurred.

1. *New memories surfaced* as a result of a trigger to past, unknown trauma.

   This new memory brought unexpected intense feelings of pain and fear, and the child relied on her previous response of dissociation to deal with these feelings. Even though strategies had been discussed to deal with such occurrences, the sudden memory and associated feelings were too overwhelming for the child to manage. The splintering of the personality may be resolved once the child is able to communicate what occurred, process it, and receive the necessary support, reassurance, and psychological protection. Reintegration with F. W.'s cases occurred rapidly once the trauma was processed.

2. *Emergence of a hidden alter* unknown to the child or the other alters that was not ready to reveal itself at an earlier time. In one of F. W.'s cases, a DID 10-year-old boy had an 18-year-old hidden alter who emerged and chased the neighborhood children with a knife. Once he was able to process his memories of sexual abuse, this alter readily joined with the child and the other fused parts.

3. *Incomplete processing of a traumatic memory* may also result in a relapse. Children may become restless with therapy or want to avoid painful memories. Although the therapist may use creative techniques to make the processing of the trauma interesting or "fun," some alters may not be ready to deal with the feelings. They may ap-

pear to be engaged in the therapeutic exercises, but only to please the therapist, parents, or other alters. Once it is apparent that integration of those alters did not occur, the therapist must review with them the short-term and long-term benefits of working through the materials and ask the other integrated parts to share with those alters how much better they have felt and the rewards they have received as a result of resolving the trauma. Brief periods of therapy breaks and negotiations for desirable activities after processing the material are techniques which may be helpful.

4. *Repeated abuse or maltreatment* may result in relapse. Therapists need to be aware of the family environment and assess the parents' ability to deal with stress, and use appropriate child management techniques. (Please refer to Chapter 13.) When there is an emergence of a new alter or a former alter, the therapist needs to inquire with the child if she has been revictimized. Referral to child protection services and intervention to stabilize and make the environment safe is necessary before the dissociative mechanism can be removed.

5. *Major environmental stressors*, such as divorce, death of a significant other, change in placement, or court appearances can cause relapse. These types of changes, particularly if they are sudden and the child does not have time to prepare for them, can cause the child to feel extremely vulnerable and overwhelmed. A previous alter who dealt with similar past changes may reappear. Once the child has the opportunity to accept changes and grieve losses in individual and family therapy sessions, the alter is more likely to rejoin with the child.

6. *Major developmental stressors*, especially during adolescence, can stimulate relapse. Adolescents normally experience various degrees of periods of anxiety, identity confusion, sexual fears, peer difficulties, and parental discord as they struggle with independence. Sexually abused dissociative children who have successfully achieved personality integration at an earlier age may need to reprocess issues during adolescence. If they continue to reside in a dysfunctional family, they are particularly vulnerable to dissociating again. One 12-year-old girl dissociated anew when she reached her teen years. She continued to reside in a dysfunctional family environment characterized by parental divorce and alcoholism and began to engage in promiscuous behavior, substance abuse, and truancy. With the pressures of adolescence and the instability of her home environment, she was not able to maintain her unified self.

In all cases of relapse, the therapist should try to uncover the underlying reasons for the setback, move to create an environment of increased safety for the patient, or help the patient with the unresolved feelings and thoughts that led to the re-fragmentation.

Post-Unification Phase

As Shirar (1996) warns, parents should not expect that personality unification will be a panacea for all the child's problems. There will be old problems, but expressed in a different way, and there will, no doubt, be new problems. Kluft (1988) discusses the importance of continued therapy for adult patients in the post-unification phase to cope with physical and psychological changes, problematic behaviors, and grieving the lost, idealized past. The therapy at this stage for children involves improving coping skills, improving interpersonal relationships, and preparing for new developmental challenges.

With many of our children who have been adopted, a major focus in this phase continues to be grieving the loss of the primary attachment figures and working on issues of trust and attachment with the adoptive parents. Each developmental milestone stimulates precarious issues of trust and identity anew. For children who remain with their biological parents, these issues are pertinent as well. As children begin to "forgive" their parents for betraying them during the time of their abuse, minor parent-child conflicts can become magnified and issues of basic trust reemerge. Providing family therapy at this stage of treatment is recommended either with the ongoing individual therapist or with an additional therapist.

In addition to issues of grief, attachment, and trust, the post-unification child must deal with developmental issues, particularly sexuality at the onset of puberty. In one case an adolescent girl's pregnancy which occurred after integration set into motion issues of trauma, loss, and abandonment, which were too overwhelming for her to handle while caring for her infant. Her extensive therapy had included thorough discussion of stopping the intergenerational abuse; consequently, she became fearful of abusing her child and released her parental rights. Ongoing followup and "check-ins" with teenagers in the post-unification phase are recommended, as adolescence seems filled with developmental crises that may require therapeutic processing. During the post-unification phase, auxiliary services such as group therapy or art therapy can help maintain gains and increase socialization (see Chapters 10 and 11).

Summary

If the therapy focus is on assisting the child to understand, accept, and treat the dissociated parts with equal importance and respect, personality integration will be a natural and accepted part of the treatment. Spontaneous fusions have been reported with many dissociative children but in some cases more formalized techniques are utilized. Techniques that foster integration for children should include a variety of sensory modalities and utilize concrete metaphors that depict the concept of unification through therapeutic creative play or other child-oriented activities. In any technique that promotes integration, it is important to emphasize to the child what will be gained through unification, rather than what will be lost.

Resistance to unification may imply that some traumatic material has yet to be processed and/or a hidden alter may need to come forward to deal with the trauma. There may be disruptions in the child's environment that interfere in the progression toward integration and maintenance of unification. Exploring with the child and care providers what may be impeding final unification is an important therapeutic task in successfully treating the dissociative child. Continuous involvement of the parents throughout all stages of treatment facilitates the resolution of attachment problems and solidifies the integration process. Post-unification therapy finalizes the treatment of the unified child by completing grief work related to attachment issues with the primary parents who abused them, learning to trust parental figures again, and developing new coping skills.

Dissociative children who have achieved successful integration may have a chance to reclaim their childhood. One teenager described her healing and integration in this untitled poem:

> I come to you now, and bring nothing in my hand.
> I bring myself to you wiped away from anger.
> I come to you today free from abuse and pain.
> I come to you now and give to you my love.
> I come to you this day showing how I changed.
> So, now that I am here empty handed,
>   but with a fulfilled heart,
> Take me under your wings and wrap me in your innocence . . .
> I am now *FREE*.

References

Albini, T. K. , & Pease, T. E. (1989). Normal and pathological dissociations of early childhood. *Dissociation, 2,* 144–150.

Bowlby, J. (1980). *Attachment and loss.* New York: Basic.

Dell, P. F., & Eisenhower, J. W. (1990). Adolescent multiple personality disorder: A preliminary study of eleven cases. *Journal of the American Academy of Child and Adolescent Psychiatry, 29,* 359–366.

Donovan, D. M., & McIntyre, D. (1990). *Healing the hurt child.* New York: Norton.

Fagan J., & McMahon, P. (1984). Incipient multiple personality in children. *Journal of Nervous and Mental Disease, 172,* 26–36.

Gil, E. (1991). *The healing power of play.* New York: Guilford.

James, B. (1994). *Handbook for treatment of attachment-trauma problems in children.* New York: Lexington Books.

Kluft, R. P. (1984). Treatment of multiple personality disorder: A study of 33 cases. *Psychiatric Clinics of North America, 7,* 9–29.

Kluft, R. P. (1985). Hypnotherapy of childhood multiple personality disorder. *American Journal of Clinical Hypnosis, 27,* 201–210.

Kluft, R. P. (1986). Personality unification in multiple personality disorder: A follow-up study. In B. G. Braun (Ed.), *Treatment of multiple personality disorder.* Washington, DC: American Psychiatric Press.

Kluft, R. P. (1988). The postunification treatment of multiple personality disorder: First findings. *American Journal of Psychotherapy, 2,* 212–228.

Kluft, R. P. (1990). Editorial: Thoughts on childhood multiple personality disorder. *Dissociation, 3,* 1–2.

Kluft, R. P. (1993). Clinical approaches to the unification of personalities. In R. P. Kluft & C. G. Fine (Eds.), *Clinical perspectives on multiple personality disorder* (pp. 101–133). Washington, DC: American Psychiatric Press.

Kluft, R. P., & Schultz, R. (1993). Multiple personality disorder in adolescence. In S. C. Feinstein & R. C. Marohn (Eds.), *Adolescent Psychiatry, 19,* pp. 259–279.

LaPorta, L. D. (1992). Childhood trauma and multiple personality disorder: The case of a 9-year-old girl. *Child Abuse & Neglect, 16,* 615–620.

McMahon, P. P., & Fagan, J. (1993). Play therapy with children with multiple personality disorder. In R. P. Kluft & C. G. Fine (Eds.), *Clinical perspectives on multiple personality disorder* (pp. 253–276). Washington, DC: American Psychiatric Press.

Piaget, J. (1962). *Play, dreams, and imitation in childhood.* (C. Gattegno & F. M. Hodgson, trans.). New York: Norton. (originally published in 1951).

Putnam, F. W. (1989). *Diagnosis and treatment of multiple personality disorder.* New York: Guilford Press.

Sachs, R. G. (1993). Use of sand trays in the beginning treatment of a patient with dissociative disorder. In R. P. Kluft & C. G. Fine (Eds.), *Clinical perspectives on multiple personality disorder* (pp. 301–310). Washington, DC: American Psychiatric Press.

Shirar, L. (1996). *Dissociative children: Bridging the inner and outer worlds.* New York: Norton.

t e n

▬

Art as an Adjunctive Therapy in the Treatment of Children Who Dissociate

Barbara Sobol and Karen Schneider

"Only through art can we get outside ourselves and know another's view of the universe which is not the same as ours and see landscapes which would otherwise have remained unknown . . ." —Marcel Proust

This chapter proposes two models of adjunctive art therapy to be used in working with children who dissociate. Both models strongly rely on the use of art as therapy and a full engagement in the art process. One model parallels the work of the primary trauma therapist, following closely the sequential pacing of the work with deepening and enriching use of the art process; the second provides a support structure through a group involvement in the art process, but with less emphasis on closely following the trauma model. Illustrations are given of how each model may work. The building of "environments"—a specific technique that can be used successfully in either model—is described and illustrated.

The Unique Place of Art in Trauma Work

Pynoos and Nader (1993) cite Piaget and Inhelder (1969) as holding that "drawing should be considered as halfway between symbolic play and the mental image" (p. 54). While a child can with ease redo or declare an end to play ("I'm not playing anymore!"), art images once made remain in the tangible world as artifacts. While images on paper are reflections of a child's mental images, they are almost always somewhat different—scarier, prettier, less accurate, or more complex—and in this altered form

We wish to thank Edward Owen for his sensitive photographs of the environments (Figures 9 and 10); Montgomery County, Maryland, Child and Adolescent Outpatient Services for its encouragement for the writing; and the many children and families who allowed the children's work to be shown.

reenter the child's internal image pool. An image developed and changed through art-making may alter or amend internal imagery. Perhaps more than other children, children who dissociate dwell in a world of images, those they have buried and those they have created in the service of emotional survival. For them, the process of art-making has special therapeutic value.

Nader and Pynoos (1990) suggest that, in drawings, a child's "perceptual experience of events may become embedded and transformed" and that drawings may also reveal "details imbued with specific traumatic meaning to a child." Thus, themes and symbols alone provide rich clues about a child's traumatic experience. Additionally, as suggested by Cohen and Cox (1995), the formal graphic elements of art expression (such as line quality or organization of space) may also be "read" and understood as corresponding to a child's internal experience. For example, two children, each encouraged to create a "home" for a plastic figure chosen from a basket of figures, may go off in different thematic and aesthetic directions. Amber, 11, creates a baroque "circus," in which a tiny plastic baby that she has painted gold is perched precariously atop a column of wood (itself insecurely attached to a cardboard base) as if about to walk off the platform onto a "tightrope" she has constructed from telephone wire. Roberto, also 11, places a red-eyed alligator in the center of a lush jungle he has made of twigs and colored feathers. He tells the art therapist that the alligator is resting, after having eaten some small and vulnerable animals and before going out for another kill. The formal qualities of the art (the shaky attachments, the suggestion of great height through proportion and placement in Amber's work; the dense and hidden qualities of Roberto's) as well as the accompanying stories bring each child's unique subjective vision into sharp focus.

Overall Goals of Therapy for Dissociative Identity Disorders in Children

Putnam and Hornstein (1992) state that in children who dissociate, preliminary studies suggest that "many symptoms and maladaptive behaviors . . . that are refractory to standard treatments . . . respond to psychotherapy addressing the dissociative fragmentation of self." Treatment goals of such therapy include: relinquishing reliance on dissociation; increasing the awareness, experience, naming, tolerance, and modulation of intense affect; developing the ability to remember and then tell his or her own life story as a continuous narrative, with a minimum of cognitive distortions; replacing internalized negative images with those of nurturance, safety,and empowerment; and learning to experience him- or herself as a whole person. In pursuit of these goals, therapists may use a variety of verbal, play, expressive, educational, hypnotherapeutic, and other techniques in a phased treatment plan (see Chapters 8 and 9). While primary therapists may—and almost certainly will—use art techniques throughout their work, the adjunctive art therapy explored here may be seen as a parallel but separate treatment, at the heart of which is the regular engagement and practice in creating art.

This paper proposes two models of adjunctive art therapy to accompany or follow the primary therapy. The first, or parallel therapy model, is the modification and natural extension of one author's (BS) work as an art therapist with traumatized children. The second, or studio model, was developed over the past two years by both authors to promote an ongoing healthy or normal use of the dissociative capacity through a thorough engagement with art.

The Parallel Therapy Model: The Art Therapist Meets the Trauma Therapist

In doing art therapy as an accompaniment to primary therapy, the art therapist follows the same phase-specific treatment sequence as the primary therapist. While this model may work most efficiently in a hospital or inpatient setting, it can work well as a collaboration between an outpatient primary therapist and an art therapist.

As a basis for such collaboration, the model relies on regular communication and on agreements between the primary therapist and the art therapist to minimize splitting and confusion and to maximize exposing the child to a system (here a system of helping professionals) in which, despite occasional differences, the parts work together in harmony. Issues to be clarified may include how the therapists present the concept of dissociation (what terms or language are to be used); what kind of hierarchy will be operating between the therapists; how regularly the therapists will exchange information; what rules or limits will be set; and how the use of art will be distributed between the therapists. The art therapist must also be willing to blend traditional art therapy principles with principles of a trauma-based model of treatment. For example, psychoanalytically trained art therapists may need to be receptive to a child's spontaneous art while finding opportunities to link behavior, thoughts, and feelings to their traumatic origins.

Ideally, a well-lighted, pleasant, and well-equipped art room should be provided for the adjunctive art therapy. It should be an inviting space where the art materials and the time, frequency, and duration of the art sessions are predictable, and where the sessions are free from disruptions.

Phase I

Children who dissociate to a pathological degree may present with a variety of symptoms (Hornstein & Putnam, 1992). Subtle developmental and cognitive considerations influence the child's attribution of meaning to perceptions and feelings, as well as the child's long range response to trauma (Pynoos & Nader, 1993; Finkelhor, 1995). Traumatized children may be engaged in an unconscious process to suppress and/or avoid feelings of terror, rage, grief, helplessness, shame, as well as physical pain, fragments of preserved perceptual memory, or intrapsychic conflict.

Each of the children discussed in this chapter had the ability to dissociate affect, sensation, and/or memory as a response to internal or external "trigger" stimuli. Each had, to a greater or lesser extent, a fragmented identity and each seemed to engage in both self and object splitting. From a panoply of figures, real and imaginary, who had passed through their lives, each had constructed idiosyncratic and often rigid internal worlds to which they would retreat when under stress. The dissociative capacity appeared in their artwork in a variety of ways as chaotic, fragmented, bizarre, or covered over imagery. Often the children seemed to be protecting their dissociative process from adult scrutiny by rationalizing an image after it was drawn, as if to give an explanation that might satisfy a worried adult. (The assessment of dissociation in children through art is outside the scope of this chapter, but the reader is referred to Sobol and Cox, 1992.)

Goals of Phase I Art Therapy

Six art therapy goals can be set for Phase I work, each of which is compatible with the goals of the primary treatment as outlined in Chapter 8. The six goals are:

1. to establish a sense of safety;
2. to support the cognitive foundations being developed in the primary therapy;
3. to provide an exploration of art media in order to discover the most pleasing as well as the most suitable media for the child;
4. to practice, through art, the ability to modulate affect and to tolerate and manage responses to "trigger" stimuli;
5. to bring to light, if possible, the child's unique internal organization of dissociated parts and processes;
6. to establish the model of cooperative "parts."

Perhaps the most important of these goals is establishing a sense of safety. Art materials themselves may be experienced as "unsafe" and overstimulating. As with Rorschach cards which provoke traumatic memory (Armstrong & Loewenstein, 1990; also see Chapter 5, this book), even an accidental image appearing on the blank page can be too strong a stimulus for the child to manage. The handling of fluid materials, exposure to color, and the invitation to create images inherently work against the child's efforts to remain "shut down." Appreciating this, the art therapist will set limited goals in support of establishing the safest possible holding environment. Some children may be unable to feel safe in any setting, but may be able to accept the setting as well as the person of the art therapist as at least benign, if not completely safe.

Methods

Art therapists who work with children often begin a course of therapy with a Kramer (Kramer & Schehr, 1983) or a Rubin (1978) art evaluation, both semi-structured, one-session procedures, well known to art therapists. Both are also meant to offer pleasure in using the art materials and to minimize anxiety, while providing a baseline understanding of the child's cognitive, emotional, and artistic development. The Kramer evaluation consists of three free-theme art tasks: a pencil or marker drawing on small (8 1/2" by 11") white paper; a tempera painting on large (18" by 24") white drawing paper; and a piece created from natural moist clay. By doing the Kramer evaluation, both child and art therapist can explore a range of materials and discover which materials will provide the greatest measure of control, pleasure, and emotional safety. Since "safety" necessarily involves the ability to modulate intense affect without slipping into dissociation, the art therapist may need to be ready from the outset to model adaptive responses to rising emotions and anxiety.

For example, during a Kramer session, a child may begin to behave in a dissociative manner (that is, "spacing out," becoming very quiet or overly focused, blocking out external stimuli, rolling eyes, etc.) or show increasing agitation. The art therapist may draw upon a range of responses based on a quick assessment of both the child's ability and his or her own ability to tolerate anxiety. The most conservative intervention with a child who begins to dissociate is to redirect the child away from the stimulating "triggers" of the art materials or themes and toward a less threatening subject or medium—acting, in traditional terms, as an auxiliary ego for the unravelling child. A less conservative approach is to allow the expression of some of this anxiety, giving the child an opportunity to recover and go on his/her own. During Phase I, the intervention that allows the greatest development of trust between child and therapist is the best intervention, and this can only be determined in the moment. The experienced therapist who has the confidence and ability to provide an anxiety-tolerant holding environment for the child will be in a better position than the novice to take the more permissive approach. In either event, the child eventually needs to be guided back to the here and now of the art session. The therapist may need to be directive and explicit, saying, for example, "Working with the clay seems to have made you 'space out' (or whatever term has been agreed upon to denote dissociative behavior). I'd like you to come back so that you and I can find something else for you to do in art right now, something that will help you not space out." And later, "I'm glad you showed me how easy it is for you to space out, because that will help us in our work." The therapist can briefly explore where the child has "gone," so that an awareness of internal process is encouraged from the very beginning, and the groundwork laid for developing self-management and responsibility.

In keeping with a commitment to the goal of decreasing dissociation, highly projective, regressive, or intrusive art activities in phase one may not be appropriate. These would include fingerpainting (regressive, stimulating), the scribble technique (Ulman, 1965) (invites projection, exacerbates lack of integration); life masks (Sivin, 1986) or life tracings (Fleming, 1989). Before the therapist knows how the child will respond to closeness and touch, techniques that require close proximity to the child may risk provoking anxiety or confusion. The child needs to trust that the therapist will protect him or her from losing control. The therapist may want to encourage the child to repeat projects that he or she has loved or has been successful with in the past, such as a technique that the child has learned at school or at camp. The therapist can demonstrate simple technical tasks, such as how to mix colors, how to join clay pieces properly, or how to construct a simple collage from magazine pictures. However, because the art work is intended to be specifically linked with the primary trauma-dissociation treatment, the art therapist may want to make that connection explicit, reminding the child that he or she can do art for fun, to learn new techniques, to express feelings or worries, to remember things, and to tell stories about his or her life.

Establishing a place where the artwork will be kept safe may be an important reassurance at this time. A child may be unable to voice the fear that using art to express hidden feelings is itself dangerous and may bring harm or punishment. If the artworks are to be photographed, it is important to ask the child's permission as well as the permission of the family or caseworker, as this may also provide reassurance that the child's privacy is respected.

Case examples

KEVIN: REDIRECTING ANXIETY

A Kramer evaluation was begun with a 5-year-old boy who had a recent history of attacking other children with sharp objects and threat-

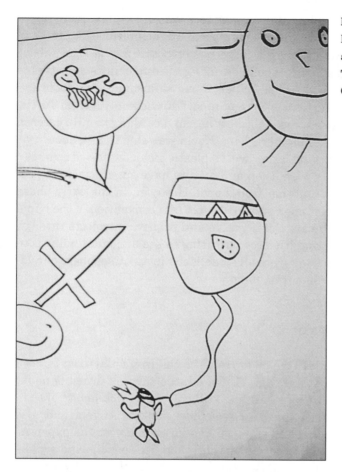

Figure 1. An anxious Kevin drew fragmented and floating Ninja Turtles in a Phase One session.

ening to kill himself. He had no ability to link these behaviors to his witnessing the near murder of his mother by his father two years earlier. During the Kramer, Kevin tried to copy a pencil drawing (hanging on the studio wall) of a sad-faced little girl standing next to a Christmas tree. He became increasingly agitated, threw down the pencil, then quickly made two paintings of large amorphous forms and sweeping directional lines, which he called "bomb" paintings. His rising agitation suggested that he was experiencing an internal reenactment of his earlier loss of both internal and external control. To redirect him, I (author BS) quickly removed the paint and suggested that we take a walk to the snack machines. Returning, we got out a set of colored pencils. Kevin, having somewhat regained his equilibrium, and able to maintain good control of this medium, showed me how he drew "Ninja Turtles." The "superempowered" persona of the Turtle seemed to calm Kevin, and before the session ended he had drawn several more Turtles. Over the next several weeks, Kevin drew a great many Turtles using only markers or colored pencils on small paper. Within the single convention, Kevin communicated widely varying states, including a state of internal threat and one of internal fragmentation (Figure 1). In his 6th session he drew on a large poster board a "life-size" (about Kevin's size) Ninja Turtle who in swinging his numchucks appeared to have hit himself on the head. When Kevin said something about the "stupidity" of the Turtle, I (BS) remarked, "But he's only a child Turtle. He's just learning and this is the best he can do." Many months later in therapy, and with his mother's help, Kevin was able to talk about trying to stab his attacking father with a plastic picnic knife—of course to no avail—and of his wish, then and now, to have superpowers to protect himself and his mother from harm. However, in the early phase one stage, simply finding a style or "voice" (the convention of the Ninja Turtle), revealing a range of negative and positive introjects through the Turtle, linking cognitive restructuring to the art, and finding control in the medium itself were all established in an atmosphere of relative safety and freedom from judgment.

ANGELA: TOLERATING ANXIETY

My (BS's) skilled intern called me into the children's playroom to see a painting made by Angela, age 11. On a large sheet of drawing paper clipped to the easel was a painting still wet with thick layers of tempera that covered the page in sweeping strokes. Angela had also painted her hands and had stamped handprints all over the paper. As the regression seemed to continue, this otherwise sensible and sophisticated girl asked the therapist to let her also paint the nearby pristine wood dollhouse. Hidden from view forever was the original image, a carefully drawn, then painted, full-body self-portrait which had looked, my intern reported, sexually developed, self-aware, and provocative. Having obliterated this self-portrait with the overlay of tempera, Angela spontaneously made a second portrait (head and shoulders only) on smaller paper and with markers. The second portrait retained the expressiveness as well as the sexuality of the first, but was rendered with great instinctive control as well as artistic flair. She continued working, going to the sand tray and creating, first, a near-empty landscape of a beach and second, a landscape overrun with snakes, rodents, insects, and dinosaurs, depicting both animal to animal violence and a baby burning in a fire in view of its parents. At the end of the session, she distanced herself from this scene by remarking that it was not a place she would like to be.

Allowing the session to run its course, with only minimal intervention, the therapist had made it possible for Angela to destroy one image of self, make a second that she could tolerate, and then repeat the sequence using the sand tray, where she had more control (was able to stay within the sturdy wood borders of the tray), and could do and undo with ease. In this session, Angela's apparent trance-like state, already underway as she worked on her first painting, was monitored by an experienced therapist who had at her disposal a number of corrective possibilities, including expressive play. As with Kevin, we could only infer that *something* was intolerable in the first painting (her beauty? her sexuality?); but here, the therapist provided a different kind of safety, that of tolerating or "holding" the anxiety so that Angela could go on to repeat and defuse the internal agitation.

Both the response to Kevin ("redirecting") and the response to Angela ("holding") were appropriate and provided safety. Each was based on the therapist's assessment of her own tolerance for anxiety and of the child's ego strength and capacity for recovery in the session.

Other Tasks and Projects in Phase I

Ideally, a mix of spontaneous projects and structured art tasks can be undertaken during phase one work. For a child who is affectively shut down, the art therapist may want to build on known techniques, such as Beverly James's "basket of feelings" exercise (1989) by making a set of 5" by 7" index cards that list a different feeling on each card. As an art project, the feelings may be represented by images that are either drawn or cut from magazines. A cigar box or school box may be decorated as both a literal and a metaphorical container for the feelings. An older, more sophisticated child might make a similar set of cards, but with lines, shapes, and colors—small abstract art works—to represent a range of feelings. A younger or developmentally less advanced child might more easily use the magazine pictures pasted onto the cards. Rather than rely on a series of ready-made projects, however, the authors prefer to simply clarify the criteria for appropriate tasks at this stage and to hold each idea up for its relevance and applicability to the particular child. Tasks that are intended to elicit difficult material from the child before the child feels safe may instead elicit defensive maneuvers and new reasons to dissociate.

Case example

CHRISSY: REPRESENTING DISSOCIATED FEELINGS

Chrissy, a fragile girl of 8, whose severe sexual and emotional abuse had begun when she was one year old, had no way to label or to discriminate among feelings. She was often overcome by waves of agitation and could not be soothed. I (BS) invited Chrissy to make sequenced cartoon stories in which emotions would be subordinate to a

Figure 2. Chrissy attempts to differentiate feeling states by line quality, color, and location in her body (Phase I).

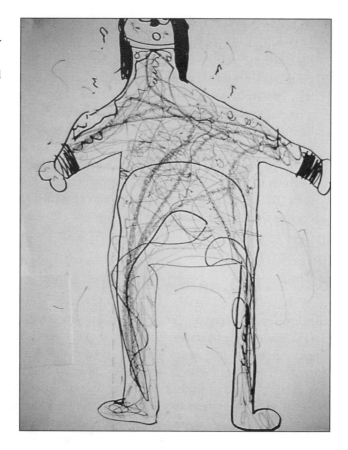

story line. At first she made only "happy" cartoons about her family. In these, she used glue and glitter liberally, which had the effect of amplifying the almost giddy mood of the drawings and also of drawing attention away from other, more disturbing elements in the drawings. Much later (in Phase II of the work), she used the same cartoon format to depict stories of her nightmares, bad memories, and bad feelings. Like Kevin, once Chrissy had found a vernacular through a combination of materials and conventions, she repeated the format over many sessions, so that the format itself served as an adaptable container for changing concerns. In Chrissy's cartoons, both color and the character of the lines served as a code through which a number of separate (unnamed) internal "parts" could give expression to otherwise dissociated feelings. On a large cartoon-like outline of a little girl (Figure 2) that we drew together on a sheet of 18" by 24" paper, she made marks in an attempt to show the nature and location of different feelings and sensations. Blue squiggles were identified as "nervous"; thin red lines as bad or "evil"; strewn glitter lines were "happy"; black question marks, "confused." Again, much later, she spontaneously used a similar technique, using shaky colored lines and arrows to show the sensation of a "floor moving" under her and her accompanying terror and disorientation. The glitter had disappeared, perhaps because Chrissy had less need to mask her darker feelings, Chrissy's ability to use structure (the cartoon strips) and to anchor her work in the graphics kept Chrissy grounded and focused in the face of much internal pressure to dissociate.

Summary of Phase I Work

In this early phase, little or no uncovering work is done; spontaneous abreaction or dissociation is gently acknowledged, then in most cases redirected until a sense of safety and trust has been established. The child learns to bring the art-making process itself and with it, metaphorically, his or her emotional life under some control and establishes themes compatible with themes worked on in primary therapy. The rudiments of safety and empowerment are established, internal parts or processes are acknowledged, and a personal, idiosyncratic "voice" or graphic vocabulary may be developed.

Phase II

For years, Richard Kluft (1986) has emphasized both the vulnerability of children who dissociate and the urgency of helping them resolve their trauma issues as early and as quickly as possible. Children who are in the second phase of treatment often will create deeply personal images from the center of their rage, grief, or pain. If the work of phase one has been successful, they will feel safe enough to give the art therapist considerable access to their imagined world and permission to act as an agent of transformation.

Goals and Methods of Phase II in Art Therapy

Because emotional flooding and dissociative flight continue in Phase II, the need to self-manage, self-soothe, and maintain physical and emotional safety also continues. There are also new and distinct treatment goals that include:

1. telling and re-viewing traumatic events and reinterpreting them through new and more mature cognitive structures;
2. expressing and transforming the hidden or dissociated aspects of self as well as negative beliefs about self;
3. identifying and reworking attachments to negative caregivers (see Chapter 8).

Ideally, a process will develop in which the work of the primary therapy and the work of the art therapy will form a continuous loop, the one enhancing, deepening, or anticipating the other. Both therapists will be striving to create a rhythm of hard work alternating with periods of rest, assimilation, and play. Both will attempt to balance a commitment to "pace and contain" expression (Turkus, 1991) and a commitment to vigorously pursue the dissociated material, so that a child will never be overwhelmed by more affect or memory than he or she can bear.

The primary therapist may use hypnosis to address a number of aspects of dissociation. Art therapists generally are not certified in clinical hypnosis; however, art-making at its deepest level is a naturally induced altered state of consciousness. Art therapists will find that some children can easily paint or draw their way into a light or a deep trance. This ability of a child to create art in such an altered state is to be welcomed; but it creates an interesting burden for art therapists who must stay within the ethical guidelines of their own field while sensitively responding to the child's "art trance."

During this phase, the art therapist more than ever needs to know the language and the pace of the primary therapist. A child who in drawing shows signs of "switching" or other dissociative response may need a reminder: "Remember that it's okay for your inside people (or whatever term the child is using for his or her internal system personae) to just 'watch and listen' from their safe places" (see Chapter 8). It is also important to review the agreements that have been made for this phase between the child and the primary therapist—for example, an agreement that no new "inside people" are to be created during the work.

In Phase II art-making may blossom and the child may create intense, focused, and profoundly meaningful works. In order for this to happen—for the images to have room to develop fully—there must be ample time given not only in each session but also from session to session so that the child may enter the art trance and return from it safely. The art session itself may require a new, expanded structure or rhythm. We have found that a natural flow of an hour's art session may now include several segments which allow pacing and recovery. The art therapist may start with a 5-minute "check-in" to determine how vulnerable the child feels or how dissociative. The next 5 minutes may be spent inviting the child to make art, collecting materials and setting them out, and letting the child settle in. The art-making itself may take one half hour or more, depending on age and attentional capacity of the child. The session may then include 5 minutes for the child to make the transition from art-making to the reality of the session. Finally, the last 5 minutes is spent on present-focused activities, such as cleaning up, summarizing the session, doing a closing "ritual" of thanks for work well done, and a "goodbye."

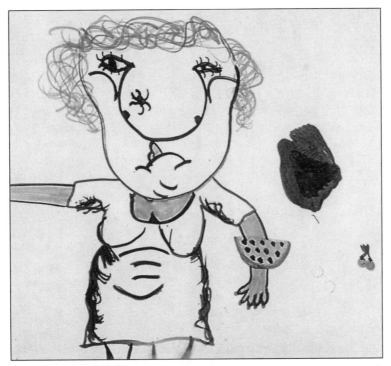

Figure 3. Serena's Phase I crude female figure with floating fruit is trance-like and self-mocking.

Case examples

Each of the children discussed below developed images touching painful core themes and making them available to the therapist's scrutiny and intervention. In two cases, the work in art therapy was successful; in the third, it failed because verbal and behavioral interventions lagged behind the outpouring of imagery, violating the need to pace the work and contain material that threatened to overwhelm the child.

SERENA: A DISCONTINUOUS IDENTITY

Serena, 11, was a child with dissociative episodes and fragmented states but not concrete embodied "alter personalities." Her fragmented presentation developed in the aftermath of two early sexual assaults by non-caregivers, but seemed to have been exacerbated by her family's concern about the issue of sexuality. Serena had engaged in the Phase I activity of establishing safety for herself by testing the art therapist's acceptance of her disintegrated, sexually explicit, and often crude paintings (Figure 3). She began her Phase II art work following a spontaneous dream she had the night before an art session. She felt com-

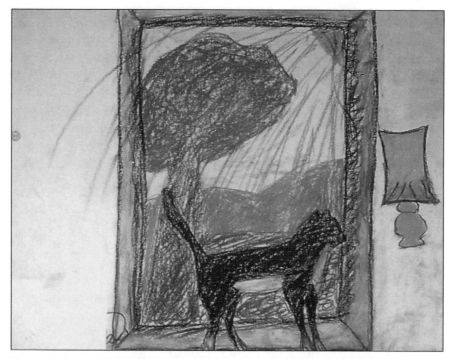

Figure 4. Serena's Phase II interior/exterior scene suggests her struggle to achieve a complex but not fragmented identity.

pelled to make a pencil drawing of the dream setting, a hotel room with high ceilings and tall windows looking out onto an ocean. At the window were fluttering curtains; but there was no sign of life other than a tiny kitten scampering away. She indicated with pencil strokes that a brilliant light was entering the room through the window. Drawing the dream seemed to invoke in Serena a deep sense of loss. Beginning with the hotel drawing, and over the course of about three months, Serena made a series of eight drawings and paintings. Each of the first seven drawings expressed an aspect of her fragmented identity, including a saintly child, a sad and weary streetwalker, and a nude pubescent girl at her bath. Each included a cat, perhaps the early embodiment of an observing, core self, and each conveyed a mysterious, almost mystical relationship between an interior scene and an exterior landscape seen through a window (Figure 4). The last drawing depicts a sailor in open air gazing at the ocean, a falcon perched on his shoulder—an identification that seemed to grant her respite from her overly eroticized childhood. The drawings were invested with a depth of focus that was remarkable, often lasting several sessions and involving a visible struggle between destroying and developing the image. As the work evolved, I began to reframe the discontinuous identity as a *complex*

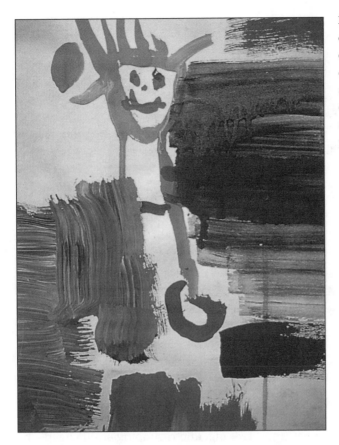

Figure 5. James's early Phase I painting of himself with unclear expression (fear, aggression, smile?) covers areas of body and scene with thick paint. (Detail)

identity and her dissociative behavior as a natural response to extreme trauma, shame, confusion, and anger.

While at the time this series of pictures was not thought of as a "book," now in retrospect this larger context could be used to "hold" or contain the series. Placing these eight artworks in a special portfolio might have given them additional definition as a single body of work, a metaphor reinforcing the concept of a single and richly complex self.

JAMES: UNASSIMILATED SEXUAL RAGE

For James, 12, the art alone could not and did not sustain the burden of the trauma work. This severely dissociative adolescent had harbored within himself a hostile personality fragment since early childhood. An early painting, done at age 5, shows a terrified, traumatized child, and James has painted over the beginning image of the sadistic "alter" (Figure 5). At age 12, over a period of several weeks, James created a pterodactyl's head, a clay sculpture that became notable for its ever-increasing size and oddness. The very making of the art—the dissocia-

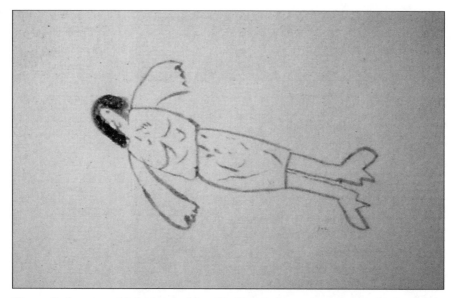

Figure 6. James, unable to manage his split-off erotic focus on women, emphasizes both breasts and slash marks, alerting the therapist to a crisis in Phase II.

tive quality of his smoothing, stroking, and reshaping of this head—reinforced James's dissociative process and with it the emergence of a hostile and malevolent "alter personality." James may have interpreted the therapist's passivity or receptivity as permission for the feelings of this "alter" to come up unchallenged. The pterodactyl sculpture was followed by a series of drawings of other sharp-taloned creatures that included both animals and sexually seductive women depicted alternately as innocent and vulnerable and as sexually predatory (Figure 6). In the absence of links between the content of the drawings and cognitive structures that could interpret, manage, or redirect the images, James's art continued to stimulate traumatic memory, sexual fantasy, and profound rage, embodied in a hostile "alter." The alter, a dissociative phenomenon not yet fully available to treatment, needed to be contained not only at the symbolic level—in the art—but also through direct behavior interventions—specific contracts not to act out the sexual rage. More aggressive interventions in the art itself (stopping, redirecting, interpreting, reframing, or creating different images) were imperative in order to help deflect James from harmful, severe acting out.

KEVIN: ABREACTION IN ART

The Ninja Turtles drawn by Kevin changed over time from aggressive and grandiose to something more appealing and hapless—a child in Ninja Turtle clothing. As the self-image aspects of the Turtle approached reality, Kevin himself became less of an automaton and more childlike in his demeanor and behavior. However, the change also evoked deep fears of helplessness and abandonment. His play shifted to repeated scenes of disaster (car accidents), failed rescue, and death, the post-traumatic play described by Terr (1981). In oral family sessions, Kevin's mother worked on giving realistic assurances of safety in their present life and on telling her account of the attack, repeating that he and she had both survived and were now safe. Changes in the external environment that might guarantee safety for Kevin were slow, and Kevin continued the aggressive reenactments. Author BS decided to have a clay session in which Kevin could pound clay, both to prepare it for art use (getting air holes out) and to get feelings out safely. Kevin, now 6, came to his session wearing old clothes as planned, and we reviewed signals we had created that would let each of us know that we needed to take a break or stop. After a tentative, nervously playful beginning, Kevin threw himself onto the clay (a 25-pound block on a drop cloth spread on the studio floor). He was quickly flooded with rage, stabbing and kicking the clay as he had attempted to stab and kick his father three years earlier. In less than 5 minutes he was exhausted and "cried out." In this transitional state, as he began to slowly reorient to the room, he pulled off a small piece of clay and shaped it quietly into two tiny dinosaurs, a "parent" and a smaller "child." (Figure 7). He called these a "father and son" at first, then a "mother and son." It seemed that he had been able to locate not only his rage at his father but also fear and rage related to his mother. Before the session ended, Kevin was reminded that he had been "only a little kid" trying to do his best when both parents were out of control.

Other Techniques and Art Tasks

Children may be invited to imagine and draw an inside person in a new role or even new clothes. They may usefully repeat making containers as "safe places" for either good or bad affect. They may be encouraged to make books that tell or retell stories that are significant to them, or to collect reminders of good or safe places, or cut out and mount magazine pictures on mat board to keep in a box as reminders of things that are soothing. Learning simple techniques (tissue collage, paper pop-ups) is also a way to take a break from the hard work of trauma resolution and may provide needed pleasure and a reminder that art may be light and playful.

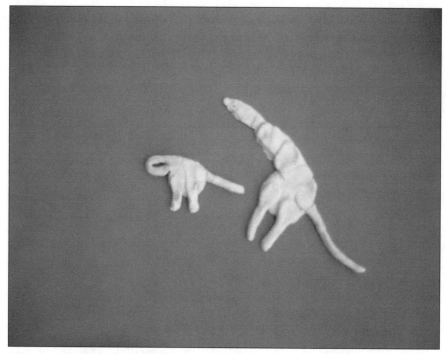

Figure 7. Kevin creates a serene parent and child dinosaur in Phase Two.

Summary of Phase II Work

Much spontaneous, personal, and intensely felt art work may be made, some in a trance-like state and some breaking through the barriers of dissociation. The art therapist must be able to help a child shut down as well as open up channels of expressed affect, to use art in a self-soothing way as well as for planned abreaction. Ethical considerations are high, since the child him or herself will tend to slip into a hypnotic state with some ease. As Phase II work comes to a natural close, the therapist should be able to see a growing lucidity in the organization and themes of the art work.

Phase III

As described in chapter 9, the treatment goals of Phase III focus on integration and making strong connections to the positive caregivers in the present. Children may spontaneously fantasize or begin to draw, dream, or talk about their unique hopes and fears about integration. These may include drawings of what it might be like to have different parts of self united, such as sharing a heart, holding hands, being like peas in a pod, living together in a house, telescoping like Russian dolls; or dropping away an outer shell to reveal a single boy or girl. Other children may convey integration more abstractly through a blending of personally significant colors, shapes, or symbols. Such images may be a way of trying out an idea that is new and possibly strange or a way to struggle with their own resistance. Stories and art about change may be combined, spontaneously or with guidance. For example, a story and picture about walking across a bridge to leave bad memories safely "in the past" may set the stage for hope and a new perspective. Art work may also be made about the present feelings. At this stage, the life mask, the life tracing, or for some children, a realistic self-portrait or portrait of the therapist or other positively connected person are probably safe to encourage or support. Containers that hold "the whole self" or that hold "all parts of the story," both the good and the bad, can be made in nearly innumerable ways, limited only by the child's creative capacity and the therapist's skill and repertoire of ideas.

Case example

CHRISSY: AT HOME IN THE PRESENT

Chrissy, the 8-year-old discussed briefly in Phase I, above, continued to make cartoon sequences in both Phase II and Phase III as she untangled her deeply embedded belief that God could not love her. Gradually, in family and individual therapy, some of her hopelessness, cynicism, and terror began to recede. Simultaneously, she began to work in clay as grounding, functional, present-oriented, and self-soothing. She appeared to take great pleasure in the physical manipulating of the medium, related, perhaps, to a growing ability to tolerate sensation in her body. The sense of creating something of substance carried over into her drawing. In a marker portrait of a beloved pet, the carefully colored-in fur gave weight and bulk to the figure and metaphorically gave substance to the feeling of security and protection. Her final work in therapy (Figure 8) was a lovingly made bowl, serene in its oval shape, yet decorated in the glittering bright colors and markings that were characteristic of her earlier work. The course of therapy had been about a year and a half. BS was able to comment on Chrissy's invested works of art by using the words and concepts of integration that were resonant with the language of primary therapy, only here specifically linked to the creation of the art. Looking at Chrissy's bowl, BS used words intended to help deepen her sense of self as a good, lovable, and worthy person: "This bowl reminds me of you. It has your sense of humor and your love of bright colors and designs, and it has some silliness too. It's got your hand and fingerprints all over it in the clay! I like

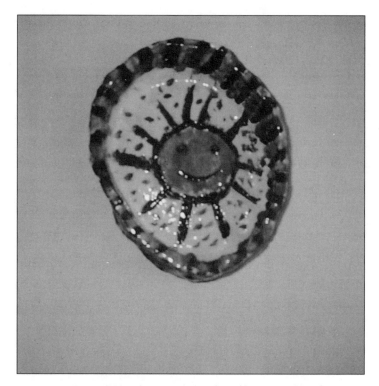

Figure 8. Chrissy's Phase III bowl is a metaphor for self as a container for many aspects of personality.

the way your bowl can hold a lot of things, just the way you are able to hold so many different parts of yourself together. And I like how solid it is; it's really here [tapping the bowl] just as you are very much here, now."

Summary of Phase III

The work of Phase III supports a strong focus on the present, while continuing to follow the child's own graphic language and imagery to deepen his or her sense of self as good, lovable, or blameless. As the work of phase three comes to an end, there may be a need for ongoing support and practice in remaining in the present. In the next section, we discuss the creation of an art support group that may continue the phase-related work or that may be an alternative model for children who are working with a primary therapist.

The Studio Model

The studio or resilience-based model emphasizes supportive therapy done in a group setting, in which the goals of the primary therapy are enhanced through an exploration of art. The link to the primary therapy is less formal and less specific, and the techniques are not as directly linked to the primary therapist's work as would be the case in the parallel model. We developed the studio model over a 2-year period. We worked first with adolescent girls from chronically troubled homes in which chaos and confusion often were the backdrop for specific traumatizing incidents. The adolescent girls' groups were created first in a public mental health outpatient setting, then developed further in a private practice setting.

The girls' groups were concurrent with the primary therapy and the girls were required to be in individual therapy throughout the duration of the group. In addition to an informal exchange of information which took place on a monthly basis, consultations took place as needed and could be initiated by either the art therapist or the primary therapist.

Goals of the Studio Group Model

Our goals were both global and specific. They were:

1. to create a sanctuary where the girls would be able to work on expressing themselves safely in pictures, words and stories;
2. to pay special attention to helping the girls modulate and regulate affect and to help them learn to tolerate their own often uncomfortable emotions without feeling the need to run away, act out or become defensive or dissociative;
3. to help the girls to tolerate their emotions long enough to symbolize them in their art work;
4. to shift the focus from trauma-specific themes to themes of resilience and the idea of reinventing the self through doing something they never thought or imagined they could do;
5. to promote the development of a vocabulary of ambivalence in order to open lines of communication among the girls through which they could discuss mixed and complex feelings;
6. to provide art activities that would be pleasant and structured, rewarding and fun, so that the girls would not want to miss them;
7. to give the girls a chance to get connected to the art work rather than over-related to each other; to foster a relationship between each girl and her own art work and de-emphasize overreliance on the therapist;
8. to help the girls to internalize the creative process so that they could continue to experience satisfaction with it on their own after the group had ended;

9. to use art to foster resilience, build self-esteem, and encourage flexibility in thinking, creativity, and self-discipline through a genuine engagement with the artistic process; and

10. to shift the use of the dissociative capacity from the pathological end of the dissociative spectrum to the adaptive and healthy end of the spectrum—that is, to teach a controlled use of and access to the dissociative process as it supports the creative imagination and a healthy, temporary, and adaptive absorption in the creative process.

Evolution of the Group

As in the parallel model of art therapy and trauma therapy, we observed that a lack of structure invited anxiety and agitation. In our first group, we offered the girls paint and paper with no instructions other than to make paintings. We found that the girls literally could not contain themselves, both in terms of their behavior—they could not refrain from touching each other and testing boundaries—and their images, which spilled over the borders or the edges of the paper.

After watching the girls' inability to cope with a free theme with no directive from the art therapists, we embarked upon a series of more structured projects which made use of contained objects, lidded boxes which were elaborately decorated, and precisely formatted surfaces (stiff white paper which was folded accordion style, then embellished by cutting window-like shapes out of it and adding collage elements). The latter project was inspired by a similarly configured, colorful invitation to an exhibition of the work of contemporary artist Lucas Samaras; the invitation card, designed by Samaras, was shown to the girls as a model for the project. The girls responded positively to the growing structure of the art projects presented, and they gradually became able to work in a more calm, focused, and sustained manner.

An important shift in the quality and the feeling tone of the sessions developed when we began to create artwork alongside the girls, so that when they walked into the studio, they found the therapists at work on their own projects. The girls' reaction became one of enthusiastic involvement, rather than a passive anticipation of didactic instruction. The adults' engagement in artmaking became a kind of gold mine for modelling an attitude toward art and life that included the ability to recover from making mistakes without self-blame. They watched and absorbed the therapists' ability to try again after making something that didn't work out as expected and to sometimes have to make several pieces before making one that was to the artists' liking.

The Environments Project

The Environments Project was an outgrowth of our studio-based approach, combined with the felicitous presence of a wide and unusual array of unconventional materials which we had to work with. Many of these materials were found objects or were given to us as donations by local frame shops, bead shops, and artists. Mat board, foam core, wood shapes, wire, fabric, sawdust, bags of beads and jewelry, pieces of vines, shells, as well as paint, markers, magazines, etc., were displayed in colorful and intriguing abundance on the studio counter and tables. We purchased an array of miniature plastic animals, birds, bird nests, eggs, and human figures, which we placed in baskets. We invited each girl to select one or two of the miniatures and create an environment for it.

Our instructions to the girls varied. We began by asking the girls to create a home for the creatures; over time, this evolved into the instruction that "you might want to make a safe place for your animal and to think about what it might need to feel safe and comfortable." We have also said "just use the materials in a way you find pleasing; you can create a realistic environment or a fantasy environment." In this and our other projects, we have found it important to include a wide range of acceptable responses, ranging from the literal to the abstract, so that each girl could respond to the instructions at her own level of ability and understanding. Each girl's environment was unique and appeared to distill and encapsulate deep aspects of the girls' inner stories.

In this and subsequent art projects, we have placed great emphasis on activities that might be described as having the correct balance of structure and flexibility, providing enough guidance to enable the child to organize his or her artistic responses and enough freedom to engage in a highly personal and creative manner to the task at hand.

Case examples

ALYSON

> Sixteen-year-old Alyson had a diagnosis that included ruling out a dissociative disorder NOS. A close relative had a diagnosis of Dissociative Identity Disorder. She had a history that included many hospitalizations and more than one suicide attempt, and although fairly stable at the time the group began, she had difficulty regulating what seemed to be a nonstop flow of ideas. She needed to use art to calm and soothe herself rather than as additional stimulation but found it difficult to do so. Although Alyson became intensely involved in her art projects and was quite productive in the group, she seemed to find the range of cre-

Figure 9. (detail). Alyson's environment, a circus for two clowns, includes a wide array of colors and patterns. Photo: Edward Owen.

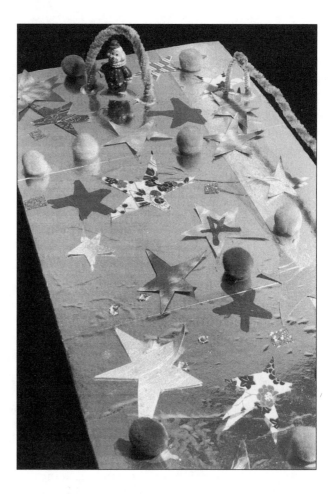

ative possibilities that were available to her to be a bit overwhelming.

For her environment, Alyson selected two clown figures, each less than an inch in height, and created a circus for them (Figure 9). Although a chaotic array of colors and patterns abounded, the piece stayed within the boundaries of its matboard base.

Alyson herself appeared to compensate for poor self-esteem with a super-competent and self-sufficient manner and with laughter. Her clown theme suggested that beneath the laughter was sadness and possibly fear and anger as well. The clown theme wove its way through her stories about her life. She tended to minimize problems. When the topic of an alcoholic uncle came up, she said of being around him, "It don't bother me none," and added that she and a friend laughed at her uncle. After completing her clown piece, Alyson missed several groups, attended a few times, and then stopped coming altogether.

In discussing Alyson's departure from the group, we wondered if the art had been too stimulating for her, engendering a need for flight. Our

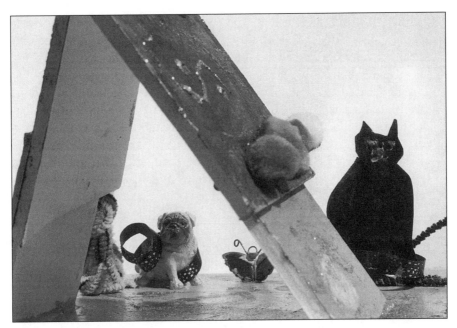

Figure 10. (detail). Jodie's environment, an A-frame house populated by animals, employs an unusual perspective. Photo: Edward Owen.

mixed experience with Alyson showed us that children's responses must be monitored carefully. It is possible that she would have fared better had we tried to limit the number of materials that she could use and further structure the projects so that she could more readily assimilate them without becoming overwhelmed.

JODIE

Jodie, 14, had a diagnosis of posttraumatic stress disorder and a rule-out diagnosis of dissociative identity disorder. She had experienced severe and ongoing abuse, both physical and sexual, throughout much of her childhood and had been placed in a series of foster homes. In the group, she often used any task as an opportunity to make a gift for her current foster mother.

Jodie worked enthusiastically on her environment, which consisted of an A-frame house populated by a cat, a dog, and a butterfly (Figure 10). Although she encountered a number of technical frustrations, she persisted and seemed pleased and surprised when one therapist remarked on her patience, a term that seemed to catch her off guard and suggest an area of possible self-esteem as yet unexplored. As she worked, Jodie told a story from a book she had read about the return of a child with severe mental and physical disabilities to her home. Jodie seemed to identify with the story, perhaps because of her own feelings of rejection by her parents and a number of earlier foster parents and because of her wish to obtain acceptance from her foster mother.

When asked to explain the project to another teenager who had arrived late for the group, Jodie said that the environments were "wonderlands" and focused on the possibilities and abundance of all the materials rather than on the overall theme of the project. Jodie, a emotionally fragile girl, often seemed preoccupied with thoughts that often spilled out into awkward behavior, inviting negative responses from other children. Many of her pieces had an unusual perspective common with children who dissociate, who may imagine themselves on a ceiling or outside a window, separate from pain or abuse, being able to imagine "that's not me" or "I am not there." Her house environment placed the viewer both above and below the horizon. The environment was one of the few projects she made that was not converted into a gift for her foster mother, perhaps because it was deeply felt and revealing and not easy to give away.

The Group Leader as Role Model

The stance of the group leaders as artist/participants along with the children in a studio atmosphere avoided the feeling of surveillance that can come up when a therapist watches a child make art. Seeing the adults make art in the group gave the girls added support for the importance of doing creative work.

The therapists' art work occasionally served as a model for touching difficult material and as permission to talk about emotionally potent events. One therapist made her own environment based on a newspaper story about a child who had been abused by creating a scene of a "safe rock" where a child and her dog could go to get away from the abuse and to comfort each other. The story captivated the girls' attention and seemed a useful way of helping them to talk about issues which they had been too uncomfortable to discuss.

Having other children's environments be visible in the studio was another valuable source of inspiration. The girls rarely copied each other's work but did get ideas from others' approaches to the materials. Interventions were often based on the artistic process. One of the girls in the group, a selective mute, usually sat quietly until the last 15 or 20 minutes of the session, when she proceeded to make work of high artistic quality in an intensely focused manner. When one of the other girls, bothered by her apparent inactivity, asked her, "Are you just going to sit there . . . and not make anything?" we could remind her how much time artists spend simply thinking or imagining the work they might like to make, looking at work already made or just sitting quietly until an idea came. They may not be making any artwork at all while engaged in these processes, but eventually everything they do leads into their work. We emphasized that many approaches to art-making were valid, from being silent and apparently inactive for long periods to using seeming "mistakes" as fodder for a new piece or new way of thinking.

As another way to inspire creativity, we showed the girls work by established artists, taking them on field trips to the National Museum of American Art to see a huge installation by James Hampton and to the National Gallery of Art to see assemblages by Joseph Cornell. It helped to validate what the girls were doing to know that adult artists had worked with similar formal problems and materials.

Summary of the Studio / Support Model

In the support group setting, where children are not expected to be working specifically on trauma issues, the opportunity is given to explore the art process and in doing so to see themselves in a new light—as people who have the capacity to create and imagine, rather than as people to whom things have happened in a passive way. The group conveys the message to children that art is something that is always available to them, something inside themselves that they can call up whenever they need it. It allows them to see themselves as real artists, that is, as people who respond to life in a creative way. For dissociative children, whose creativity has been poured into coping with overwhelming events, creative energy can be restored to a more healthy purpose and direction.

References

Armstrong, J. G., & Loewenstein, R. J. (1990). Characteristics of patients with multiple personality and dissociative disorders on psychological testing. *Journal of Nervous and Mental Diseases, 178,* 448–454.

Cohen, B. M., & Cox, C. T. (1995). *Telling without talking: Art as a window into the world of multiple personality.* New York: W.W. Norton.

Finkelhor, D. (1995). The victimization of children: A developmental perspective. *American Journal of Orthopsychiatry, 65* (2), 177–193.

Fleming, M. (1989). Art therapy and anorexia: Experiencing the authentic self. In E. Baker and L. Hornyak (Eds.), *Experiential approaches to the treatment of eating disorders.* New York: Guilford Press.

Putnam, F. W., & Hornstein, N. L. & (1992). Clinical phenomenology of child and adolescent dissociative disorders. *Journal of the American Academy of Child and Adolescent Psychiatry, 31* (6), 1077–1085.

James, B. (1989). *Treating traumatic children.* Lexington, MA: Lexington Books.

Kluft, R. P. (1986). Treating children who have multiple personality disorder. In

B. G. Braun (Ed.), *Treatment of multiple personality disorder.* Washington, DC: American Psychiatric Press.

Kramer, E. & Schehr, J. (1983). An art therapy evaluation session for children. *American Journal of Art Therapy, 23 (*October 1983), 3–12.

Nader, K., & Pynoos, R. S. (1990). Drawing and play in the diagnosis and assessment of childhood post-traumatic stress syndromes. In C. Schaefer (Ed.), *Play, diagnosis and assessment.* New York: Wiley.

Piaget, J., & Inhelder, B. (1969). *The psychology of the child.* New York: Basic Books.

Pynoos, R. S., & Nader, K. (1993). The impact of trauma on children and adolescents. In J. Wilson & B. Raphael (Eds.), *The international handbook of traumatic stress syndromes* (535–657). New York: Plenum Press.

Rubin, J. A. (1978). *Child art therapy.* New York: Van Nostrand Reinhold.

Sivin, C. (1986). *Maskmaking.* Worcester, Mass.

Sobol, B., & Cox, C. T. (1992). Art and childhood dissociation: Research with sexually abused children. American Art Therapy Association Conference.(Casette recording no. 59–144.) Denver, CO: National Audio Video.

Terr, L. (1981). Forbidden games: Post-traumatic child's play. *Journal of the American Academy of Child Psychiatry, 20,* 741–760.

Turkus, J. (1991). Psychotherapy and case management for multiple personality disorder: Synthesis for continuity of care. In R. Lowenstein (Ed.), *Psychiatric Clinics of North America, 14,* 649–660.

Ulman, E. (1965). A new use of art in psychiatric diagnosis. *American Journal of Art Therapy, 30* (February, 1992), 79. (First described in Cane, F. (1951). *The artist in each of us.* New York: Pantheon Books.)

eleven

███████ Supportive Group Psychotherapy
for Adolescents with
Dissociative Disorders

Bethany Brand

Adolescent cases of dissociative disorders are thought
to be more refractory and difficult to treat than are childhood cases (Dell
& Eisenhower, 1990; Silberg, Stipic, & Taghizadeh, in press). Although
there is a growing literature suggesting that individual psychotherapy
(Bowman, Blix & Coons, 1985; Dell & Eisenhower, 1990; Kluft, 1985) and
inpatient hospitalization (Hornstein & Tyson, 1991) can be beneficial for
adolescents with dissociative disorders, nothing has been written about
group psychotherapy with these patients. This absence of literature suggests that few, if any, clinicians have attempted to conduct groups with
dissociative adolescents and that little is known about the potential impact of such groups. This paper is pragmatic in orientation and outlines a
rationale for a group for dissociative adolescents, its history and format,
a summary of the common themes and difficulties encountered, and patients' reactions to the group. The results reported here are considered
preliminary (the group has only been in existence for one year) and of possible potential benefit as a pioneering attempt to extend the literature on
the treatment of dissociative adolescents.

The author first considered creating a psychotherapy group for dissociative youth when deluged by a number of requests for diagnostic and
therapeutic consultations with outpatient and inpatient children and
adolescents at a hospital well-known for its specialization in treating dissociative disorders (Sheppard and Enoch Pratt Hospital, Baltimore). The
number of children and adolescents diagnosed with dissociative disorders, most frequently dissociative disorder not otherwise specified
(DDNOS) and dissociative identity disorder (DID, formerly known as
multiple personality disorder) suggested a need for specialized treatment

for these patients that outstripped the hospital's and community's available services. At least as important, these children and adolescents often felt very alone, "crazy," and stigmatized by their disorder and the trauma which they had endured.

Our successful experience with adult group psychotherapy supplements a small body of clinical literature which suggested that group psychotherapy for dissociative adults is beneficial (Coons & Bradley, 1985; Courtois & Turkus, 1994; Hogan, 1992; Karfgin, 1994). It was hoped that by adapting the techniques used successfully in dissociative adult group psychotherapy, dissociative teenagers could be helped. This group was formulated as an informal experiment to test its potential efficacy, to extend the available resources, and to offer the isolated adolescents the hoped-for benefit of decreasing their isolation and stigmatization via sharing stories of similar experiences with peers in a group.

The group was intended to be supportive, educational, and structured in its format to avoid provoking disruptive symptoms such as flashbacks and uncontrolled switching to unmanageable alter personalities. It was viewed as an adjunct to individual psychotherapy with specific goals of increasing the girls' knowledge about their symptoms, enhancing self-esteem, and decreasing the girls' sense of "craziness" and isolation.

The sparse literature (Silberg et al., in press) recommended homogeneous group therapy for adolescent DID patients only during "the most stable periods of their treatment." Although this recommendation is wise, the nature of many of the referrals (many came from an inpatient setting) presented a dilemma about which patients to admit. It was impossible to admit all the dissociative adolescents due to their wide range of functioning, degree of potential dangerousness to themselves or others, and degree of discomfort with discussing their diagnosis or personal issues within a group format.

Creation of the Group

The first step in creating the group was discussing it as a possibility in consultation with clinicians familiar with treating dissociative adolescents and adults. Referrals were sought by announcing the group at a conference on dissociative disorders and by mailing flyers to in-house therapists and to treatment centers and clinicians in the community who specialize in treating traumatized patients.

Initially it was unclear whether the group would be for males or females, adolescents or children. Because all the referrals were female and most of them were adolescent, a fairly homogeneous group was created by selecting female adolescents between the ages of 12 and 18 who were diagnosed with a severe dissociative disorder (DDNOS or DID). To qualify for the group, the girls had to voluntarily agree to participate and had to be in individual psychotherapy with a therapist who endorsed the addition of group psychotherapy. Outpatients required family or guardian support and inpatients required support of the inpatient team.

Although it was hoped that the majority of members would be able to attend the group for several months or more, this was not often possible. Many of the girls had sudden shifts in placements or had financial or transportation constraints. Financial assistance was available for some of the girls through the hospital. Without this assistance it is unlikely the group could have survived, due to the financial limitations faced by most of the biological or foster families or the girls' custodial guardians, such as the Department of Social Services.

Most of the adolescent girls who were diagnosed with DDNOS or DID at the hospital were initially welcomed into the group, but experience suggested that some newly diagnosed adolescents were too afraid of the diagnosis and peers who shared this illness to comfortably join the group. Furthermore, it was decided that only girls who would be able to attend the group for at least several months should be included, due to the disruption to the already established group process. Newly diagnosed adolescents did find the group helpful in addressing their initial concerns and questions about their diagnosis. The more senior members of the group often seemed to enjoy sharing their knowledge and experience with the new referrals although there was occasional hesitancy to self-disclose due to issues of trust.

The trauma literature suggests significant benefit from the use of a co-therapist for survivor groups (e.g., Cole & Barney, 1987; Courtois 1988; Herman & Schatzow, 1984; Sprei, 1987). The benefits of co-therapy teams in leading groups for trauma survivors include mutual support, shared observation and processing, and the potential for decreasing the intensity of counter-transference reactions (Courtois, 1988). Female-female co-therapy teams have been recommended by some authors (Herman & Schatzow, 1984; Sprei, 1987).

The co-therapists in the adolescent dissociative group were female, which seemed to help the members feel more trust and fostered identification with the leaders. One of the co-therapists was Caucasian and the other was African-American, which may have helped girls from different ethnic and racial backgrounds feel more comfortable. One of the co-therapists was a nurse manager within the hospital and had considerable experience in leading adolescent groups, while the other had experience in leading adult dissociative psychotherapy groups and in providing individual psychotherapy with dissociative children, adolescents, and adults. The co-therapists' differences have been beneficial in providing different perspectives on group dynamics, styles of intervention, and a wider base of knowledge and skill.

It was essential during difficult moments in the group to have both co-therapists present to help manage the girls and process interactions. For example, occasionally one of the members reported feeling self-destructive during the group. Having two co-therapists present allowed one of them to escort the girl back to the inpatient unit after the group or to meet with the girl to discuss a plan for helping her remain safe. Only rarely was it necessary to refer the girl to her individual therapist for an emergency phone call or therapy session. Because most of the girls are chronically suicidal or self-destructive, it was assumed that acting-out behavior would occur on occasion before, during, or after the group. The co-therapists implemented limits and structure the group so as to minimize the frequency of unsafe behavior.

Group Format

The group was conceptualized as primarily supportive and educational in nature. Initially it was carefully structured around concrete paper and pencil exercises (adapted from Golden Mandell & Damon, 1989, and Spinal-Robinson & Easton Wickham, 1992) and art projects. For example, the girls made collages depicting specific feelings and drew "what it feels like to be inside your head with your alters." These concrete activities helped to decrease the members' anxiety, facilitated group sharing, deterred acting out, and increased self-awareness through exploration and expression of feelings. As the members learned to trust each other and the co-therapists more, they became willing to admit problems and spontaneously asked the group for help. Thus, structure came increasingly from the members. For example, one girl told the group that she had "lost time" so frequently in the prior month that she was unaware of the causes of changes in her relationships with her classmates. The group spent the session discussing ways to decrease amnesia and increase cooperation among the alters who were interfering with her relationships. Additionally, group dynamics have begun to unfold which have been crucial to address, such as testing limits, competition for attention and control, and collaborative resistance (MacLennan & Dies, 1992). Thus, the group has become less structured and at times it resembles a therapy group more than a support group (Yalom, 1985).

The group met every other week for one hour, at the request of the girls. Some were concerned about the long commute and wanted to have "some nights off from therapy" so they could participate in sports and social activities. The group room was in the outpatient section of the hospital and had a small table around which chairs were gathered. Each group began with introductions if needed and updates on important events that had taken place since the last group. The "updates" were initiated after it was realized that the girls were often preoccupied with important real life occurrences such as changing foster care placements and court proceedings against their abusers. Beginning the group with an opportunity to discuss these complicated issues helped build cohesion and a sense of being important and cared about, as well as giving the group a focus for starting discussion. Prior to instituting this structure, it had been difficult for the girls to reconnect to the group after having not met for two weeks.

In each girl's initial session, they were invited to decorate a folder with stickers, markers, and glitter pens, which they could use to keep the group exercises, drawings, and journaling. This afforded newcomers a way to slowly enter into the group and decrease their anxiety. This was a favorite activity. One girl who had a particularly tragic history of deprivation and abuse asked repeatedly to create new folders, which was permitted because it seemed to give her such a sense of importance and self-nurturance.

A closing ritual evolved in which each girl identified what she hoped for herself or wanted to work on until the next group. This structure was initiated after the group twice ended on a pessimistic note with one or more girls discussing how depressed they felt. It was hoped that ending on a more forward-looking note would help the group be more supportive of safety and growth.

Group Rules

The co-therapists formulated guidelines to encourage a cohesive group with safe limits. These guidelines were initially repeated at the beginning of the sessions but then were reiterated only when a new member joined the group. The rules were:

1. No graphic talk about details of the abuse. This rule was created to prevent destabilization, flashbacks, and potential "contamination" regarding types of abuse the girls reported having experienced.
2. Attempt to avoid switching to alter personalities, especially destructive or child alters, which may be disruptive to the group.
3. Be respectful of other members. No one is allowed to ridicule another's feelings, thoughts, behaviors, or treatment.
4. Tell the group if you are having any internal difficulties. This rule gives the girls permission to discuss internal conflicts such as alters telling them not to talk or trying to distract them. Encouragement to discuss these issues was crucial for the group process because so much of what the girls experience was difficult to decipher from body language and because for so much of their lives their feelings and internal experiences had been shrouded in secrecy.
5. If you are disruptive after being given notice that your behavior is not acceptable, you may be asked to leave the group for a time-out. This rule was instituted because members were occasionally unable or un-

willing to control their behavior, despite efforts to process this. Sometimes inappropriate behaviors appeared to be caused by rapidly switching between alters or uncontrolled affect. Taking a time-out outside of the group room helped members calm down and decreased the switching. The hope was that as the group developed, verbal confrontation alone would be sufficient in helping the girls contain themselves.

Discussion Topics

The co-therapists created a list of discussion topics based on their experience of common issues that dissociative adolescents discuss in individual therapy and issues that dissociative adults discuss in group therapy. The topics are listed in the order of presentation in the group, although these topics frequently surfaced during the course of group discussions. This was interpreted as an indication that these concerns were of significant concern for dissociative adolescents. The following outline details the issues, frequently asked questions, and exercises used to encourage discussion and self-reflection.

1) Dissociation:

What is it? When do members dissociate? Are there good times and not such good times to dissociate? How do people react when members dissociate? The consensus regarding how to manage dissociation in the group was to call the person's name repeatedly until the girl became reoriented to the group. The girls were embarrassed about their potential for dissociating in the group and were quite sensitive about how this would be managed. The girls were encouraged to define dissociation in their own words and to give examples of how they look and behave when dissociating.

Exercises:
- Draw where you are, what is happening, or what you are thinking about when you dissociate.
- List the feelings that trigger dissociation.

2) Dissociative Identity Disorder:

What is it? Is it good or bad? How did you find out you had parts inside? How do you refer to your parts (e.g., as personalities, parts, inside children, alters, feelings, etc.)? What were your reactions to the diagnosis initially and over time? How do your family, friends, and therapist react to your diagnosis? What did you think this diagnosis meant at first? Now?

The co-therapists often mentioned that a common strength the girls shared was having survived scary things by using their minds creatively. Helping them reframe their disorder as a creative way to survive a situation which many people would not have been able to survive decreased shame. They were encouraged to think about their inner strengths, including alters, which enabled them to survive.

Many of the girls became animated during these discussions as they related how they had lost many friends and relationships with family members due to people's misperceptions about DID. This often led to a discussion of the media's treatment of the disorder, prejudice and discrimination, and famous people who were alleged to have DID or to be victims of childhood abuse.

This topic brought up both ambivalence about having revealed the abuse and ambivalence towards alleged abusers. The co-therapists believed that the repeated discussions of variations around this topic were the most helpful aspect of the group in decreasing the girls' sense of shame and isolation.

Exercises:
- Take turns reading preselected excepts from books about dissociation, including *Can I Look Now?* (Downing, 1992), and from *Multiple Personality Disorder from the Inside Out* (Cohen, Giller, & W., 1991).
- Draw what it feels like to have inside parts.

3) Trust:

How can you tell if someone is trustworthy? How do you respond when you initially meet someone? Is it better to trust all at once, gradually over time, or never to trust? What effect does it have on you if you do not trust anyone? Whom do you tell about your diagnosis and abuse? Can you get better if you do not trust your therapist? How can we build trust in this group?

Exercise:
- The whole group can draw one big poster of the extremes of trusting no one versus immediately trusting someone completely. Create in the center of the picture what a "middle ground" approach to trust might be.

4) Feelings:

How can you identify feelings? Are there certain feelings that are more difficult to identify? Which feelings are more difficult to deal with safely? What are good ways and not such good ways to deal with anger, loneliness, helplessness, sadness, happiness, guilt, shame?

This topic was one of the more perplexing issues for the girls. They often mislabeled the feelings which people in magazines depicted. For example, a child who looked scared was described as excited. They had difficulty even recognizing feelings so we often repeated this topic at a basic level.

Exercises:
- Create a group collage depicting three different feelings (e.g., fear, happiness, anger) from magazine pictures.
- Complete a survey about the frequency with which you experience a list of feelings (adapted from Spinal-Robinson & Easton Wickham, 1992). Discuss the situations which cause you to feel these feelings.
- Create a group list of safe ways to deal with different feelings.

5) Safety:

What does it mean to be safe? Have you ever felt safe? Would you like to feel safe? Do some of your alters seem to prefer to be unsafe? Why do they do that? What places or people are safe? Discuss whether self-harm is safe or not.

Some girls reported having alters who believed that "hurting yourself is an okay way to deal with feelings." The girls were encouraged to think through such cognitive distortions by asking them the long-term pros and cons of self-harm. The group discussed what steps members had taken to get safer. The concept of internal safe places (see Kluft, 1989) was discussed. If someone in the group had already learned how to make an internal safe place, we asked her to describe how she did it and how it helped her.

Exercise:
- Would any of your parts like to have an inside safe place? Make a collage or drawing of what each girl would want inside her safe place. Encourage the girls to use all five senses to help make her safe place more "real" and therefore helpful during times of stress.
- Encourage girls to practice getting alters to safe places for homework or with their individual therapist.

6) One System, One Inside Family, One Body:

How do your parts interact? Are they lonely, afraid, frequently fighting, or working together as a team? Do any of your parts feel different emotions, like different things, do different jobs? Do your parts realize they share one body? Do you think they are separate from you? How do you make decisions when there are different points of view inside?

Some members thought they would cease to exist if other parts took over, or that somehow they magically had different bodies due to not feeling pain, having amnesia, or hallucinating that their body looked differently according to which alter was "out." We found it important not to force members to change their ideas. Rather, members were encouraged to try to be open to different explanations from peers and co-therapists. This discussion often led into the next topic.

7) Group Decision Making and Compromising:

How do you handle it when different parts of you want to do something wrong or different from what you want to do? How can everyone inside feel that their needs, feelings, and points of view are important? What are examples of how members have negotiated compromises with parts?

Exercise:
• Make a group list of how to handle inside disagreements. (See list below for ways to handle conflicts that the group created.)

How To Balance Things Inside
1. Find a common goal.
2. Have each part give in partially.
3. Voice your opinion.
4. Give yourself time to cool off.
5. Rationalize things. (The girls meant that they should try to understand each part's point of view and needs.)
6. Agree on a way to meet a part's need that is more agreeable to your needs.
7. Find out by talking or journaling if someone inside is upset.
8. Get hold of your therapist in an emergency.
9. Go to a safe place or a safe person as soon as possible.
10. Stay away from situations that cause you to be suicidal.

Things Not To Do in a Compromise:
1. Be stubborn.
2. Give in completely (because then you will get mad later).
3. Give the others the silent treatment.
4. Have a large argument over it.
5. Agree to do something that makes you uncomfortable.
6. Take it out on your body.

8) Posttraumatic Stress Disorder:

What is it? What are its symptoms? How can you manage flashbacks, body memories, nightmares, and extreme fear? What things scare you? What are good and bad ways to handle being afraid? How do you tell if something is real or not when you are afraid of it (e.g., hallucinations of past trauma)?

This discussion often required more than one group sessions. Girls were taught containment techniques such as turning down feelings as you would the volume dial on a stereo. Flashbacks were imagined as if on a television screen connected to a VCR machine, and clients were taught to turn off the picture and sound, eject the tape with all thoughts, feelings, and sensations related to memory recorded on it, and put the tape in an imagined internal secure place such as a bank vault. (For more containment techniques, see Hammond, 1990; Kluft, 1982, 1983, 1985b, 1989.)

Exercises:
- Make a group poster listing examples of extreme ways to deal with fear: "jumping into it" and "jumping away from it." (See lists below for examples that the dissociative adolescents created.) This exercise is a helpful way to present the biphasic nature of PTSD in easy-to-understand language.
- Create a list of "middle of the road" ways to deal with fear.
- Practice containment techniques for homework (alone or with your individual therapist), progressing from neutral stimuli such as cartoons to slightly anxiety-producing stimuli, until you feel confident about being able to put away disturbing memories.

Ways to Respond to Fear

"Jump Into It"
1. Wallow in fear. Think about what happened to you all the time.
2. Watch scary movies and read scary books.
3. Talk about what happened to you a lot.
4. Do dangerous or risky things like speeding, cutting classes, stealing.

"Middle of the Road"
1. Have other people around. Talk with friends about your feelings.
2. Take medication as prescribed.
3. Tell yourself calming things.
4. Have your parts tell you calming things.
5. Tell yourself the flashbacks are not real now because they happened long ago.

6. Tell jokes.
7. Remind yourself of the good things about people.
8. Talk on the phone.
9. Watch comedies.
10. Do inside safe places.
11. Do feelings dials.

"Jump Away from It"
1. Pretend you are not present (i.e., dissociate).
2. Get out of your body (i.e., out of body experience).
3. Run away literally.
4. Distract yourself by staying on the phone all night, watching TV constantly, joking all the time.
5. Act weird, crazy.
6. Forget it happened.
7. Space out.
8. Use drugs or alcohol.

Special Problems

Group Dynamics

Dissociative patients have a variety of "traumatic transferences" in therapeutic relationships (Loewenstein, 1993; Wilbur, 1988). Feelings and behavioral sequences that trauma survivors experienced during the abuse tend to get played out with others, including with therapists and group members. While the group was intended primarily for support rather than for therapeutic interpretation of trauma reenactments, an understanding of these dynamics contributed to an appreciation of the group dynamics. At times the group process was sufficiently exaggerated or disruptive that ignoring the dynamics would have been detrimental to the functioning of the group. Terror, helplessness, and identification with the aggressor were traumatic transference reactions which were observed by the co-therapists in the group.

The girls in this group had more difficulty than usual confronting each other and talking assertively about their views and feelings. Most of the girls quickly became passive if a peer began to act out. They began to dissociate or became quiet, seemingly falling into a role of passive child "victim" while the unruly "perpetrator" adolescent got out of control. The co-therapists felt a pull to watch silently in surprise as the acting out member was not confronted by her peers (i.e., reenacting the "unprotective mother" role) or to jump in to save the victim (i.e., reenacting the "rescuer" role). (See Messler, Davies, & Frawley, 1994, for a discussion of these roles.)

Scapegoating was not only directed at group members. Often therapeutic staff in general or more explicitly, the co-therapists, were seen as unhelpful, uncaring, "uncool," or uninformed. The co-therapists became the targets of anger displaced from abusers, from therapists who misdiagnosed the girls or who were in some way unhelpful, or from family and friends by whom the girls feel betrayed. These interpretations were not offered in the group. Instead, if a girl was appropriately expressing her feelings, she was allowed to do so and was often given support for safely expressing herself as long as she was not detracting from the group focus. It was hoped that as the group matured, the concept of displaced anger could be explained and explored, but in the meantime such an attempt would have been wounding or summarily dismissed.

Roles developed in the group, one of which was to act out against authority. The girls were encouraged to consider what impact this behavior was likely to have in the long run. A girl may have bragged, for example, of being oppositional at school. Only very gradually were girls in this role able to admit that this behavior made them lonely and isolated.

Family Issues

The degree of family and parents stress had an important impact on the girls. A parents' group was eventually created and offered at the same time as the girls' group to assist the girls' parents in understanding their daughters' behaviors and disorder and to help encourage positive, supportive interactions amongst the families. This group was led by a psychologist with expertise in treating dissociative children and adolescents. To decrease the girls' fears regarding confidentiality and to thwart potential power struggles amongst the parents and children, the girls were informed of the group and asked to discuss their feelings about it before it was offered. Because their feelings were considered and their concerns dealt with openly, all the girls agreed to allow their parents to participate. They were given the opportunity to authorize their parents' participation by signing the following "permission slip":

> "I hereby give permission for _____ *(parent's name)*
> to participate in the parents' group. I understand that my parents will
> not use the group to discuss details of my history and other confiden-
> tial information. I understand that the purpose of the group is to learn
> general guidelines about how to help kids with my kinds of problems.
> I understand that my parents may occasionally tell accounts of my be-
> havior and how I was dealt with for the purpose of helping other par-
> ents deal with their kids. I understand that my parents will not share
> with me information learned in the group about other kids. Signed
> _____ *(daughter's signature)* "

The parents' group was quite popular amongst the parents (all mothers) who were able to attend, although many parents were not able to come due to work and child care obligations. The group validated the parents' struggles with managing the diagnosis and helped diffuse feelings of anger, guilt, and helplessness among the parents (Silberg, personal communication).

Group Cohesion

One of the most difficult aspects of conducting the group was that of creating a cohesive group. A number of variables contributed to this including the wide variation in cognitive and psychological sophistication amongst the girls, the severity of their symptoms which often impeded their concentration and frequently required hospitalization, the disruptive influence of quick turnover in membership due to placement changes, and the girls' fear of getting hurt by opening up intense feelings or by being disliked or rejected by the group. To improve attendance, a rule was instituted in which families were responsible for paying for more than two missed sessions in six months. Referrals were also screened more carefully to determine who might be likely to attend infrequently or drop out soon.

To address the common fear of feelings and potential rejection, the group became somewhat more process oriented. Maladaptive defenses that prevented the girls from getting better were gently discussed. For example, sometimes girls became silly and disruptive when difficult issues were addressed. The co-therapists nicknamed this behavior "wearing a shield" so that attention could be called to the dynamic and the underlying reason for girls' behavior. When therapists attempted to resolve disputes which sometimes occurred between group members, the issue of favoritism emerged. On one occasion, this led to an important discussion in which each girl shared that she felt herself to be the least "liked" in some way by the co-therapists and the other girls. The members were surprised to hear how pervasive was the sense of inferiority in the other girls. This provided an opportunity for discussing that low self-esteem is a normal consequence of having been abused. The girls could see that, in reality, all of them could not be the "worst," so their cognitive distortion about their lack of worth was confronted.

Developmental Tasks of Adolescence

Another challenge in leading this group has been finding a balance between educating about and focusing on illness and symptoms and focusing on strengths and normal adolescent issues. The group leaders were sensitive to not overly pathologizing the patients or having them become overly invested in their dissociative diagnosis. This was accomplished by emphasizing normal aspects of development and providing a role model. The role model was an articulate dissociative college student who was further along in her treatment than were the group members. As a guest speaker, this young woman openly discussed with the girls her struggle with symptoms related to her DID and PTSD over five years of therapy. She shared ways she had increased her inner communication and cooperation. This guest appearance of a beautiful and obviously "not crazy" young woman helped some of the girls become more motivated in their treatment and encouraged them to set higher goals for themselves.

The girls requested that the group celebrate birthdays together after they discovered how many of them had had holidays marred by abuse or disappointment. Thus, we celebrated each girl's birthday by having a special treat and making a birthday card in the group. The group also began by briefly discussing important events that occurred between groups. This was often a time when the members discussed how relationships were going at school and with their boyfriends. This gave the girls time to simply enjoy and share the normal ups and downs of adolescence. This was important because they had rarely had the chance to innocently enjoy the simple pleasures of their childhoods.

Conclusion

The co-therapists believe that the group helped the girls feel better about themselves, their disorders, and other people. At times it was extremely challenging to lead, due to the severity of the girls' symptoms, the fragility of some of their families or placements, and the transference issues which were played out in the group. Most of the girls reported that the group was enjoyable and helpful. When asked what was most helpful about the group, the girls usually said they found it most helpful to learn that they were not alone with their problems and feelings. The sense of universality in the group challenged their secret fear that they could not be helped, liked, or understood. Perhaps the lessons learned from this group will encourage other clinicians to experiment with group psychotherapy for dissociative adolescents. It remains to be seen how such groups will fare over time and which dissociative patients will most benefit from group psychotherapy.

References

Bowman, E. S., Blix, S., & Coons, P.M. (1985). Multiple personality in adolescence: Relationship to incestual experiences. *Journal of the American Academy of Child Psychiatry, 24,* 109–114.

Cohen, B. M., Giller, E., & W. L. (1991). *Multiple personality disorder from the inside out*. Lutherville, MD: Sidran Press.

Cole, C. H., & Barney, E. E. (1987). Safeguards and the therapeutic window: A group treatment strategy for adult incest survivors. *American Journal of Orthopsychiatry, 57*, 601–609.

Coons, P. M., & Bradley, K. (1985). Group psychotherapy with multiple personality patients. *Journal of Nervous and Mental Disease, 173*, 515–521.

Courtois, C. (1988). *Healing the incest wound: Adult survivors in therapy*. New York: Norton.

Courtois, C. A., & Turkus, J. A. (1994, June). *Group therapy with dissociative disorder clients*. Paper presented at the Sixth Annual Eastern Regional Conference on Abuse and Multiple Personality, The Psychiatric Institute of Washington, DC.

Dell, P., & Eisenhower, J. W. (1990). Adolescent multiple personality disorder. A preliminary study of eleven cases. *Journal Academy of Child and Adolescent Psychiatry, 29*, 359–366.

Downing, R. (1992). *Can I look now? Recovery from multiple personality disorder*. Baltimore: Educational Recovery Communication.

Golden Mandell, J., & Damon, L. (1989). *Group treatment for sexually abused children*. New York: Guilford.

Hammond, C. (Ed.). (1990). *Handbook of hypnotic suggestions and metaphor*. New York: Norton.

Herman, J., & Schatzow, E. (1984). Time-limited group therapy for women with a history of incest. *International Journal of Group Psychotherapy, 34*, 605–616.

Hogan, L. C., (1992). Managing persons with multiple personality disorder in a heterogeneous inpatient group. *Group, 16*, 247–256.

Hornstein, N. L. & Tyson, S. (1991). Inpatient treatment of children with multiple personality/dissociative disorders and their families. *The Psychiatric Clinics of North America—Multiple Personality Disorder, 14* (3), p. 631–648.

Karfgin, A. (1994, September). *Inpatient and outpatient group psychotherapy for dissociative identity disorder*. Paper presented at Dissociative Disorders: Rigorous Assessment and Responsible Treatment in the 1990s, The Sheppard and Enoch Pratt Hospital, Baltimore, MD.

Kluft, R. P. (1982). Varieties of hypnotic interventions in the treatment of multiple personality disorder. *American Journal of Clinical Hypnosis, 23*(4), 230–240.

Kluft, R. P. (1983). Hypnotherapeutic crisis intervention with multiple personality disorder. *American Journal of Clinical Hypnosis, 26*(2), 73–83.

Kluft, R. P. (1985a). Childhood multiple personality disorder: Predictors, clinical findings, and treatment results. In R.P. Kluft (Ed.), *Childhood antecedents of multiple personality* (pp. 167–196). Washington, DC: American Psychiatric Press.

Kluft, R. P. (1985b). Hypnotherapy of childhood multiple personality disorder. *American Journal of Clinical Hypnosis, 27*, 201–210.

Kluft, R. P. (1989). Playing for time: Temporizing techniques in the treatment of multiple personality disorder. *American Journal of Clinical Hypnosis, 32*(2), 90–98.

Loewenstein, R.J . (1993). Posttraumatic and dissociative aspects of transference and countertransference in the treatment of multiple personality disorder. In

R. P. Kluft & C. S. Fine (Eds.), *Clinical Perspectives on multiple personality disorders* (pp. 51–85). Washington, DC: American Psychiatric Press.

MacLennan, B. W., & Dies, K. R. (1992). *Group counseling and psychotherapy with adolescents* (2nd ed.). New York: Columbia University Press.

Messler Davies, J., & Frawley, M. G. (1994). *Treating the adult survivor of childhood sexual abuse: A Psychoanalytic perspective.* New York: Basic Books.

Silberg, J. L., Stipic, D., & Taghizadeh, F. (in press). Dissociative disorders in children and adolescents. In J. Nosphitz (Ed.), *Handbook of Child and Adolescent Psychiatry*. New York: John Wiley & Sons.

Spinal-Robinson, P., & Easton Wickham, R. (1992). *Cartwheels: A workbook for children who have been sexually abused.* Notre Dame, IN: Jalice Publishers.

Sprei, J. E. (1987). Group treatment of adult women incest survivors. In C. M. Brody (Ed.), *Women's therapy groups* (pp. 198–216). New York: Spring Publishing.

Wilbur, C. (1988). Multiple personality disorder and transference. *Dissociation, 1*(1), 73–76.

Yalom, I. D. (1985). *The theory and practice of group psychotherapy* (3rd ed.). New York: Basic Books.

twelve

Psychopharmacologic Interventions for Children and Adolescents with Dissociative Disorders

Elaine D. Nemzer

Dissociative identity disorder (DID), previously called multiple personality disorder (MPD), is a chronic, complex form of dissociative disorder, characterized by disturbances in memory and identity. Retrospective case histories of adult and child DID patients have found that DID is associated with severe, repetitive trauma or abuse during early childhood (Putnam, 1989). In childhood, DID may present in a more preliminary form—"incipient multiple personality disorder" (Fagan & McMahon, 1984), currently diagnosed as dissociative disorder, not otherwise specified (DDNOS). For the ease of discussion, the DDNOS child and adolescent will be included under the general heading of DID, as the medication issues are identical.

As the post-traumatic roots of DID have become better understood, the considerable overlap between DID and post-traumatic stress disorder (PTSD) is more apparent. Loewenstein (1991) described DID as a "post-traumatic dissociative developmental disorder" and found that 80% of dissociative patients also met DSM-III criteria for PTSD. Dissociative disorders share many features with PTSD. Putnam (1994) reports that approximately 50% of adult PTSD patients have pathological levels of dissociation. Hornstein and Putnam (1992), in a study of child and adolescent dissociative disorders, found that 80–90% of DID children had post-traumatic symptoms, including hypervigilance, hyper-startle reactions, traumatic nightmares, and intrusive thoughts.

Dr. Nemzer is grateful to David Scandinero, M.D., for his background information and helpful discussions which contributed to the preparation of this chapter.

Research in the neurobiology and psychopharmacology of adults and children diagnosed with PTSD (which has been more extensively studied than DID) provides insights into the pathophysiology of dissociation and possible treatments for it.

This chapter focuses on the use of medication for dissociative disorders. Unfortunately, we do not currently have medications that treat the most problematic core symptoms of dissociative disorders: amnesias, instability of consciousness, and identity alteration (switching). Psychopharmacology is not the primary therapeutic approach for these symptoms or for dissociative disorders in general, and medications should not be used as the sole treatment modality. Many children with dissociative disorders do not need medication and should not be exposed to the potential side effects unnecessarily. Dissociative children without clearly targetable symptoms or syndromes (e.g., sleep problems, hyperarousal, depression, ADHD, etc.) should be treated exclusively with psychosocial and psychotherapeutic interventions.

However, medications can be helpful as an adjunct to psychotherapy and as part of a comprehensive treatment program. Medications can be useful in alleviating specific symptoms (such as overwhelming anxiety or severe insomnia) that may interfere with daily functioning and with progress in psychotherapy. Medications can also be used to treat common co-morbid conditions in a child with DID, such as attention deficit/hyperactivity disorder (ADHD) and major depression. See page 266 for guidelines on when to use which drugs and page 267 for a list of generic and trade names.

With both adult and child dissociative disorder, the diagnostic issues of co-morbidity are complicated. In general, when treating adults who have DID, symptoms that involve mood, anxiety, or personality should be assumed to be secondary to the dissociative disorder and not treated as separate disorders (Loewenstein, 1991; Putnam, 1989). This principle may not be as applicable to children with DID. For example, given the high prevalence of ADHD in pediatric populations, it is likely that a very active and distractible child with DID may also have ADHD and stimulant medications would be beneficial.

I will discuss the neurobiology of acute and chronic trauma, and review the theoretical rationale for currently and potentially useful pharmacological interventions. Special emphasis is placed on clinical issues in the use of medication for children and adolescents with dissociative disorders.

The information presented here is based on the adult and child DID literature, child psychopharmacology research and the author's clinical experience. There are few double-blind, placebo-controlled studies on the medical treatment of PTSD or DID in children or adolescents. Most published work is open-label in small series or anecdotal case reports. Many of the uses of medications discussed in this chapter differ from the indications or age groups that the FDA has formally approved to be advertised as safe and effective. Many of these "off-label" uses of medication are commonly accepted medical practice, some non-approved uses are less widely accepted, and some are still in the clinical research phase. The suggestions discussed here should be viewed as preliminary and are offered in the spirit of furthering the currently meager literature on the psychopharmacology of childhood DID. It is assumed that medication will be prescribed by trained psychiatrists with a specialty in child work and that no recommendations here will be applied to specific children without a thorough physical and psychological assessment, careful consideration of all of the options, and informed consent of the caregivers.

Neurobiological Basis for PTSD and Dissociative Disorders

An examination of current research and theory in the neurobiology of dissociation and PTSD will lay the ground work for a better understanding of psychopharmacological issues. Since the early 1980s, research into the neurobiology of humans and animals has greatly advanced our understanding of the abnormalities induced by acute and chronic stress. Acute traumatic stress activates a complicated set of interrelated processes in a reaction termed the "alarm" or "flight or fight" mechanism. This mechanism, which is highly adaptive for individual survival in situations of immediate danger, affects a number of body systems, including central nervous system neurotransmitters, the peripheral autonomic nervous system, the hypothalamic-pituitary-adrenal (HPA) axis, and the endogenous opioid system (van der Kolk & Fisler, 1993).

The alarm reaction sensitizes catecholamine neurotransmitters and receptors to subsequent stimulation. Neural networks involved in sensations, perceptions, and memory processing become attuned to react quickly to future threats of danger. This normal reaction to trauma usually promotes an individual's survival, but in cases of special vulnerability or when the stressor is prolonged or intense, an excessive maladaptive response can occur, producing post-traumatic stress symptoms. This mechanism leads to the PTSD symptoms of hyper-reactivity and hyper-arousal. Through feedback inhibition this sensitization may also produce symptoms of hypo-reactivity, such as avoidance and numbing (Schwarz, 1994).

The autonomic arousal associated with PTSD is manifested as elevated resting heart rate, systolic blood pressure, and muscle tone. Clinically this is seen as hypervigilance, excessive startle reaction, and over-reactivity to traumagenic stimuli. Increased production of catecholamines (as measured in urine), a marker for autonomic dysfunction, has been documented, both in veterans with combat-related PTSD (Yehuda, Southwick, Giller, Ma, & Mason, 1992) in sexually abused children (DeBellis, Lefter, Trickett, & Putnam, 1994).

Traumatic stress also affects the hypothalamic-pituitary-adrenal axis in complicated ways. An acute stressor initiates the process by which corticotropin-releasing hormone (CRH), produced in the hypothalamus, stimulates pituitary ACTH secretion, which triggers the adrenal release of gluco-corticoids or cortisol. Excessive production of cortisol can inhibit growth, reproduction, and immune inflammatory response (DeBellis & Putnam, 1994).

While the effects of even acute time-limited stress on a mature nervous system are dramatic and can lead to PTSD, severe, repetitive traumatic stress can cause alterations of brain physiology and anatomy. Prolonged stress in a young child, whose nervous system is still rapidly developing, can have profound effects in terms of neural growth, migration, and differentiation (Perry, 1994b). These effects may be part of the neurophysiological basis of pathological dissociation. Ornitz and Pynoos (1989) suggest that alterations of brain stem circuits, due to chronic trauma, may be responsible for excessive startle reflex in children with PTSD. Maturation of these brain stem circuits is completed around the age of eight years, so younger children are especially vulnerable to physiological brain changes caused by traumatic stress. This aspect of neuro-development is consistent with the observation that DID rarely develops in individuals whose trauma began after the age of eight.

Several recent magnetic resonance imaging (MRI) studies of the brain, focusing on centers critical to memory processing, have shown the hippocampal volume to be smaller than average in women subjected to sexual abuse as children (Stein, 1995), and in combat veterans with PTSD (Bremner et al., 1995). The proposed mechanism is that the high level of endogenous cortisol secretion associated with the stress reaction has a neurotoxic effect on the hippocampus. Stein (1995) found an inverse correlation between severity of Dissociative Experience Scale scores and size of hippocampus on MRI. Actual degeneration of hippocampal neurons has been observed in the brains of monkeys following psychic stress (Sapolsky, Uno, Rebert, & Finch, 1990). Difficulty with the retrieval of memory (a hallmark feature of dissociative disorders) may be related to this anatomical abnormality.

Acute and chronic trauma can also cause abnormalities of endogenous opioids. The alarm mechanism affects the body's production of endogenous opioids and may be the basis of the alterations in sensory experience and pain perception that occur in PTSD and DID. Resting pain threshold is lowered, i.e., minor pain is felt more acutely. In contrast, severe acute pain in PTSD patients induces significant analgesia. The stress-induced analgesia is reversed experimentally by naloxone (an opiate-blocker), strongly suggesting that the opioid system is involved in these PTSD symptoms (Pittman & van der Kolk, 1990). Cutting or other self-injury is a common behavior in DID patients. These maladaptive behavior patterns may be reinforced by triggering endogenous opioids. This may be a conditioned response to opioid release during childhood abuse. That is, a child who has been subjected to repeated episodes of severe pain followed by endogenous opioid release learns to evoke this process by self-inflicted pain.

In contrast to the hypercortisol state associated with acute trauma, repetitive or chronic stress produces alterations in receptor sensitivity, resulting in a negative feedback situation. This leads to long term hypofunctioning of the HPA axis and low levels of cortisol secretion.

Studies using biological probes have uncovered dysregulation of a number of neuroendocrine systems in individuals with trauma histories. Besides the HPA axis, abnormalities have been detected in thyroid function, growth hormone, and sex hormones (DeBellis & Putnam, 1994). Although physical stress may cause delayed puberty, a few studies suggest that sexual abuse can trigger earlier onset of puberty (Putnam & Trickett, 1993). These processes are complex and not completely understood.

Sleep and dream abnormalities are frequently present in traumatized children and adults. This includes difficulty falling asleep, increased awakenings, less time in stage 4 (deep) sleep, increased body movement, and traumatic nightmares (Inman, Silver, & Doghnamji, 1990). Children with PTSD and DID experience an increased frequency of both nightmares, primarily in REM sleep, and night terrors in stage 4 sleep (Pynoos, 1990). Although the neuropathology of sleep disorders is not well-understood, these deficits could be related to physiological hyperarousal or neurotransmitter dysfunction.

Recent studies on drug-induced dissociation have greatly added to the research on the neurobiology of the dissociative process. Short-acting barbiturates, lactate, yohimbine, and MCPP (m-chlorophenylpiperazine) can all trigger flashbacks, panic attacks, and intrusive memories in individuals with panic disorder or PTSD (Krystal et al., 1994). Dissociative symptoms can be triggered even in normal subjects by marijuana, LSD, mescaline, and most notably ketamine (an anesthetic). Krystal et al. (1994) reported that the administration of sub-anesthetic doses of ketamine most closely models dissociative experience in healthy subjects. It acts through the excitatory amino acid (EAA) receptor system, a neurotransmitter system that is involved in sensory processing, learning, memory, sleep, and executive functions. The proposed action is through non-competitive antagonism of the N-methyl-D-aspartate (NMDA) receptor. Krystal suggests that a substance that would facilitate NMDA receptor function could be effective in treating dissociative symptoms. However, no such medication is currently known.

In summary, research is beginning to document that trauma (particularly repetitive early trauma) produces long-standing significant physiological changes. The multiple symptoms of abused children and adolescents—hyperarousal, abnormal pain response, self-injury, sexual precocity, memory problems, sleep problems and even dissociation may result from these neurobiological alterations. It follows that medications that have clear neurobiological effects may produce some symptom relief. Clearly the exact pathways for symptom reduction are not well understood. Further research to elucidate the neurobiological changes associated with trauma will help us develop more advanced understanding of these processes.

Differential Diagnosis

The first step in the pharmacotherapy of dissociative disorders is accurate diagnosis. In my experience as a consulting child psychiatrist, few children with dissociative disorders are appropriately recognized as such before they are evaluated for treatment with medication. Often the history of past or ongoing abuse is unknown and children come to the psychiatric evaluation with long-standing or preliminary diagnoses of more well-known conditions, such as attention deficit/hyperactivity disorder (ADHD), depression, conduct disorder, eating disorder, borderline personality disorder, or psychosis. Occasionally a diagnosis of post-traumatic stress disorder (PTSD) has been given, but in general, recognition of dissociative and trauma-induced symptomatology is still low among most mental health professionals.

Clinicians should explore the possibility of DID in every child who is evaluated, no matter what the nature of the presenting problem. Typically a child or adolescent is referred for psychiatric evaluation because of being "resistant to treatment," having severely disruptive behavior, or engaging in self-injury. Psychotic-like symptoms, such as auditory and visual hallucinations or experience of passive control, may prompt a psychiatric consultation.

The diagnosis of DID is often a challenge requiring a high index of suspicion and astute clinical skills as similar or identical symptoms and behaviors occur across a number of diagnostic categories. A skilled clinician can usually sort these out by noting subtle differences in the mental status exam and asking detailed questions about motivation and thought processes as well as sleep and mood.

A detailed family, developmental, and psychosocial history is essential for accurate diagnosis of any psychiatric disorder. Questions regarding family history will help with differential diagnosis, as many child psychiatric disorders have a genetic component (e.g., ADHD, bipolar and other mood disorders). A detailed psychosocial history may help uncover details about abuse or other traumatic life events. While PTSD can occur in traumatized individuals at any point in the life span, DID is highly correlated to severe or repeated trauma or abuse before the age of eight years. Questions regarding age of onset may help differentiate among ADHD (early childhood), depression or mania (school age or older), and schizophrenia (late adolescence or early adult). Certain DID symptoms must be distinguished from neurological disorders. Dissociative trance states can resemble petit mal or temporal lobe seizures. Pseudoseizures in adults have been shown to be strongly correlated with dissociative disorders (Bowman & Markand, 1996). Video-electroencephalographic monitoring is invaluable in differentiating pseudoseizures and dissociative trance states from epilepsy.

However, diagnostic categories are not mutually exclusive, as DID patients often have co-morbid disorders. A typical dissociative patient may meet diagnostic criteria for DID, ADHD, and major depression (Hornstein & Putnam, 1992; Dell & Eisenhower, 1990). When treating DID patients, the clinician should decide on a primary diagnosis and consider symptoms that may be part of a co-morbid psychiatric disorder. When considering medications, it is important to see features of the co-morbid condition in more than one personality state. For example, if dysthymia is present across the personality system, with many or most alters affected, it is more likely to respond to antidepressant medication. If most personality states are hyperactive, the diagnosis of ADHD (and a positive response to stimulants) is more likely. See the diagnosis guide (page 264) for some common child psychiatric symptoms and some recommendations for their differential diagnosis.

After a thorough diagnostic evaluation of the child or adolescent identifies dissociative and/or post-traumatic symptoms, a comprehensive treatment plan should be put into place. If severely impairing symptoms or behavior continue despite appropriate psychosocial and psychotherapeutic interventions, a trial of medication should be considered. In every case, the risks of drug treatment need to be weighed against the likely course of the disorder if untreated, and its impact on the child's development.

Case example: need for careful assessment

Brenda was a pretty 15-year-old girl, the daughter of professional parents. Previously a good student, her grades had deteriorated in recent years. She made several suicide attempts and had violent temper outbursts. Seen for weekly individual psychotherapy, she appeared very different from session to session. Sometimes she arrived cheerful and lively, dressed in colorful clothes, with blonde hair. Other times she wore all black, dyed her hair brunette, and appeared vegetatively depressed.

Brenda's behaviors were puzzling. She reported that once she had skipped school and dressed in her mother's business suit and, briefcase in hand, had attended a museum meeting. She couldn't explain why she did this. She had rapid mood changes. After one unremarkable therapy session, she left with calm demeanor but was found 30 minutes later in the clinic restroom, bleeding from self-inflicted cuts on her wrists. Brenda had strong conflicts with her parents, who themselves had serious marital problems. A talented artist, she sketched mostly unhappy drawings. One was of a young nude female, crying inside a glass cube.

Because of her drastic mood swings, the tentative diagnosis was bipolar disorder. Several medications were tried, including antidepressants, lithium, and valproic acid, with no significant benefit.

After six months of minimal progress, she suddenly improved in mood, behavior, and academic work. This major improvement coincided with her parents separating and her father leaving the home. She then revealed that she had been the victim of years of physical and sexual abuse perpetrated by her father. Brenda also described in detail her experience of having six alters with distinct names and personalities. The diagnosis of DID explained all of her baffling symptoms. She continued in therapy and was doing well at one-year followup.

Target Symptoms

The initial choice of psychoactive medication depends on both co-morbid diagnosis and target symptoms which are interrelated but not identical. Sometimes the diagnosis will determine which medication or class of medications to prescribe, while at other times the target symptoms are more important in choosing the medication. For example, if the symptom is hyperactivity, medication should be appropriate for the diagnosed syndrome (such as ADHD or childhood mania). However, incapacitating symptoms, such as sleep problems, need to be addressed as such whatever the diagnosis. When a syndrome (e.g., ADHD) is being treated, a specific target symptom such as impulsivity should be monitored to measure the patient's response to treatment. Treating these target symptoms can alleviate suffering, facilitate therapy, and lead to improved control over the core symptoms of DID. The following review of target symptoms will discuss medications briefly, but a more in-depth treatment of medications and research based justifications is contained in the following section.

Attention Span Problems

Dissociative children are often inattentive and impulsive, and short attention span is frequently a cause of significant academic problems. Their trance-states that can make them look "spacey" and "out of it" can resemble ADHD, ADD without hyperactivity, autism, or petit mal epilepsy. ADHD children and adolescents usually are aware that they are inattentive and their mind wanders. In my experience, many dissociative children are not aware of attentional problems; they think they are paying attention, but they have memory gaps ("lost time"). Neurological evaluation, including an electroencephalogram, may be necessary to rule out seizure disorder. Autistic children do not show the extreme fluctuation in relatedness seen in dissociative children.

Differentiating attention deficit disorder from dissociative disorder can be difficult as many DID children also have co-morbid ADHD. Fortunately, the distractibility and short attention span problems of ADHD respond well to stimulant medications such as methylphenidate, dextroamphetamine, and pemoline. Clonidine (oral or transdermal patch) has also been found useful for ADHD symptoms such as the hyperactivity and impulsivity. Clonidine has special advantages over stimulants in underweight children, in whom the appetite suppressing effects of stimulants should be avoided. Hyperactive children with Tourette's or tic disorders benefit considerably from clonidine, which also helps alleviate tics.

Aggression and Impulsivity

Aggressive outbursts, often without clear precipitants, are especially troublesome behaviors in the dissociative child or adolescent (Hornstein & Putnam, 1992; Riley & Mead, 1988; Dell & Eisenhower, 1990). Lithium, anticonvulsants, antipsychotics, benzodiazepines, buspirone, propranolol, and clonidine have been tried with varying success for these symptoms (Stoewe et al., 1995). Impulsiveness due to underlying ADHD may be treated with stimulants. Impulsiveness due to underlying mood disorder may be treated with antidepressants or mood stabilizers. Trazodone, being a selective serotonergic agent may be of special benefit for treating aggression (Stoewe, Kruesi, & Lelio, 1995). Abnormal EEG findings in these cases can give more justification for a trial on anticonvulsives such as a carbamazepine or valproic acid. Lithium has been found useful for explosive behavior and aggression in a wide range of patients, even those without an affective component (Rosenberg, Holttum, & Gershon, 1994).

Affective Symptoms

Mood symptoms, including irritability, tearfulness, and feelings of worthlessness, may indicate affective disorders, which seem to have a particularly high rate of co-morbidity with childhood dissociative disorders (Dell & Eisenhower, 1990; Hornstein & Putnam, 1992). These mood symptoms may respond to antidepressants, especially if associated with vegetative symptoms of depression such as sleep and appetite problems. If major depression is present and risk of self-harm is significant, the antidepressants of choice are selective serotonin reuptake inhibitors (SSRIs), since they have a high margin of safety in case of overdose.

However, I have found that suicidal thoughts and self-injury in DID patients are often not due to affective disorder but may be manifestations of dissociative symptoms such as conflict among alters which need to be addressed in psychotherapy.

Sleep Problems

Sleep problems are a frequent complaint of DID children and their care-givers. Nightmares, often with traumatic content, can be intrusive and repetitive and lead the child to fear going to sleep. For many sexually abused children, darkness, beds, and bedrooms can trigger association to terrifying recollections of abuse. The more exhausted and sleep-deprived the child becomes, the more likely they will have a REM rebound and vivid nightmares, causing a vicious cycle. Sleep deprivation itself may exacerbate dissociative symptoms (Gainer and Torem, 1994), and medications that help promote restorative sleep are very beneficial. Sleep disturbances include traumatic nightmares, restless or fragmented sleep, and difficulty falling or staying asleep. Antidepressants (especially trazodone), benzodiazepines, clonidine, and antihistamines can be effective in promoting more restful sleep.

If the sleep problem is primarily difficulty falling sleep, my preference for children under age ten is clonidine. If clonidine is not helpful, an antihistamine such as diphenhydramine can be tried. Low dose trazodone, an atypical antidepressant, is often used in older children and adolescents with sleep onset problems and may be helpful for anxiety as well.

If the problem is primarily fragmented sleep or traumatic nightmares, then antidepressants are helpful. These include the tricyclic antidepressants (TCAs) such as imipramine, as well as selective serotonin reuptake inhibitors (SSRIs), and trazodone. Night terrors and excessive sleep walking are effectively treated with low dose, short-term benzodiazepines.

Hyper-arousal and Anxiety Symptoms

Hyper-arousal and anxiety symptoms of traumatized children include hypervigilance and exaggerated startle reflex (Perry, 1994a). These are helped significantly by a number of medications, including benzodiazepines, buspirone, antidepressants, antihistamines, clonidine, and propranolol (Bernstein & Perwien, 1995). Oral clonidine or the clonidine patch are especially helpful in hyperarousal problems in young children.

Anxiety symptoms and panic attacks may be treated with antianxiety medications, such as antihistamines, buspirone, and benzodiazepines

(BZDs), or adrenergic agents (propranolol and clonidine). Tricyclic and SSRI antidepressants are also useful. A long-acting BZD such as clonazepam, used frequently for adult DID (Loewenstein, 1991) is thought to have less potential for abuse, and if carefully monitored can be helpful on a short term basis for severe, overwhelming anxiety.

Intrusive Symptoms

Flashbacks and intrusive thoughts are the most likely PTSD and dissociative symptoms to respond to medications (Putnam, 1994). Various kinds of antidepressants are beneficial: tricyclics, selective serotonin re-uptake inhibitors (SSRIs), and mono-amine oxidase inhibitors (MAOIs). Antianxiety agents, especially benzodiazepines (BZDs), adrenergic agents such as propranolol and clonidine, and anticonvulsants have also been reported to reduce these symptoms (Sutherland & Davidson, 1994). TCA and SSRI antidepressants are good first choices for these symptoms.

Hallucinations

Hallucinations and thought disorder symptoms, such as the experience of passive control and hearing voices arguing in one's head, can be dramatic in dissociative disorder patients. Often these patients are misdiagnosed as having schizophrenia, and so are treated with antipsychotics, which are usually not effective for these symptoms (Putnam, 1989). Some very disorganized dissociative children may respond to antipsychotics with decrease in thought disorder symptoms. However, it is unclear whether the benefits are due to a specific anti-psychotic effect or to generalized sedative (and anti-anxiety) effects. Recently the newly introduced risperidone has been thought to be helpful in some cases with fewer side effects than conventional antipsychotics.

A further discussion of each of the most commonly prescribed medications will assist with the careful analysis of what medications to choose in a specific case.

Medications

The main classes of medications that are applicable in treating children and adolescents with DID are stimulants, antidepressants, adrenergic agents, antianxiety medications, lithium carbonate, anticonvulsants, and antipsychotics. The "Quick Guide" at the end of this chapter gives an overview of the use of these classes of medication for various diagnosed syndromes.

Stimulant Medication

Stimulant medications, especially methylphenidate, dextroamphetamine, and pemoline, are very effective in treating children and adolescents with Attention-Deficit/Hyperactivity Disorder (ADHD). This is a vast subject, beyond the scope of this chapter. For details see Greenhill (1995) or Rosenberg et al. (1994).

Case example: ADHD and depression

Adam, a 7-year-old boy on methylphenidate 5 mg BID, was referred by his pediatrician because of four episodes of apparent seizures. He would shake and fall to the floor but did not lose consciousness. One episode occurred in the pediatrician's office and was diagnosed as a psychogenic pseudoseizure. A full workup revealed no abnormalities except for hyperactivity and attention span problems.

Adam was a bright, creative, but socially awkward child. He attributed the "bad nerves" episodes to a "brain friend" who first came to him at age three when he was locked in a room by a baby-sitter.

Adam's ADHD symptoms were not adequately controlled by his current dose of methylphenidate. Increased to 10 mg TID, his grades improved and his behavior problems diminished. Adam continued to be irritable, self-critical, and dysphoric with frequent crying spells. The addition of the antidepressant sertraline 75 mg greatly improved his mood and behavior. Family therapy was helpful in improving parent-child communication. Adam had no further episodes of pseudoseizures, and has done well in followup. Adam explained that "the brain friend went away."

Case example: ADHD

Barry, a 9-year-old boy from an intact middle-class family, had been referred for routine evaluation of ADHD. History was consistent with ADHD, but a few things did not fit. He was episodically aggressive and was caught engaging in sex play with a younger child. The teacher noted that often after a reprimand Barry would appear genuinely surprised that he was doing anything wrong. Mental status was noteworthy in that he frequently contradicted himself. Routine inquiry about hearing voices led to his volunteering in detail about his "four inside people," including one responsible for the aggression and another for the sex play.

It was unclear how many of his behavior problems were due to DID and how much to ADHD. Since there was potential benefit from medication and even a negative outcome would help clarify the diagnosis, a four week trial on methylphenidate was started.

Barry showed a dramatic improvement with methylphenidate, consistent with ADHD uncomplicated by DID. His grades and behavior improved at school, and parents noted improvement at home as well. On followup, Barry reported that his "inside people are nice now" and not getting him into trouble any more. He and his parents continued to participate in psychotherapy.

In both the cases of Barry and Adam, the stress of problems related to co-morbid conditions (ADHD in Barry; ADHD and depression in Adam) exacerbated their dissociative symptoms. When the co-morbid disorders were treated, the dissociative symptoms improved.

Antidepressants

Antidepressants are a mainstay of treatment of both the anxiety component of PTSD and DID symptoms and the often co-morbid major depression. Types of antidepressants include the tricyclics (such as imipramine, desipramine, and clomipramine), mono-amine oxidase inhibitors (such as phenelzine), selective serotonin reuptake inhibitors (such as fluoxetine, sertraline, paroxetine), and atypical antidepressants such as trazodone and bupropion. All have documented efficiency for depression and panic disorder and have been tried with some success for PTSD symptoms in adults (Sutherland & Davidson, 1994). Few child or adolescent studies have been reported, but clinical experience supports the benefits of antidepressants in children with dissociative disorder who manifest targetable symptoms.

For a given individual, the choice of which antidepressant to prescribe depends on many factors: side effect profile, drug interactions, formulation (liquid, pill, or capsule), dosage schedule (once a day vs. 3 times a day), cost, reliability of caregivers to administer appropriately, risk of overdose, previous trials on medications, the family's positive or negative views (based on personal experience or reports from others or the media), accessibility of EKGs, willingness of the child to have blood tests when needed (and of the parents to take the child for blood tests). Another factor is the setting in which the child is receiving treatment. Inpatient and residential settings with 24-hour medical supervision, safely allow for more rapid titration and higher dosage ranges than an outpatient setting.

Tricyclic antidepressants (TCAs) have the advantage of being the best studied in children and have the longest track record. Imipramine is approved by the FDA for use in children 6 and over for bed-wetting and in children 12 and over for depression. Imipramine has been used clinically in children for enuresis, depression, school phobia, ADHD, panic disorders and sleep terrors (Rosenberg et al., 1994).

TCAs are generally well tolerated by children. However, they can cause dry mouth, constipation, orthostatic dizziness, and rebound vomiting.

Cardiac toxicity is a concern at higher doses and in overdose. Even at therapeutic serum levels, cases of sudden death have been reported (Kye & Ryan, 1995). Baseline and periodic EKG monitoring are recommended. Serum levels are useful in measuring compliance, and in documenting the attainment of levels in the therapeutic range. Doses above 5 mg/kg are not recommended.

Because of the risk of hypertensive crises and the need for dietary restriction, MAO inhibitors are not recommended for children and adolescents. The memory problems of DID patients complicate compliance with a diet and make the use of MAOIs especially risky in this population.

For a child who needs an antidepressant, imipramine is a good first-line agent, especially if the child is 7 years or younger. Its side effects are well-known and it is the only antidepressant approved by the FDA for use in children as young as 6 years. If imipramine is not effective, or if side effects are troublesome, the patient may be switched to bupropion or an SSRI such as fluoxetine or sertraline. I have found that bupropion is particularly beneficial if there is co-morbid ADHD or disruptive "externalizing" behaviors. The SSRIs are especially useful if there is co-morbid "internalizing" disorder such as generalized anxiety, social phobia, or obsessive-compulsive disorder.

Trazodone is an atypical serotonergic antidepressant which does not have the anticholinergic or antiarrhythmic effects of tricyclics. Trazodone is very sedating and in rare cases can cause priapism. In adults, it has proved beneficial in low doses for sleep problems (Schatzberg & Nemeroff, 1995). Although little has been published about the effect of trazodone on children or adolescents, clinical experience with adolescents has shown trazodone to be helpful in improving sleep.

Bupropion, another atypical antidepressant, has some properties in common with stimulants. Barrickman et al. (1995) found bupropion to be as effective as methylphenidate in the treatment of ADHD in children. In my experience, buproprion is often beneficial for children with conduct disorder with or without ADHD. Overall, it has relatively few side effects, is not sedating, and causes minimal cardiovascular effects. Because of a slightly increased risk of seizures, it should be not be used in patients with a history of seizure or eating disorders.

Selective serotonin reuptake inhibitors (SSRIs) are a relatively new class of antidepressants. Currently available SSRIs include fluoxetine, sertraline, paroxetine, and fluvoxamine. The first of these, fluoxetine, has been marketed in the United States since 1990. SSRIs have many advantages over TCAs, due to improved safety in overdose and benign side effect profile. Gastrointestinal side effects, such as nausea and diarrhea, are common but usually transient. In addition to being effective in treatment of depression, SSRIs are also helpful for obsessive-compulsive symptoms and trichotillomania (hair pulling), which may be seen in some dissociative patients. SSRIs are being used in adults with DID (Putnam

& Loewenstein, 1993), PTSD (Sutherland & Davidson, 1994), and depersonalization disorder (Hollander et al., 1990). SSRIs pose a risk of behavioral activation (insomnia and increased motor activity) which may be a
side effect or may reflect a switch to mania in predisposed individuals.

All types of antidepressants can precipitate mania. Depressed adolescents and children are more likely than depressed adults to have occult
bipolar disorder and are more likely to become manic when treated with
antidepressants (Kye & Ryan, 1995). Children and parents should be educated about how to recognize manic symptoms, but careful assessment
of whether the observed behavior change is mania or "alter interference"
is important. Interviewing the child about the subjective experience of the
onset of the change in behavior, mood, or cognition is the best way to assess this. For traumatized children, who may have co-morbid bipolar disorders as well as dissociative symptoms, this discrimination is far from
easy. Some dissociative children with bipolar manifestations have been
helped with mood stabilizers such as lithium carbonate, valproic acid or
carbamazepine.

Case example: severe PTSD

Paul, a 6-year-old boy, attended a day treatment preschool program
and lived in a therapeutic foster home. He was removed from his
mother's care at age four, due to substantiated extreme physical abuse
perpetrated by his mother's boyfriend. The abuse included beatings
and being tied up and left in a basement. When removed from the
home he had multiple rope burns on his wrists and ankles.

Paul's mother may have had a dissociative disorder herself. As a
child she had been a victim of physical and sexual abuse, and saw the
murder of her father when she was 10. She was labile in her moods
and often demonstrated unpredictable and explosive anger.

An emotionally fragile child, Paul had a hypervigilant, haunted
look. He was constantly on the lookout for danger, easily startled, and
his play was preoccupied with violent themes. He had frequent
tantrums, during which he was self-abusive, hitting and scratching his
face. His sleep was often interrupted by traumatic nightmares. He also
pulled out his hair at night while lying in his bed.

Paul often regressed to the level of a 2- or 3-year-old, whimpering
and hiding under furniture. These regressed episodes were usually
triggered by a reminder of the perpetrator: a man who looked like him,
or any unfamiliar man. Even the sight of the female social worker who
took him for visits to his mother's house came to be associated with regression. The stress of supervised visits with his mother would result
in a "total shutdown" in which he would sleep for 20 hours straight,
several days in a row.

Paul talked about a part of himself named "Bat" that was "mean" and came out to pull his hair at night. His foster mother identified several "Pauls": the age-appropriate 6-year-old, the regressed baby, and the violent, self-abusive one.

He had difficulty functioning even in the supportive setting of the day treatment program. Medication was indicated for some relief of his severe PTSD, especially the hyperarousal, sleep problems, and intrusive thoughts. A meeting was held to obtain the staff's observations of Paul and attain a consensus on use of medication. His teachers, therapist, protective services worker, foster mother, and biological mother were all involved in the decision-making process along with the child psychiatrist.

Initially tried on clonidine, Paul showed some improvement in sleep onset and had fewer startle reactions. With the addition of imipramine, there was significant decrease in nightmares, hypervigilance, and tantrums. His mood and overall functioning improved. After several months, the imipramine stopped being helpful, and consideration was given to obtaining a serum level. There was concern that the act of having blood drawn, which included the use of a tourniquet, would trigger memories of the abuse. It was decided to continue the clonidine but switch from imipramine to fluoxetine liquid. Within two weeks, the foster mother noted improvement in sleep and more consistent appropriate daytime functioning. The regressive and self-abusive episodes greatly decreased. Paul's play, both in therapy and at the therapeutic preschool, was noted to be less violent. Despite improvement, neither he nor his mother is thought to be ready for reunification. He continues to reside in a foster home.

Case example: cutting

Lucy, a 15-year-old girl, presented with a 4-month history of sleep problems, tearfulness, and three episodes of cutting her wrists. Lucy reported feeling depersonalized. She was entranced by watching blood drip down her arm "as if it belonged on someone else." She revealed memories of being sexually abused by an ex-stepfather when she was 6 to 8 years old and had not previously told anyone about this abuse. Lucy scored very high on the Adolescent Dissociative Experience Scale (see Appendix). Sertaline greatly helped her crying spells, sleep, and mood. She made rapid progress in individual therapy, especially after a 7-year-old alter recounted the abuse in detail. After this session, Lucy said "I feel more whole."

In family therapy she was able to reveal her secret to her parents, who were supportive. She stopped cutting herself and her grades and social functioning improved. The antidepressant helped alleviate the vegetative symptoms of major depression. This enabled Lucy to more fully engage in psychotherapy.

Adrenergic Agents

Clonidine and propranolol are two adrenergic agents that have been especially useful in ameliorating PTSD and DID symptoms. Clonidine, an alpha-2-noradrenergic agonist, was originally marketed as an antihypertensive. In recent years it has been widely used for a number of medical and psychiatric conditions including Tourette's disorder, ADHD, mania, opiate withdrawal, and migraine. Clonidine has also been of benefit for hyperarousal symptoms in adults with PTSD, panic disorder, bipolar disorder, and psychotic agitated states (Hunt et al., 1990). Braun (1990) reported clonidine and propranolol to be useful in decreasing rapid switching in adult DID patients. In adults with PTSD, Friedman (1991) found clonidine to be of significant benefit for sleep, startle, and intrusive recollection symptoms. Perry's (1994b) study of the use of clonidine in 17 children with PTSD included a few who had "pre-psychotic and psychotic symptoms." It is likely that the children with "pre-psychotic" symptoms were dissociative. In this small open-label study, the positive response to clonidine (up to 0.4 mg per day) was dramatic, with improvement in impulsivity, anxiety, concentration, arousal, and mood. Basal heart rate and measures of autonomic arousal fell to near normal levels.

Clonidine can be administered orally, or in a transdermal patch (which is postage stamp sized). For adults the patch lasts 7 days, but for children the patch lasts only 5 days. Sedation is a common side effect of clonidine and in some children, the patch causes contact dermatitis. If clonidine is discontinued, it should be tapered down gradually to avoid rebound hypertension. Blood pressure should be checked regularly in children taking either form of clonidine.

I have found that clonidine (in dosage of 0.05 to 0.40 mg per day) has been the most reliably helpful pharmacological agent for PTSD and dissociative disorders, used either alone or in combination with other medications such as an antidepressant or stimulant. In some dissociative children, clonidine has alleviated symptoms such as sleep problems, hyperactivity, impulsivity, aggressive behaviors, intrusive thoughts, and hyperarousal. Especially helpful for problems falling asleep, it causes no morning grogginess.

Guanfacine is an alpha-2-noradrenergic agonist similar to clonidine, but with a longer duration of action. It may provide similar benefits with the convenience of once- or twice-daily oral dosing. It is also reported to cause less sedation and hypotension than clonidine (Hunt et al., 1995).

Case example: clonidine

Jasmine, a 6-year-old girl, was brought to the guidance clinic by her guardian because of hyperactivity, poor sleep with nightmares, and oppositional behaviors alternating with clingy, babyish behaviors. She and her older sister had been sent to live with the guardian after their mother was incarcerated for the beating death of a 4-year-old child. The older daughter had experienced sexual abuse. The extent of Jasmine's exposure to violence and abuse was unknown.

Jasmine often insisted on being called other names. Over the course of several sessions, a number of personality states appeared. A lively, outgoing personality that sang lewd songs and danced in the office was named "Princess Jazz." A whining, very regressed and clingy personality was called "Jaslin." One personality wrote in neat, legible print. Another wrote in mirror writing. All personality states were impulsive and distractible, although activity level varied from one alter to another. The guardian's major complaints were the patient's extreme impulsivity and poor sleep.

Clonidine (up to 0.1 mg at bedtime) greatly improved her sleep. One-quarter tablet twice a day helped daytime behavior. She continued to be very impulsive, whiny, and attention seeking. Because of her moodiness and a strong family history of affective disorder, a trial on an antidepressant was indicated. She was tried on a low dose of an SSRI. Unfortunately, she developed a manic-like behavioral activation effect, so it had to be discontinued after two weeks. Her activity level returned to baseline but was still problematic. A trial on methylphenidate was successful in improving concentration and lowering impulsivity and other ADHD symptoms.

On one occasion, the patient pointed out that I had written "the wrong name" on the prescription. I explained that the insurance company knew her as Jasmine and I had to use that name. She did not object. Maintained on clonidine 0.1 mg 1/4 tablet twice a day and one tablet at bedtime, and methylphenidate 5 mg three times a day, she is making gains in group and individual therapy.

Propranolol is a beta adrenergic blocking agent which was originally developed as an antihypertensive. It is used for the treatment of panic attacks, performance anxiety, aggression, and neuroleptic and lithium side effects (Rosenberg et al., 1994). Famularo et al. (1988) reported beneficial response to propranolol in children with acute PTSD secondary to abuse. Propranolol has been used in PTSD children and adolescents with marked improvement in clinical hyperarousal symptoms (Scandinero, 1995). Side effects include sedation, brachycardia, and orthostatic hypotension. Because of its effects on bronchi, propranolol is contraindicated in patients with asthma.

Case example: propranolol

Ben, age 16, was admitted to a residential treatment center after being arrested for assaulting a male teacher. In the previous few years he had become increasingly oppositional and explosive at home and in school. He found himself full of rage and acting as if he were "someone else." To deal with his inner anxiety, pain and feelings that he was "changing" he tried street drugs and exercise to no avail. Once he pedalled his bicycle for 20 miles in a daze, only to discover that he had damaged his knees and was unable to walk for 2 days.

Ben had been sexually abused at age 5 by a male neighbor and at age 7 by an uncle. Though beginning to reveal his memories in the residential setting, he continued to be explosive, especially with male staff. He reported that "an evil side" came out. He exhibited mild features of attention deficit/hyperactivity disorder and learning disorders, and was also diagnosed with "dissociative disorder, not otherwise specified."

His resting pulse was elevated at 120 beats per minute, and showed a marked increase with orthostatic challenge. Because of this evidence of autonomic hyperarousal, a therapeutic trial of propranolol was initiated. After one week on propranolol, titrated up to 2.5 mg/kg, he reported better control over internal feeling states. He became less volatile and was able to work more effectively on memories of his abuse.

Antianxiety Medication

Antianxiety medications include the benzodiazepines, antihistamines, and buspirone. The benzodiazepines (such as diazepam and alprazolam) have been used widely in adults with anxiety disorders and are considered generally safe and beneficial in that population (Schatzberg & Nemeroff, 1995). Clonazepam in particular has been studied in adults with DID and shown to be of benefit for their PTSD symptoms (Loewenstein et al., 1988). A controlled study of clonazepam in children with anxiety disorders produced mixed results (Graae et al., 1994). Since substance abuse is common in DID patients, including adolescents, potentially abusable medications such as the benzodiazepines should be used with caution. BZDs also can cause disinhibition, cognitive dulling, and amnesia, which are all particularly problematic side effects in DID children. BZDs, if used at all in children and adolescents, should be at low dose and short-term.

The antianxiety agent buspirone and antihistamines such as diphenhydramine and hydroxyzine are not abusable and may be of value in some cases for generalized anxiety symptoms. The antihistamines in particular have a large margin of safety but can cause anticholinergic effects such as dry mouth.

Lithium Carbonate

Lithium carbonate is a cation salt that is efficacious in the treatment and prophylaxis of bipolar disorder in adults and children. It has also been used successfully for severe aggression and explosive behavior in children with a range of diagnoses, including conduct disorder, neurological problems, and mental retardation (Stoewe et al., 1995). Van der Kolk (1987) reported that lithium produced significant improvement in a small series of adult PTSD patients. It has been tried in DID in adults with little documented benefit (Loewenstein, 1991). At this time, lithium should be reserved for DID patients with co-morbid bipolar disorder or severe aggression.

Anticonvulsive medications

Anticonvulsives are sometimes prescribed for DID patients because dissociative trances, amnesias, and pseudo-seizures can resemble the symptoms of seizure disorder. Electroencephalogram (EEG) data are important but it should be noted that abnormal EEGs are not uncommon in DID patients (Putnam, 1989). Anticonvulsive medications are known to interfere with kindling (van der Kolk, 1987), and may be helpful in PTSD and DID. PTSD and dissociative symptoms have responded to carbamazepine in adults (Devinsky, Putnam, Grafman, Bromfield, & Theodore, 1989; Coons, 1992) and in children (Looff, Grimley, & Kuller, 1995), and to valproate in adults (Fesler, 1991). Carbamazepine and valproate are often beneficial for aggressive behaviors and co-morbid bipolar disorder. These agents require close monitoring with serum levels, complete blood counts, and liver function tests to avoid toxicity.

Antipsychotic Medication

Antipsychotic medications are sometimes prescribed for DID patients because of symptoms such as visual and auditory hallucinations (also called pseudo-hallucinations) and passive control experiences. Aside from some anxiolytic response due to sedating side effects, conventional antipsychotic medications have little benefit for dissociative hallucinations. There can be significant neuroleptic side effects, such as acute dystonias, akathisia, and the risk of tardive dyskinesia. Thioridazine may be helpful occasionally for acute agitation or, in low doses, for severe sleep problems.

Some clinicians have found the recently introduced antipsychotic risperidone beneficial for severely disorganized DID children (Silberg, personal communication).

Opiate Blocker

Naltrexone, an oral opiate antagonist, is an effective treatment for acute opiate toxicity. It counteracts the effects of heroin and morphine-like agents, and is also thought to block the effects of endogenous opioids. Naltrexone has been studied in adults with various disorders in which dysregulation of endogenous opioids is hypothesized to play a role, such as alcoholism (Volpicelli et al., 1992), eating disorders, autism, and self-injuring behavior by the mentally retarded (Rosenberg et al., 1994).

Although current studies are preliminary, some children with autism have responded to naltrexone with decrease in social withdrawal, hyperactivity, and self-stimulatory behaviors (Campbell et al., 1996). Naltrexone has shown promising results in decreasing self-injury behavior of dissociative adults (Loewenstein, personal communication). Further research will determine if naltrexone will ameliorate the self-injuring behavior of DID children and adolescents.

Treatment Problems and Strategies

Pharmacotherapy can be valuable as one component of a comprehensive treatment plan for the challenging DID child or adolescent. As discussed above, medications can be particularly useful for drug-responsive symptoms and can facilitate the psychotherapy. However, this treatment population presents many unique treatment challenges including problems with alliance, compliance, differential alter response to medication, and alter conflicts. Family problems related to acceptance of the diagnosis, management of the difficult DID child, or psychiatric impairments in the parents can all affect the success of medication trials. The effectiveness of psychopharmacological interventions can be enhanced by sensitivity to these problems, which will be discussed below.

Establishing an Alliance

Children with DID usually have experienced abuse by caregivers and they have reason to distrust adults. Developing a trusting therapeutic relationship with a DID child may be difficult, but is essential to any successful treatment, whether with psychotherapy or medication. Ideally the treating psychiatrist provides both the psychotherapy and medication treatment for a DID patient. In a setting where this is not feasible, the psychiatrist should communicate often with the therapist, especially at times of crisis. The prescribing psychiatrist needs to have a good understanding of DID phenomenology and principles of therapy.

Dissociative children often have unique and colorfully descriptive ways to talk about their inner sense of dividedness and multiplicity. Examples include: "my inside people," "imaginaries," "The Wolfman," "brain friends," as well as given names which are sometimes variants of the child's first or middle name. Acknowledging the reality of these constructs for the child facilitates the establishment of rapport. Speaking to the DID child with his or her own terms helps foster the sense of being understood.

It is important for the child or adolescent to be a full participant in the decision to take medication. For younger children, ask if they have mastered the art of swallowing pills. Show them a picture or scaled drawing of the pill or capsule. If possible, give the child choices about the form of medication: whether liquid, capsule, coated or chewable tablet, even the color or size of pill. Inquire about which potential side effects the child finds tolerable and which not. In this way the child will feel more invested in the decision. Handouts about the medicine written at an age-appropriate level may be useful.

When talking with the child about his or her symptoms, identify target symptoms that the child wants to improve, which may not be behaviors or symptoms that the parents and doctor would choose. A child might not be bothered by poor grades, but may want a better attention span for football plays or video games.

Many DID children and adolescents are suspicious of medication. They may see how adversely their parents are affected by illicit drugs, alcohol, misused prescription or over-the-counter medications. They are understandably reluctant to take anything that they think will affect their mind or personality. They may have had the anti-drug message "Just say no" hammered into them at school. The clinician needs to be sensitive to these issues, acknowledge and address their concerns, and clearly point out, in language they can understand, the difference between street drugs and appropriately prescribed and used medication. A child may be reluctant to take medicine at school for fear of stigma or being labeled. Long-acting stimulants or once-a-day antidepressants can eliminate the need to take a midday dose.

A sensitive exploration of the reasons behind a child's reluctance to take medication can often lead to valuable historical or psychodynamic information. One teenage girl was perfectly willing to try a tricyclic antidepressant until she heard that constipation is a possible side effect. She then adamantly refused the medication. This extreme fear of constipation became a clue to uncovering one of the family secrets. One of the ways that her abusive mother (who had DID) mistreated her was by administering coercive enemas.

The following describes explanations of drug effects that may be useful in encouraging the patient to see the benefit of the proposed medication trial.

1. To a child who fears that taking medication means a loss of control: "The (symptoms or behaviors) are now out of your control. Taking the medicine will help you get back in control. It will help you do what you want to do. You can choose to behave better or not, but it will be your choice."

2. To a child with severe mood swings: "You told me how your mood goes up and down, like riding a roller coaster. This medicine can be like having brakes and a steering wheel so that you have more control over your own mood and behavior."

3. To a child with attention problems: "You see that having a short attention span is causing you problems in school. Your parents and teachers might think you are not trying. You are trying hard, but your concentration problem gets in your way. It has been hard for you to focus your brain power. It's like running a race with a ball and chain on your ankle. Or it's like trying to read without the right glasses; this medicine can be like a new set of glasses to help you focus clearly on the work so that you can do your best. This medicine can make a big difference for you if you give it a chance."

4. To a patient who is aware of several alters: "Another benefit of this medicine is that it can help your (parts/inside people) work together better."

5. To a patient who is not willing to make a firm commitment: "Let's make an agreement together. You take the medicine for the next four weeks, the way it is prescribed. After four weeks, if you don't see any benefit, or if there are side effects that bother you too much, we will stop it then. I'll write a letter to your teacher asking for her observations, and to give you another chance to make up your work."

6. To a child who is depressed, empathize: "I know it's hard to behave well when you don't get a good night's sleep. It's miserable to feel cranky all the time. This medicine can help you sleep better, feel less grouchy, and not have so many nightmares. I hope you will give it a try. Some people find that it causes a feeling of a dry mouth, or a stomachache. If that happens to you, tell your mom to call me."

Case example: a reluctant patient

Sam was a very oppositional and depressed 10-year-old. He finally agreed to take an antidepressant after lengthy discussion and looking at pictures of the options in the *Physicians' Desk Reference*. He was given a choice of sertraline tablet, fluoxetine capsule, or fluoxetine liquid. He chose the capsule because he didn't want to have an unpleasant taste and he liked the colors. We negotiated a 4-week trial period. He agreed to take the medicine cooperatively for 4 weeks. Afterwards we would reevaluate. He could choose to stop it at that point if he felt the side effects outweighed the benefits. After 4 weeks on fluoxetine, Sam was much improved in sleep, mood, and behavior, with minimal side effects. He had forgotten the 4-week contract. When I reminded him that he could choose to stop now, he said "Why would I do that? I don't want to feel crappy again."

In monitoring the ongoing effect of medication with dissociative children and adolescents, psychiatrists must be sensitive to these patients' high levels of suggestibility. Dramatic placebo responses and extreme sensitivity to side effects are common. Placebo responses can generally be distinguished from genuine medication responses by noting how closely the response parallels known and expected pharmacological outcomes. Major deviations from known medication effects should prompt skepticism that the medication is actually "working" for the DID patient. This suggestibility works to the patient's benefit as well, since patients may respond to postive hopeful messages, or more formal hypnotic suggestions that help alleviate distressing symptoms.

Differential Responses and Alter Conflicts

One of the most challenging aspects of pharmacotherapy for DID patients is the well-documented observation that various alters may respond quite differently to the same medication (Putnam 1989, Braun 1986). This is an intriguing and poorly understood phenomenon which may be due to physiologic differences among various ego states or the alters' need to be different from each other. It can be confusing to a clinician if at one session the patient seems to be doing well on a certain medication and the next session an alter appears and reports a long list of intolerable side effects. One alter may demand that the medication be changed or stopped, but another alter insists the medicine is helping and should be continued.

If communication can be facilitated between alters, usually some compromise can be reached. "If Jackie agrees to put up with the dry mouth problem, will Stephanie stop bothering her at night?" It is helpful to tell the patient that some alters may be more sensitive than others to various effects of the medication. Emphasize that "everyone" should work toward the well-being of the whole personality system.

In older DID children and adolescents, conflict among alters over compliance with medication is not uncommon. It can be handled in a manner similar to the resolution of other inter-alter disagreements. Cooperation and consent for medication should be elicited from all parts of the personality system. Each alter should be given the opportunity to air opinions about the medication. Sometimes one alter has a reason against taking medication that is a key to a psychotherapeutic issue. Perhaps the aversion to taking medication stems from memories of a perpetrator using drugs to sedate the child during sexual abuse. An adolescent alter may want to be off medication so that she can get pregnant. One alter fears the host will overdose and cannot be trusted. As much as possible, each alter's issues should be addressed. Often the clinician's acknowledgment that the alter's concerns are valid is enough to foster trust and cooperation.

The therapist might say something like this. "I want all of the (sisters/parts/inside people) to listen while I talk about benefits and side effects of taking this medication. You are having a lot of (flashbacks/crying spells/nightmares). I think this medicine may help you. After you have taken it for a few weeks you will see the improvement. Meanwhile, you may notice side effects such as (constipation/diarrhea/dry mouth). Many young people with these problems have benefitted from this medication. We will work together to find the right dose for you. If you are bothered by side effects, I want you to tell me about them. If this does not work for you, we will try to find something else that will. Please discuss this among yourselves and make a united decision. I will be happy to answer any questions."

Adolescent and adult DID patients with a co-morbid eating disorder may have an unusual compliance problem. The host may be dutifully taking the medication as prescribed, but be amnestic for an alter who vomits up the pills. This possibility should be considered in such patients when the medicine "stops working" at the same time that there is evidence of flare-up of bulimic episodes or weight loss. If the patient can comply with keeping an accurate timed log of medication, food ingestion and vomiting episodes, this problem can be monitored.

Parents and Other Caregivers

The therapeutic alliance should be established between the child and the treating physician, as well as between the parents and the physician. The care of DID children often involves dealing with many caregivers and professionals including parents, step-parents, adoptive parents, foster parents, teachers, therapists, protective services workers, respite care providers, pediatricians, psychologists, and psychiatrists. A collaborative relationship with mutual respect and cooperation is essential for optimal treatment outcome. For DID children, this kind of treatment team alliance also provides a model of cooperation that fosters internal integration.

Parents or caregivers of child and adolescent patients must be fully informed about potentially serious medication side effects and give their consent for treatment. Written handouts for families to refer to at home are very valuable. If a medication is prescribed for a non-approved use or age group, the physician should fully document the decision and inform the caregivers.

Some parents are looking for a "quick fix" and try to pressure the psychiatrist into prescribing certain medications. It is important to acknowledge their frustration and explain what treatment modalities are being used for their child. If parents insist on a particular medication, after potential benefits and side effects are carefully described, and medication is not contraindicated, a brief time limited trial with clearly defined target symptoms can be done. As teachers and therapists participate in monitoring the child's response to medication, the use of symptom rating scales can be valuable for assessing the helpfulness of the medication.

Conversely, some parents may deny the need for medication with justifications such as "I had a rough childhood, too. I learned to live with it. I didn't need drugs"; "He never acts up around me. Everyone else lets him get away with stuff"; "He just needs discipline, not medicine." These parents can sometimes be convinced to try a medication such as methylphenidate for their child only during school hours. After seeing the benefits at school they may agree to have their child be medicated at home as well.

Many parents of traumatized children are reluctant to acknowledge the extent or duration of their child's trauma. Whether out of guilt, fear of being blamed, denial, or lack of knowledge, many parents minimize the abuse history or dismiss the possibility that trauma could be the cause of their child's serious emotional and behavioral problems. Parents are often unwilling to accept PTSD or DID as the diagnosis, preferring a non-trauma related diagnosis such as oppositional/defiant disorder or bipolar disorder. Since many dissociative children are treated for years for other diagnoses without their dissociative symptoms being recognized, this adds to the parents' resistance to the diagnosis. Educational brochures, articles, and symptom checklists such as the Child Dissociative Checklist (Putnam, Helmers, & Trickett, 1993) can be particularly useful in educating parents about the disorder (see Chapter 13 and Appendix A).

Reluctant parents should be educated about potential benefits and side effects of a medication trial, and the likely course if the medication is not used. The psychiatrist should carefully explore the parent's opinion, past experiences with medication, and knowledge base, which often comes from sensationalized media reports. Providing accurate information and answering questions honestly promotes the therapeutic alliance. Once trust is established, parents usually go along with professional recommendations.

DID and PTSD children often come from unstable homes where multigenerational dysfunction is common, and so the reliability of caregivers must be considered when planning treatment with medications. There is a high rate of dissociative disorder in the parents of DID children (Braun, 1985; Coons, 1985). A mother who herself is subject to dissociative amnesias may be unable to consistently administer medication to the child. If the parent or caregiver has a history of chemical dependency, the physician should be wary, especially when prescribing medications that have abuse potential. As stimulants and benzodiazepines might be abused by the parents or sold on the streets, it is important to carefully monitor the quantities prescribed. Given the potential of parental unreliability, there are special advantages to once-a-day preparations that can be given at school or to transdermal patches that are easily verifiable. Helping the parent to set up a weekly compartmentalized pill box can also improve compliance.

Psychiatrists who work with children and adolescents often have to deal with the problem of lack of agreement between the child and parents, or among various caregivers and professionals involved with the child. Even with non-dissociative children, it takes a highly skilled and experienced clinician to sort out how much credence to give to a child's version of events and symptoms versus the testimony of adults. Careful negotiation of these issues is important to avoid escalating parent-child conflict. With dissociative children the problems of disagreement regarding observed behavior are greatly compounded due to the child's memory difficulties and behavioral inconsistency. For example, a teacher may be the only adult to see an aggressive alter who presents at school to deal with bullies; a baby alter may only come out for the mother; a female psychiatrist or therapist might not see a sexualized alter that appears only around men.

Since variability is a hallmark of dissociative identity disorder, the clinician should be aware that the DID child will behave differently when with different people in different settings, and even with the same people in the same settings! The clinicians and caregivers should pool their observations and work as a team for the child's benefit.

In general, it is best to weigh more heavily the child's version of subjective symptoms and sleep problems. The parents may not be aware of the child's "inner life," including the dissociative symptoms of hearing voices, having imaginary playmates, or feeling a sense of multiplicity or depersonalization. Sleep difficulties may also go unnoticed by parents unless the child wakes them up at night.

On the other hand, it is best to give more credence to caregivers' description of externalized behaviors, such as apparent lying, stealing, tantrums, aggression, and oppositional behavior. These are behaviors for which the child may be amnestic or reluctant to acknowledge. Making decisions in these cases can be complex. It is important to evaluate judiciously all sources of information, and synthesize them with the clinician's own observations of the child's mental status, such as affect, behavior, dissociative symptoms, play themes, and projective drawings.

Some families may use medication as a new battleground for parent-child conflicts. It is important to prevent the use of coercive tactics, threats, or punishments to get children to take medication. Caregivers should not trick the child into taking medication by sneaking medication into the child's food without his/her knowledge. As these are children who have been mistreated by caregivers, trust in adults is fragile, and the precedent should be set for open and trusting parent-child interactions. If parents are in favor of medication and the patient is opposed, this may reflect an underlying parent-child conflict, which should be addressed directly in a therapeutic setting. Medication will be more successful if the child chooses to take the medication to help him- or herself, not to please a parent or therapist.

Beyond Medication

No medication will be effective for dissociative or PTSD symptoms if the child is in an unsafe environment. Threats to a child's sense of security and personal safety will cause dissociative defense mechanisms to be activated. Exacerbation of a child's behavior problem may have more to do with an environmental stressor than the dose or type of medication.

Case example: symptom escalation

Victor, an 8-year-old boy whose aggressive outbursts had decreased significantly after starting sertraline, began to be violent again. His mother felt "the medicine stopped working" and insisted on a change to another medication. The treatment team (a psychiatrist, therapist, and teacher) met to review the situation. The consensus was that Victor's regression was due primarily to his father's relapse into the use of crack cocaine and verbally abusive behavior. A switch of medication was unlikely to be helpful while the father was still in the home. Under pressure from the family, the sertraline was stopped and the child was started on fluoxetine. As predicted, little benefit was noted. The home situation continued to be highly stressful.

Case example: interpreting the symptoms

Jenny was a 6-year-old girl with blonde hair, the only child of divorced parents. She lived with her mother and saw her father on weekend visits. Jenny had violent rages, night terrors, sexualized play, and severe separation anxiety. She often asked her mother to call her "Julie" and acted like a baby at those times. She played a game in which she was the leader of a group of five imaginary sisters, who had different ages and hair colors. The "baby sister" was called Julie. The sisters' game often involved angry play in which Jenny would make stabbing motions and say "we are going to kill the baby's daddy." Jenny's mother was loving and devoted, but was frustrated and puzzled over Jenny's behavior. She sought professional help. Despite a year of weekly play therapy, a 3-week inpatient hospitalization, and numerous medication trials (including stimulants, antidepressants, and mood stabilizers), the diagnosis remained unclear and Jenny's serious behavior problems continued. The night terrors and sleep difficulties had improved somewhat on low-dose trazodone. After transferring to a new therapist, Jenny revealed "the secret" that she was being sexually abused by her father on weekend visits. All contact with her father was stopped, and over the next several weeks she gradually improved. The rage outbursts ended. Taken off all medication except low dose trazodone for ongoing sleep problem, Jenny is continuing to make progress in a therapeutic school setting. Now much of her spontaneous play involves "keeping her babies safe." She no longer asks to be called Julie, and no longer plays the "five sisters game."

Jenny's case illustrates a number of issues common in the treatment of DID children. Diagnosis was delayed by the complexity of the presentation. The dissociative symptoms should have been a red flag for trauma or abuse history. Finally, this case shows that any treatment modality (psychotherapy or pharmacotherapy) is inadequate if the child is still being exposed to physical, sexual, or psychological abuse.

Conclusion

Confusing multi-symptomatic presentations are the norm with dissociative disorders. A child with DID may have a heavy genetic loading for psychopathology and prenatal drug and alcohol exposure, have been a victim of a one or more neglectful and/or abusive caregivers, and have been subjected to multiple forms of abuse by numerous perpetrators. Experienced clinicians will humbly acknowledge that we don't always know exactly what we are treating with pharmacotherapy. The medication of each dissociative patient is an empirical trial with a sample size of one (Ross, 1989).

We can err either by being overly confident about what medication can do for the patient, or conversely by being too quick to rule out medication as an option. A cautiously open-minded approach is best (Kluft, 1984). Further research, both basic and clinical, is needed to advance the current rudimentary knowledge in this field, and lead to better treatments for both adult and childhood dissociative disorders.

A Quick Guide to Differential Diagnosis for DID

1. ATTENTION AND MEMORY PROBLEMS

ADHD: Consistently distractible, short attention span, very sensitive to non-specific external stimuli (a tiny sight or sound).

DEPRESSION: Morbid preoccupations, slowed thinking, poor short-term recall such as remembering details of a story. Preoccupied with internal thoughts or rumination.

MANIA: Racing thoughts, can't process, can look inattentive if responding to internal stimuli. Flight of ideas.

PTSD: Hyper-vigilant, anxious, scans environment for danger, cues from adults, overreacts to perceived threats, may have flashbacks and intrusive memories.

DID: Amnesia too extensive for ordinary forgetfulness. Memories absent or highly variable. Personal information may not be intact. Often self-contradictory, can appear disorganized. Trance states are common. Can seem to be "in own world." Inconsistently inattentive.

SCHIZOPHRENIA: Disorganized thought processes; personal information may be delusional.

2. AGGRESSION (fighting, injury to others)

ADHD: Impulsive, reacting to the moment.

DEPRESSION: Explosive temper, deliberate, intentional, "holding a grudge," irritable.

MANIA: "Wild and crazy," grandiose, reacting to violent or racing thoughts, irritable.

PTSD or DID: "Out of character," aggressive alter, abrupt switch in and out, may be amnestic for it, may appear deliberate and unprovoked.

SCHIZOPHRENIA: Reacting to paranoid or delusional thoughts.

3. RISK-TAKING (reckless disregard of danger)

ADHD: Impulsive, fails to assess the risk. For example, runs into street after ball, jumps out of tree during game.

DEPRESSION: Deliberate risk-taking. Accurately assesses danger but doesn't care about personal safety. Walks into traffic. Quasi or overtly suicidal.

MANIA: Grandiose, sees risk but thinks of self as invulnerable. Takes dares, e.g., to jump off a high wall to impress peers or hang out of second story window to get attention.

PTSD or DID: External traumatic stimuli may trigger conditioned dissociative response, including passivity, numbing, altered time sense. Minimizes the perception of pain or danger. Blocks out conscious awareness of risk, e.g., soldier in battle or child in abusive family.

SCHIZOPHRENIA: Fails to assess risk due to delusional thinking. For example, leaps out of moving car to escape Martian-controlled radio waves.

4. SELF-INJURY

ADHD: Impulsive, soon regretted. No true suicidal intent. Goal is attention-seeking or anger-driven.

DEPRESSION: Premeditated, may have true suicidal intent. Long-standing self-harming thoughts. Goal is relief from psychic pain.

MANIA: Due to delusional or grandiose thinking, e.g., believes can defy gravity. Showing off, e.g., putting hand in fire.

PTSD or DID: May be due to a punishing alter personality, goal is relief of tension or numbing. Often feels detached from event as if happening to someone else.

SCHIZOPHRENIA: Usually due to paranoid or delusional thinking.

5. MOOD AND MOOD LABILITY

ADHD: Mood is generally OK, but can be quick to anger and quick to resolve. Mood cycles measured in minutes. Tantrums are generally short (less than 30 minutes).

DEPRESSION: Depressed or irritable. Mood cycles in days or weeks. Tantrums may be long (more than 60 minutes).

MANIA: Euphoric, sometimes irritable. Mood cycles in days or weeks.

PTSD: Variable, often anxious. Mood can change quickly with exposure to trau-magenic stimuli.

DID: Variable mood, can change abruptly, within seconds.

6. SLEEP PROBLEMS

ADHD: Hard to settle down to sleep, may be physically active in sleep, but sleeps soundly and is alert in the morning.

DEPRESSION: Trouble falling asleep and staying asleep, light, restless, non-restorative, or excessive sleep. Groggy in the morning.

MANIA: Decreased need for sleep compared to same age peers.

PTSD or DID: Fragmented sleep, traumatic nightmares, night terrors. Sleep-walking is common.

7. ANXIETY AND HYPERAROUSAL

ADHD: High activity level, but usually not anxious.

DEPRESSION: May have low energy level, look sleepy, or have psychomotor retardation. May be anxious.

MANIA: Can be hyperaroused, due to flight of ideas, violent or racing thoughts.

PTSD or DID: Very anxious and hyper-reactive. Hyper-vigilant, startles easily. May panic at the sight of any person who resembles the perpetrator.

SCHIZOPHRENIA: Anxiety is related to paranoid or delusional thinking.

(continued)

Differential Diagnosis for DID (continued)

8. THOUGHT DISORDER (hallucinations, passive control)

DEPRESSION (with psychotic features): Hallucinations or delusions involve dysphoric mood-congruent themes of worthlessness, punishment, or guilt. May have impaired reality testing.

MANIA: Hallucinations or delusions involve grandiose themes; may have impaired reality testing.

DID: Auditory hallucinations heard as coming from within; identifiable voices; reality testing is intact.

SCHIZOPHRENIA: Auditory hallucinations heard as coming from outside; voices may be whispering or not intelligible; reality testing impaired.

A Quick Guide to Medications for Children with Dissociative Disorders

1. If there are no drug-responsive target symptoms or co-morbid conditions, then use psychotherapy only (no medication).
2. If patient has PTSD, identify the main symptoms.
   (a) For intrusive thoughts, avoidance, numbing, sleep maintenance problems or nightmares: consider SSRI or TCA.
   (b) For hyperarousal, consider clonidine, guanfacine, or propranolol.
   (c) For sleep-onset problems, consider oral clonidine, antihistamines, or trazodone.
   (d) For night terrors, consider short-term low dose TCA or BDZ.
3. If patient has ADHD, consider stimulants, clonidine, buproprion, or TCA.
4. If patient has a major depression or dysthymia, consider SSRI, buproprion, or TCA.
5. For co-morbid bipolar (manic-depressive) disorder, consider lithium, valproic acid, or carbamazepine.
6. For anxiety or panic disorder, consider SSRI, TCA, buspirone, short-term BZD, or antihistamine.
7. For obsessive-compulsive disorder or eating disorder, consider SSRI or clomipramine.
8. If patient is aggressive, consider clonidine, propranolol, lithium, or anticonvulsants.
9. If patient is disorganized or psychotic, consider an antipsychotic such as risperidone.

A Quick Guide to Generic/Brand Names by Category

Stimulants
  dextroamphetamine (Dexedrine®; Adderall®)
  methylphenidate (Ritalin®)
  pemoline (Cylert®)
Antidepressants
  bupropion (Wellbutrin®)
  clomipramine (Anafranil®)
  desipramine (Norpramin®)
  fluoxetine (Prozac®)
  fluvoxamine (Luvox®)
  imipramine (Tofranil®)
  paroxetine (Paxil®)
  phenelzine (Nardil®)
  sertraline (Zoloft®)
  trazodone (Desyrel®)
Adrenergic agents
  clonidine (Catapres®, Catapres TTS1®)
  guanfacine (Tenex®)
  propranolol (Inderal®)
Antianxiety agents
  alprazolam (Xanax®)
  buspirone (BuSpar®)
  clonazepam (Klonopin®)
  diazepam (Valium®)
  diphenhydramine (Benadryl®)
  hydroxyzine (Vistaril®, Atarax®)
Lithium carbonate
  (Eskalith®, Lithobid®, Lithane®, Lithonate®)
Anticonvulsive agents
  carbamazepine (Tegretol®)
  valproate/valproic acid/divalproex (Depakote®)
  valproic acid (Depakene®)
Antipsychotics
  risperidone (Risperdal®)
  thioridazine (Mellaril®)
Opiate blockers
  naloxone (Narcan®)
  naltrexone (Revia®)

References

Barrickman, L. L., Perry, P. J., Allen, A. J., Kuperman, S., Arndt, S. V., Herrmann, K. J., & Schumacher, E. (1995). Bupropion versus methylphenidate in the treatment of Attention-Deficit Hyperactivity Disorder. *Journal of the American Academy of Child and Adolescent Psychiatry, 34,* 649–657.

Bernstein, G. A., & Perwien, A. R. (1995). Anxiety disorder. *Child and Adolescent Psychiatric Clinics of North America, 4,* 305–322.

Bowman, E. S., & Markand, O. N. (1996). Psychodynamics and psychiatric diagnoses of pseudoseizure subjects. *American Journal of Psychiatry, 153,* 57–63.

Braun, B. G. (1985). The transgenerational incidence of dissociation and multiple personality disorder: A preliminary report. In R. P. Kluft (Ed.), *Childhood antecedents of multiple personality disorder* (pp. 127–150). Washington, DC: American Psychiatric Press.

Braun, B. G. (1986). *Treatment of multiple personality disorder.* Washington, DC: American Psychiatric Press.

Braun, B. G. (1990). Unusual medication regimens in the treatment of dissociative disorder patients: Noradrenergic agents. *Dissociation, 3,* 144–150.

Bremner, J. D., Randall, P., Scott, T. M., Bronen, R. A., Seibyl, J. P., Southwick, S. M., Delaney, R. C., McCarthy, G., Clarney, D. S., & Innis, R. B. (1995). MRI-based measurement of hippocampal volume in patients with combat-related PTSD. *American Journal of Psychiatry, 152,* 973–981.

Campbell, M., Schopler, E., Cueva, J. E., & Hallin, A. (1996). Treatment of autistic disorder. *Journal of the American Academy of Child and Adolescent Psychiatry, 35,* 134–143.

Coons, P. M. (1985). Children of parents with multiple personality disorder. In R. P. Kluft (Ed.), *Childhood antecedents of multiple personality disorder* (pp. 151–165). Washington, DC: American Psychiatric Press.

Coons, P. M. (1992). The use of carbamazepine for episodic violence in multiple personality disorder and dissociative disorder not otherwise specified: Two additional cases. *Biological Psychiatry, 32,* 717–720.

DeBellis, M. D., Lefter, L., Trickett, P. K., & Putnam, F. W. (1994). Urinary catecholamine excretion in sexually abused girls. *Journal of the American Academy of Child and Adolescent Psychiatry, 33,* 320–327.

DeBellis, M. D., & Putnam, F. W. (1994). The psychobiology of childhood maltreatment. *Child and Adolescent Psychiatric Clinics of North America, 3,* 1–16.

Dell, D. F., & Eisenhower, J. W. (1990). Adolescent multiple personality disorder: a preliminary study of eleven cases. *Journal of the American Academy of Child and Adolescent Psychiatry, 29,* 359–366.

Devinsky, O, Putnam, F., Grafman, J., Bromfield, E., & Theodore, W. H. (1989). Dissociative states and epilepsy. *Neurology, 39,* 835–840.

Fagan, J., & McMahon, P. P. (1984). Incipient multiple personality in children. *Journal of Nervous and Mental Disease, 172,* 26–36.

Famularo, R., Kinscherff, R., & Fenton, T. (1988). Propranolol treatment of childhood post-traumatic stress disorder, acute type. *American Journal of Diseases in Children, 142,* 1244–1247.

Fesler, F. A. (1991). Valproate in combat-related post-traumatic stress disorder. *Journal of Clinical Psychiatry, 52,* 361–364.

Friedman, M. J. (1991). Biological approaches to the diagnosis and treatment of post-traumatic stress disorder. *Journal of Traumatic Stress, 4,* 67–87.

Gainer, M. J., & Torem, M. S. (1994). Sleep and dissociation—new findings. *International Society for the Study of Dissociation News, 12,* 8 (August).

Graae, F., Milner, J., Rizzotto, L., & Klein, R. (1994). Clonazepam in Childhood Anxiety Disorders. *Journal of the American Academy of Child and Adolescent Psychiatry, 33,* 372–6.

Greenhill, L. L. (1995). Attention-deficit hyperactivity disorder: The stimulants. *Child and Adolescent Psychiatric Clinics of North America, 4,* 123–168.

Hollander, E., Liebowitz, M. R., DeCaria, C., Fairbanks, J., Fallon, C. & Klein, D. F. (1990). Treatment of depression with serotonin reuptake blockers. *Journal of Clinical Psychopharmacology, 10,* 200–203.

Hornstein, N. L., & Putnam, F. W. (1992). Clinical phenomenology of child and adolescent dissociative disorders. *Journal of the American Academy of Child and Adolescent Psychiatry, 31,* 6.

Hunt, R. D., Arnsten, A. F. T., & Asbell, M. D. (1995). An open trial of guanfacine in the treatment of ADHD. *Journal of the American Academy of Child and Adolescent Psychiatry, 34,* 50–54.

Hunt, R. D., Capper, L., & O'Connell, P. (1990). Clonidine in child and adolescent psychiatry. *Journal of Child and Adolescent Psychopharmacology, 1,* 87–102.

Inman, D. J., Silver, S. M., & Doghnamji, K. (1990). Sleep disturbance in post-traumatic stress disorder: A comparison with non-PTSD insomnia. *Journal of Traumatic Stress, 3,* 429–437.

Kluft, R. P. (1984). Aspects of treatment of multiple personality disorder. *Psychiatric Annals, 14,* 51–55.

Krystal, J. H., Karper, L. P., Seibyl, J. P., Freeman, G. K., Delaney, R., & Bremner, J. D. (1994). Subanesthetic effects of the NMDA antagonist, ketamine, in humans: Psychotomimetic, perceptual, cognitive, and neuroendocrine effects. *Archives of General Psychiatry, 51,* 199–214.

Kye, C., & Ryan, N. (1995). Pharmacologic treatment of child and adolescent depression. *Child & Adolescent Psychiatric Clinics of North America, 4,* 261–281.

Loewenstein, R. J. (1991). Rational psychopharmacology in the treatment of multiple personality disorder. *Psychiatric Clinics of North America, 14,* 721–740.

Loewenstein, R. J., Hornstein, N., & Farber, B. (1988). Open trial of clonazepam in the treatment of post traumatic stress symptoms in MPD. *Dissociation, 1,* 3–13.

Looff, D., Grimley, P., Kuller, F. (1995). Carbamazepine for PTSD [letter]. *Journal of the American Academy of Child and Adolescent Psychiatry, 36,* 6.

Ornitz, E. M., & Pynoos, R. S. (1989). Startle modulation in children with PTSD. *American Journal of Psychiatry, 147,* 866–870.

Perry, B. D. (1994a, November). Dissociation and physiological hyper-activity as persisting adaptions in response to childhood trauma. Paper presented at the 11th International Conference on Dissociative States, Rush-Presbyterian-St. Luke's Medical Center, Chicago.

Perry, B. D. (1994b). Neurobiological sequelae of childhood trauma: PTSD in children. In Murburg, M. M. (Ed.), *Catecholamine Function in PTSD* (pp. 233–255). Washington, DC: American Psychiatric Press.

Pittman, P. K., van der Kolk, B. A., Orr, S. P., & Greenberg, M. S. (1990). Naloxone-reversible analgesic response to combat-related stimuli in post-traumatic stress disorder. *Archives of General Psychiatry, 47,* 541–544.

Putnam, F. W. (1989). *Diagnosis and treatment of multiple personality disorder.* New York: Guilford Press.

Putnam, F. W. (1994, November). Psychopharmacology of post-traumatic stress and dissociative disorders. Paper presented at conference sponsored by the Foundation for Advanced Education in the Sciences, Inc., Bethesda, MD.

Putnam, F. W., Helmers, K., & Trickett, P. K. (1993). Development, reliability, and validity of a child dissociation scale. *Child Abuse and Neglect, 17,* 731–741.

Putnam, F. W., & Loewenstein, R. J. (1993). Treatment of multiple personality disorder: A survey of current practices. *American Journal of Psychiatry, 150,* 1048–1052.

Putnam, F. W., & Trickett, P. K. (1993). Child sexual abuse: a model of chronic trauma. *Psychiatry, 56,* 82–95.

Pynoos, R. S. (1990). Post-traumatic stress disorder in children and adolescents. In B. D. Garfinkel, G. A. Carlson, & E. B. Weller (Eds.), *Psychiatric disorders in children and adolescents* (pp. 48–63). Philadelphia: W. B. Saunders.

Riley, R. L., & Mead, J. (1988). The development of symptoms of multiple personality in a child or three. *Dissociation, 1,* 41–46.

Rosenberg, D. R, Holttum, J., & Gershon, S. (1994). *Textbook of pharmacotherapy for child and adolescent psychiatric disorders.* New York: Brunner/Mazel.

Ross, C. A. (1989). *Multiple personality disorder: Diagnosis, clinical features, and treatment.* New York: Wiley.

Sapolsky, R. M., Uno, H., Rebert, C. S., & Finch, C. E. (1990). Hippocampal damage associated with prolonged glucocorticoid exposure in primates. *Journal of Neuroscience, 10,* 2897–2402.

Scandinero, D. (1995, March). *Psychophysiological consequences of abuse and potential psychopharmacologic intervention strategies.* Presentation at March meeting of Child and Adolescent Psychiatrists of Central Ohio.

Schatzberg, A. F., & Nemeroff, C. B., Eds. (1995). *The American Psychiatric Press Textbook of Psychopharmacology.* Washington, DC: American Psychiatric Press.

Schwarz, E. D., & Perry, B. (1994). The post-traumatic response in children and adolescents. *Psychiatric Clinics of North America, 17,* 311–326.

Stein, M. B. (1995, May). *Neuroanatomic and cognitive correlates of early abuse.* Paper presented at American Psychiatric Association Annual Meeting, Miami, FL.

Stoewe, J. K., Kruesi, M. J. P., & Lelio, D. F. (1995). Pharmacology of aggressive states and features of conduct disorder. *Child and Adolescent Psychiatric Clinics of North America, 4,* 359–379.

Sutherland, S. M., & Davidson, J. R. T. (1994). Pharmacotherapy for post-traumatic stress disorder. *Psychiatric Clinics of North America, 17,* 409–423.

van der Kolk, B. A. (1987). The drug treatment of post-traumatic stress disorder. *Journal of Affective Disorders, 13,* 203–213.

van der Kolk, B. A., & Fisler, R. E. (1993). The biological basis of post-traumatic stress. *Primary Care Clinics of North America, 20,* 417–432.

Volpicelli, J. R., Alterman, A. I., Hayashida, M., & O'Brien, C. P. (1992). Naltrexone in the treatment of alcohol dependence. *Archives of General Psychiatry, 49,* 876–880.

Yehuda, R., Southwick, S., Giller, E. L., Ma, X., & Mason, J. W. (1992). Urinary catecholamine excretion and severity of PTSD symptoms in Vietnam combat veterans. *Journal of Nervous and Mental Diseases, 180,* 321–325.

Part Three

Management

thirteen

███████████ Parents as Partners
in the Treatment
of Dissociative Children

Frances S. Waters

Effective treatment of the traumatized dissociative child includes engaging the child's family to facilitate the child's ongoing recovery from trauma. As demonstrated repeatedly (Dell & Eisenhower, 1990; Fagan & McMahon, 1984; Silberg & Waters, Chapter 6, this volume), dissociative children who make the most gains from appropriate therapy are the ones in a safe and nurturing environment with consistent parents. Consistent parenting promotes healthy attachment, provides affect modulation and containment, and helps to counteract the pessimism and demoralization learned from the child's abusive experiences. Providing the ideal environment for dissociative children is a challenge, as their behavior may be provocative, rejecting, and out of control. Many parents report that these children may seem uncaring or unattached, and parents are embarrassed by their child or adolescent's unpredictable behavior. Families are hungry for any clues that might help them understand, manage, and normalize their child's behavior. The therapist's task is to stimulate parental involvement in treatment and to provide guidance and support to parents in their difficult role. Therapists need to spend considerable time with parents of dissociative children, particularly in the initial stage of treatment, to engage them as collaborators and supporters of their child's therapy. Parents need to be viewed as the "in home treatment providers" of their child since they are more likely to be present when he/she abreacts traumatic memories, has nightmares, switches personalities, and has extreme mood changes. This chapter presents a review of the parenting challenges these children present, suggestions for therapeutic approaches to parents, and some behavior management strategies appropriate for families with dissociative children and adolescents.

In my experience, most families I have encountered are cooperative, engaged, and eager for direction and support. However, the traumatic background of these at-risk children dictates that the first task with families is always to assess if the child is safe. Severely pathological environments of dissociative children characterized by abuse, neglect, and conflicting demands have been described by Dell and Eisenhower (1990), Fagan and McMahon (1984), and Kluft (1986). Krugman (1987) has described an intergenerational pattern of family violence characterized by impairment of attachment, in which child maltreatment reflects ongoing environmental stressors and parental frustrations. In cases of extreme family pathology and child endangerment, involvement of protective service agencies is essential. The setting of firm, carefully enforced limits with abusers and refusal to collude with a family presentation of "face-saving falsehoods" are essential strategies (Kluft, 1986). Krugman (1987) emphasizes interventions for abusive families within a multi-modal, coordinated treatment plan that addresses the full ecological system. In these cases, addressing the dissociative aspects of the child's pathology in therapy is ill-advised, as the child retains the need for these defenses as long as danger is perceived.

Fagan and McMahon (1984) advise that the assessment of the family environment should include both the family's willingness to cooperate with treatment recommendations and the severity of the child's acting-out potential. Dissociative children can be extremely provocative with angry alters or pseudo-mature adult alters who test parental authority. They can exhibit sudden destructive or challenging behaviors that place intense demands on parents and require them to exercise self-control and employ appropriate child management techniques. If these parents have unresolved trauma issues themselves, the child is at high risk for retraumatization. Given this precarious atmosphere, it is imperative that the parents' mental health status and child's safety be continually evaluated, particularly if the child is residing in the family of origin of the trauma. However, the therapist should not disregard the need to assess these issues in foster homes or adoptive homes as well. While I have worked with numerous stable and committed placement homes, one of my DID patients was sexually abused by her adoptive father shortly after placement, and others have experienced other forms of retraumatization.

In order for the therapist to take a firm stance in being the child's strongest advocate and manage the treatment process of a child at risk, the therapist should collaborate with the criminal justice system and its personnel, the school environment, protective service agencies, health personnel, and placement agencies. If available in the community, the therapist might join an interdisciplinary team of professionals specializing in facets of child abuse. This team can assist in crisis management and long term monitoring of abusive families. Effective child treatment in these cases must synchronize interdisciplinary efforts on behalf of the child.

I have found a straightforward approach in working with abusive families to be effective. Limits are set with expressed sincerity, understanding, and empathy to chaotic families, who are desperate for relief. A detailed family genealogy that tracks abuse history, substance abuse history, and mental illness can suggest problematic areas in the family constellation that may influence the child's recovery and course of treatment. Appropriate referral of family members who have a history of emotional, physical, or sexual abuse or substance abuse problems may avert a crisis from occurring, e.g., further maltreatment of the child or mental deterioration of a parent which requires hospitalization and placement of the child.

The techniques and recommendations described in the remainder of this chapter are most appropriate when working with families that are not abusive or in severe turmoil. These are families that may have crises, temporary disruptions, or lapses in judgment, but these families are characterized by stability, commitment, and availability to the child during recovery.

The Challenges of the Dissociative Child

Traumatized children have multiple deficits in cognition, affect, interpersonal relationships, impulse control, and vegetative function (Eth & Pynoos, 1985). These deficits may impede their learning and adjustment to family routines. Dissociative children present other unique challenges which further compound these trauma-based developmental problems. A dissociative child is amnestic periodically to intense and sudden behaviors and feelings, exhibits varied developmental needs due to alters' different ages, and has sudden flashbacks of traumatic memories (Hornstein & Tyson, 1991). These dissociative features complicate the parenting of the child and place considerable strain on the parents and other family members to manage the child effectively and intervene appropriately.

When a dissociative child lives in a family with siblings, parents have the added burden of deciding when to intercede to protect younger siblings from harm and when to allow the siblings to resolve what appears to be a normal squabble. Parents need to be vigilant to step in quickly and effectively to prevent the dissociative child or other family members from being hurt by alters who may contain anger or hatred and express homicidal or suicidal feelings. Minor irritations with a sibling, e.g., conflict over a toy, could result in the sibling becoming seriously harmed by an alter who spontaneously emerges. One mother reported that her 2-year-old son enjoys singing at the breakfast table but her 9-year-old dissociative daughter became very angry at her brother's singing and lashed out at him repeatedly. The mother had to arrange for the two children to eat their breakfast at separate locations to prevent further harm to her 2-year-old.

Many parents of children who were diagnosed with a DID (Dissociative Identity Disorder) have described a typical scenario at a family gathering: The mother turns her back when her children are playing satisfactorily. Her dissociative child, Johnny, suddenly picks up a stick and swings it at his younger sister, who begins to wail. Johnny's mother intervenes to reprimand him. Johnny appears perplexed about what happened and adamantly denies he is responsible. Upon further exploration with Johnny by his therapist, it is learned that his angry alter had emerged momentarily to hit his sister; Johnny himself was amnestic to this event.

These incidents are very challenging for the parent who may feel that normal parental interventions, such as grounding or taking away privileges, are ineffective in preventing further incidents from occurring. The usual parenting strategy of grounding both siblings until the responsible party admits to the incident may not be effective. A dissociative child who is amnestic to his behavior may not be able to admit to his behavior unless he has coconsciousness and awareness of his alter's offending behavior. My experience with dissociative children indicates that while behavioral interventions need to be in place, they have minimal impact on the child's ability to control himself and learn from the consequences. Effective therapeutic approaches (as described in Chapter 8) will ultimately enable the child to control his destructive impulses and benefit from appropriate child management techniques.

There are many other trying incidents parents of dissociative children have to face. A parent may be called from work or home to pick up the child at school for an unprovoked attack on a child or teacher. At other times, the school will call to report that the child is dazed or unresponsive. The child's shifting academic profile makes scholastic planning difficult, and some settings may not be willing to keep the child in the school program.

The everyday routines of eating, dressing and sleeping may become battlegrounds as alters vie for control, display changing preferences, or experience traumatic triggers. Dinner may be interrupted because the dissociative child switches alter states and refuses to eat what is prepared because the alter does not like the meal. One parent of an 8-year-old DID girl reported to me how she had to be constantly aware as to what alter was present in the morning and to adjust her schedule and developmental expectations of her child accordingly. Mornings were often slow periods, in which decisions made the previous night as to what the child wanted to wear were changed in the morning if another alter who had a different preference was dominant. If a younger alter was out, then the mother would have to assist her in picking out the appropriate school clothes. Also, this younger alter would easily get sidetracked and require more supervision and direction to brush her teeth and hair. A parent may be awakened during the night to attend to a child who is abreacting a traumatic memory. A tired parent watching their child "relive" abusive episodes may become confused, frightened, or impatient. These daily challenges require the parents to be adaptable and tolerant.

Oftentimes parents of an undiagnosed dissociative child are, at best, perplexed by their child's denial of unacceptable behavior or repetitive destructive behavior. Their child appears sincere, confused, and angry at being unfairly accused. Parents wonder if their child is lying to manipulate the situation or to blame others to avoid consequences. The parents are angry and exhausted by their child's frequent outburst of unprovoked, assaulting, and destructive behavior. These parents may even think that they are "losing their minds" when they observe their dissociative child act out and the child totally denies what they had witnessed.

These are some of the daily challenges facing parents of dissociative children. However, as challenging as these children are, they need a safe and supportive family environment with parents who have stamina and stability. If at all possible, it is important to maintain the child in a home environment and provide the child with the opportunity to have consistent nurturing and understanding from capable parents, siblings, and extended family members. It is imperative that therapist work closely with parents and provide them with guidelines to assist them in understanding and managing these provocative children.

These tasks and guidelines are derived from working with parents and care providers of approximately 50 dissociative children (dissociative identity disorder and dissociative disorder not otherwise specified) from my clinical practice and from consultation with other therapists treating dissociative children (Hornstein & Waters, 1995; Silberg & Waters, 1995; Waterbury & Waters, 1992).

Therapeutic Strategies for Parents

The challenges discussed above may seriously strain the parents' marriage or the child's sibling relationships. The child's continued placement in school may be in jeapordy, and issues related to protective service reports may result in further intrusions and disruption to the family. The therapist who works closely with the family can provide support during these difficult times, guidance in decision-making, and advocacy for the child. In this team approach, the parent provides weekly feedback to the therapist regarding the child's behavior at home, at school, and in the community, and the therapist informs the parent of the progress of his child's therapy. Usually I see the parent briefly at the beginning of the scheduled child's session. Confidentiality with the child is respected, but I may request permission from the child to inform the parent about the child's dissociative states, traumatic incidents, or feelings and thoughts, as these may help the parent achieve an ongoing understanding of their child's behavior. Preferably I will have supportive and understanding parents join the sessions as the child tells them about his/her alters, trauma, feelings, and thoughts throughout the course of treatment. During particularly difficult times for the parents, they may require a session devoted to only them as tactical management approaches are planned together.

Below are concrete therapeutic strategies designed to help parents accomplish the goal of successfully maintaining their child at home and supporting the child's treatment. These approaches may apply to biological, adoptive, or foster parents.

1. Educate the parents about the child's dissociation.

Education is a most important task which occurs throughout the treatment process. Providing parents with the knowledge of trauma and its impact, information about the dynamics of dissociation, and the stages of treatment will assist the parents in knowing what to expect and enable them to become a part of the treatment team. At each stage of treatment the parents will need to know obstacles which they may encounter and become prepared to deal with them. The parents will need to know how to respond to the particular issues during the treatment stages, and how to provide the necessary adjustments in their home to manage the child's intense feelings, thought, and behaviors as traumatic memories are surfacing. Providing written materials about dissociation will aid the parents in learning about the dynamics related to dissociation and the process of treatment (see Appendix B).

2. Explain to the parents about the importance of structure and predictability when managing the dissociative child.

Children who have suffered traumatic events that were sudden, unpredictable, or frequent may become accustomed to using dissociative defenses. This learned coping style may be used in mildly stressful circumstances as well. One 8-year-old DID patient would "blank out" (dissociate) when a stranger to the child—but friend to the parents—would come to the house. These children have conditioned themselves to dissociate because of their distrust of adults and their environment and their fragile personality makeup. Dissociation has become a conditioned and routine response to minor stresses. Providing predictability and structure may help to defeat this conditioned response.

While it is impossible to provide constant structure and predictability in a family's life, the parents need to be aware that any simple change in the schedule may cause a switch in the personality of the child or the child may become easily agitated. Knowing this, parents may prevent these events from escalating by discussing in advance any anticipated changes in the schedule. When there has been an unanticipated change in the schedule, it is wise to explain to the child the situation and ask him or her (and the alters, if known) for their cooperation. This can be an opportunity for the parent to educate the child about learning to trust in changes and that changes in the family schedule do not mean harm to the child.

Structure and predictability can also help to manage the sometimes embarrassing appearance of an alter. For example, the therapist may help the family contract with the child to allow a baby alter to come out at bath time or bedtime to avoid appearing in school. Many dissociative children have an alter of the opposite sex. Providing toys, such as trucks desired by a male alter of a female child, seems to negate gender-based resentment and competition over activities. Although some professionals have expressed fears that this could result in more separation of the personality, I have found that allowing alters to get their needs met at appropriate times actually erodes boundaries and sets the stage for successful integration.

However, as a cautionary note, parents need to be judicious in eliciting alters for special occasions or special treats or catering to an alter's wants and desires. Such treatment can cause jealousy and internal power conflicts. The child's whole personality system needs to be the focal point and it may not be advantageous to obtain special gifts. Parents and therapist should discuss this issue and carefully decide to what degree the parent should meet a specific request by an alter, using the guiding rule, How might it benefit the child's total personality system, and the child's overall recovery? The therapist and parents should also discuss the appropriateness of a parent's initiating communication with a specific alter. In my clinical cases, a parent might call for a particular alter related to an explicit behavior problem or request assistance from an alter to solve a problem. Additionally, alters spontaneously emerge at home to work on traumatic memories with the parent and to receive attention to deal with developmental needs.

The child, therapist, and parents should discuss the issues of time, activities, toys, food and clothing preferences, and negotiate with the alters over such matters respecting time constraints and limited resources. In most cases, increasing the child's awareness that toys are common possessions is better than a toy belonging to one alter. If the therapist is constantly working towards coconsciousness and sharing of experience, all parts of the personality will enjoy the special moments that have been prearranged for a designated alter to emerge. Kluft (1985a) and McMahon and Fagan (1993) have also described this outcome. A general rule for alters' appearance is that they occur in the home, and after the child has completed homework.

3. Explain to the parents about the importance of establishing and maintaining family rituals.

Many of my dissociative patients have reported that they were abused in a ritualistic manner and during holidays or birthdays. Ritual abuse is defined by Bryant, Kessler, and Shirar (1992) as ". . . any kind of abuse done in a ceremonial or systematic form by a specific group." The report of the Ritual Abuse Task Force of the Los Angeles County Commission for Women (1994) gives some reported examples of ritual abuse (psychological abuse, physical abuse, and sexual abuse) which describe the scope of brutality a child may have endured.

Parents need to be aware that children can have anniversary reactions to trauma on those holidays, birthdays, or special events for years after the original traumatic event. These anniversary reactions may include post-traumatic nightmares, recurring and intrusive memories, and thoughts and feelings associated with the trauma. In order for parents to be prepared for those anniversary times, the therapist and parents should discuss the rituals associated with the abuse and the special times or dates when the trauma occurred. Parents are much better at coping with and adapting to a child's flashbacks to a traumatic event if they expect it and prepare for it. The parents are advised how to respond to the child's reactions and establish new rituals on anniversary dates.

In family therapy session therapist and parents discuss with the child in advance the forthcoming anniversary memory and assist the child to process it cognitively, emotionally, and spiritually. They work out a plan of how that day can be structured differently. The child can have input as to what he would like to do on that day to make the memory for the next year overshadow the memory of the original traumatic event. Much open discussion about the details of the day, even what the menu will be for the event, is frequently repeated. In preparation of the day, the parents, child, and therapist develop techniques to be employed at home for the child to deal with the intense feelings toward the abuser which may surface. (Any of the modified treatment techniques described under #7, Child Management Guidelines, page 291, may be useful.) Preparation for anniversary reactions is the key to minimizing the negative influence of the original trauma.

Due to dissociative children's sensitivity and vulnerability to simple changes, it is wise to repeat family rituals yearly if feasible. One highly anxious 10-year-old DID patient requested that the same 4-course Christmas dinner be served each year, as she feared dissociating if there were any variations in the menu.

Bedtime Rituals. Traumatized children have reported being sexually abused in bed or at bedtime and will frequently have sleep disorders. They will resist going to sleep because bedtime is a reminder of the trauma, or they will fear recurring nightmares. An exhausted 5-year-old DID girl would literally hold her eyelids open to keep herself from falling asleep because she had been abused at bedtime and had terrifying nightmares. To minimize anxieties about bedtime, the parent should set a routine bedtime ritual in which the child and parent spend rewarding time together.

It is best to discuss traumatic memories earlier in the evening, if possible. One set of adoptive parents would set a 7:00 p.m. time for such discussions, which allowed the child to deal with disturbing feelings earlier in the evening and be calmer at bedtime. This helped her to go to sleep on a positive note. Parents need to frequently remind and encourage their dissociative child to discuss feelings and memories at the prearranged time.

Even if an earlier time was arranged for discussion of feelings, it is common for children to have memories surface as they climb into bed. Therefore, parents need to be alert to such occurrences and set an early time for bedtime preparation in the event that their child needs to talk before it is late, and the parents are too exhausted.

Reading children's books in the early evening which deal with values or conflict resolution can help the child discuss issues relevant to him- or herself (see Appendix B). The *Berenstain Bears Series* (1987) contains excellent examples of universal conflicts with which families struggle and can open a discussion for the child and parents. Storytelling by the parents with the theme of a child or animal overcoming some struggle that parallels the child's difficulties can be therapeutic for the child. With young children, parents can hold and rock the child at bedtime. Although traumatized children may have difficulty with receiving or giving hugs, parents can offer hugs but respect their child's limits. Parents need to make references to hugging and loving all those parts of the child. From my clinical experience, this actually encourages cooperation and coconsciousness among the alters and decreases jealousy within the personality system. Parents need to reassure their child that they care for him or her and are there to help. Ending the night with a positive talk with the child about his or her qualities and something good the child did that day can overshadow a difficult day and encourage positive reframing of the child's negative self-perception.

I have made tapes for dissociative children to listen to at bedtime that can contain a "safe place" for the child (see Chapter 8), messages about cooperation and coconsciousness within the personality system, cooperation with the child's family, and soothing symbols and metaphors designed to encourage sleep.

4. Discuss homework and academic concerns and set realistic goals.

Frequently parents' greatest struggle with their child is assisting the child with homework. Until the personality system is known and there is internal cooperation, the child may not be able to consistently complete assignments and turn the homework in on time. This concern brings up important questions which the parent needs to address. What should the school know about my child and his or her diagnosis? Who in the school should know? What special arrangements need to be made on behalf of my child? These questions are resolved on a case-by-case basis depending on the type of school, the quality of the school environment, and the relationships of the parents to the school personnel.

Further questions to clarify these concerns are: How understanding is the teacher toward children with special needs? What is the current relationship between the teacher and child, and between the teacher and the parent? Are there concerns about maintaining confidentiality regarding the child's problems and diagnosis? Does the school principal demonstrate flexibility and commitment to children with special needs and willingness to make exceptions to the rules? What are the special services that would be available to the child, e.g., an aide or a learning resource room? What are the laws pertaining to the school's responsibility for arranging special services for emotionally or behaviorally impaired students, and what are the federal or state agencies monitoring the enforcement of these laws? The therapist should have information readily available to help parents confront and resolve these issues.

Ultimately, parents make the decision about how much information the school should have about their child's problems. Whether the school is notified about the specific diagnosis or not, the therapist should advocate regarding the child's needs and collaborate with the school personnel to develop a plan. In most cases of dissociative children in the primary grades who were experiencing severe learning and behavioral problems, the parents and I have agreed to notify the teacher and school social worker about the child's past history and resulting dissociative disorder. In these clinical cases, the school social worker, the teachers and other school personnel have been most helpful in modifying the child's schedule and lowering expectations regarding completion of assignments and evaluations of the child's performance. Meetings have occurred with therapist, teacher, school social worker, principal, and learning resource specialists to map out a plan. One highly dissociative 8-year-old DID child, who had uncontrollable switching of personalities, was assigned an aide to sit with her in the classroom. Because of her extreme distractibility, a screen was placed by her desk so she could keep her focus on the work and not distract the other children; this allowed her to be mainstreamed in a regular classroom.

In another school an 8-year-old DID girl, Susan, who had masculine and aggressive alters, would frequently exhibit disruptive and behavioral problems in the classroom and on the playground. A series of school meetings occurred in which a partial day program was temporarily arranged until her dissociative features were under control. A tutor came to her home in the afternoons to supplement her learning. The school social worker would coordinate her therapy with the author and see Susan weekly in school and periodically at her home to observe her and provide support and guidance to her mother. Over a 4-month period Susan eventually returned to a full day at school.

With dissociative teens in middle and high school who have many teachers, it is advisable that only a select group of people know about the child's diagnosis and scope of trauma, to help maintain confidentiality and prevent stereotyping. Generally the school social worker/counselor may have more information about the teenager's problems, while the teachers may have only general information that the teen has problems affecting learning and behavior. It is advisable to provide just enough information to the school personnel to be helpful in modifying the school curriculum and expectations for the teen.

Success of a specialized academic program for a dissociative child is dependent on educating the school system about dissociation. Therapists can provide an inservice with the school personnel to alert them to indicators of childhood dissociative disorders and provide an overview of intervention strategies in managing these children in school. In cases where this has occurred the schools became more receptive, flexible, and committed to the dissociative children. When schools are educated about childhood dissociative disorders and treated as a respected partner with the therapist and parents, they become crucial partners in the child's recovery.

Once the school has some understanding about the child's problems, realistic expectations for the child and a program designed to meet those expectations can occur. Regular coordination and communication between parents, therapist, and school personnel is necessary. My experiences with schools have been a positive joint partnership as specialized programs were developed. (See Chapter 15.)

5. Advise parents to keep a journal of their child's behavior.

Keeping a daily journal regarding the dissociative child's emotional and behavior states is a most valuable tool in monitoring many aspects of the child. It helps the parent monitor the child's struggles and progress and track the child's dissociative features (times in which alters were present, child's amnesia to behaviors, etc.). A daily journal can demonstrate a pattern the child may have regarding certain problematic behaviors the child or alters may exhibit over a period of a week or a month. One parent used a large monthly calendar to note her DID adoptive daughter's personality system and associated behavioral problems. She realized that one of her daughter's alters would have difficulty on Fridays and Saturdays, which were the former visitation days at the mall with her biological mother.

Once there was a connection made between those days and the disturbing memory, the adoptive mother and therapist worked with that alter to sort out her feelings of unresolved attachment to her biological parent. An environmental change was made in which Friday and Saturday visits to the mall were avoided and other structured activities were arranged on those days. These strategies helped the alter resolve the conflicts she experienced at those times. Maintaining a daily journal provides useful information about significant triggers and patterns of behaviors by the child and the alters which otherwise may be missed.

6. Parents are introduced to the child's alters and they "adopt" each other.

It is common for parents to be familiar with the child's alters while living with the child, but not understand that they are alter personalities. The parents are confused by the child's sudden change in food, taste, or behavior. Parents express relief at finally being able to make sense out of their child's many contradictory and perplexing behaviors when they become formally introduced to the alter personalities. One parent was enlightened when she was formally introduced in a family therapy session to a male alter of her 13-year-old DID daughter who liked to dance for hours, contrary to the quiet birth personality who spent time reading in her room.

It is important for the parents to be formally introduced in family therapy session to their child's alters and to learn the origin of the alters, their likes, dislikes, thoughts, and feelings. Parents and therapist should not assume that the alter personalities perceive the child's parents as their parents. In my clinical cases, some of the alters did not perceive themselves as having parents, and some perceived themselves as having different parents from the child. The goal of the therapy is to help the alters and parents learn about each other, accept each other, and adopt each other. (See Chapters 8 & 9.)

Parent or Adult Alters. One common challenge for parents to contend with is conflicts over alter personalities who are adults or "parents" to the child. A 9-year-old adopted DID child had an adult alter who did not want to give up her control and authority. The therapist persuaded the adult alter that the parents were present now to protect the child and that she did not need to continue to assume that role but could begin to enjoy life. Finally the adult alter agreed to work with the parents in carrying out appropriate expectations for "their child." However, until conflicts over control and authority are resolved between the maternal or adult alters and the parents, alters need to understand that the parents are in charge of the home and managing the child. As the mother or adult alters view the parents as advocates and protectors, then they are more likely to relinquish their parental or adult authority. Family therapy sessions with a child and his/her alters talking with the parents about their respective feelings and thoughts regarding traumatic events, and conveying mutual respect will pave the way for a "formal adoption." In the above example of the 9-year-old, after several family therapy sessions the adult alter consented to being adopted by the child's parents and spontaneously regressed to the child's age. The challenge over control among the parents and adult alter was resolved through mutual respect and understanding of their perspective roles, acceptance, and lastly, "adoption" of each other. The adoption between alters and parents can be a simple exchange of acceptance of each other in the therapy session or a more formalized ritual or party.

7. Refer parents for individual or couples therapy as required.

As discussed in the early part of this chapter, if the biological parents of dissociative children were the abusers of the child, they most certainly need to be assigned to their own therapist and receive the appropriate therapies. It is important to assess the parents for a possible dissociative disorder since there has been some research suggesting a multigenerational history of dissociation (Braun, 1985; Coon, 1985; Kluft, 1986; Waters, 1990). Benjamin and Benjamin (1994) describe a detailed family treatment model in working with children of dissociative families. If the biological parents were not the abusers, they may need to receive therapy to deal with guilt or blame they feel which could interfere in their ability to be firm with their child.

Adoptive parents of a dissociative child may also need to receive psychotherapy if the dissociative child's behavior triggers unresolved issues of abuse in their past. One adoptive mother of a DDNOS (Dissociative Disorder Not Otherwise Specified) teenage girl began to have flashbacks of horrendous physical abuse rendered by her own biological mother when her adoptive daughter physically assaulted her. The daughter, who was afraid of attaching, was temporarily placed in foster care and received psychotherapy. The adoptive mother entered individual therapy to resolve her own issues pertaining to her early physical abuse. The adoptive mother's successful recovery appeared to be the most effective intervention in the eventual return of her daughter, who had made only minimal gains in foster care and in her individual therapy sessions. The adoptive mother was able to maintain control and calmness when her daughter attempted to intimidate her during family therapy sessions and visits. The mother was loving, patient, rational, and consistent in saying to her daughter that she belonged at home with her family. The daughter realized that her manipulations to set up her parents to reject her were no longer working, and she agreed to return home. On followup she appeared to have successfully attached to her adoptive family, and she and her mother joked about the daughter's past "shenanigans."

Therapists need to evaluate for abuse in parents' history regardless of whether the parents are biological or adoptive parents. The therapist needs to determine if the parent's past history of trauma is affecting her ability to deal with her child's history of abuse. Providing parents with needed psychotherapy so they can deal with their own issues of trauma can be crucial to the parents' ability to effectively deal with their traumatized child. Treating the traumatized parent may be the determining factor in holding the family together while the dissociative child is recovering.

8. Assist parents in receiving respite care.

Parents of a dissociative child may feel as though they are psychologically dealing not only with one child but with a group of children. Great demands are placed on the parents emotionally, physically, and financially, and the burnout rate is high. To avoid total parental burnout, which would threaten the home placement and/or place the child at risk for maltreatment, the therapist should explore with parents respite care options at the time of diagnosis. Some options may be relatives, college students majoring in social work, psychology, or related fields, and community mental health centers with respite care programs. I have met with college students who agreed to provide respite care. I have educated respite care providers about the child and have given specific guidelines on structuring activities and dealing with potential problems with the child. Respite care providers are a necessary link in the chain of helping families with dissociative children.

9. Provide a parental support group

A parental support group of parents with dissociative children can be an invaluable support system. Monthly meetings with the parents and the children's therapists sharing struggles and solutions can enlighten and strengthen the parents' resolve to "hang in there," particularly when they are feeling hopeless or extremely frustrated. Rules of confidentiality are set. Parents can share phone numbers, if they agree. My parental support group became a creative vehicle for developing problem solving techniques. They were able to laugh and cry together. Their experiential sharing of what it was like living with a dissociative child could not have been provided in any other way. Brand (Chapter 11) describes a helpful parenting group for parents of teen dissociative patients, for which the teen must give formal permission.

Child Management Guidelines

It is difficult to anticipate the unusual family problems that may arise, with the constant interaction of patients and their alters with parents, siblings, friends and extended family. Clinicians and parents must be flexible in responding to the individual challenges of each unique dissociative child. However, the guidelines below are viewed as universally applicable to all dissociative children and may provide a framework for resolving management questions.

1. Use only non-physical forms of discipline.

A dissociative child who has been traumatized sexually or physically is very susceptible to tactile triggers related to early memories of abuse, even if the touch is an appropriate one. Incidents such as a sudden tap on the child's back may initiate a profound startle reaction, and parents may become accustomed to avoiding unexpected touches. It is important to stress to parents that purposeful hitting, pushing, spanking, or slapping are never acceptable forms of discipline for a dissociative child. These assaults to the child's body can set off a full blown abreaction to early physical forms of abuse and strengthen the child's dissociative defenses. These children have learned aggression from their maltreatment, and physical forms of discipline may increase these aggressive and retaliatory tendencies.

Because these children are very provocative, they require parents who are well versed in appropriate child management techniques and can work out an agreed plan with the child in advance for appropriate rewards and consequences for chores and problematic behaviors. As with normal children, it is important to give consequences soon after the inappropriate behavior if possible and to employ grounding for a reasonable period of time. However, until there is co-consciousness in which the child and the alters share information and are all attentive, the parent should not expect the child to learn immediately from the behavioral interventions such as grounding and removal of privileges.

2. Use a calm, low voice when the child is out of control.

Traumatized children may have been emotionally and verbally abused by screaming, shouting, and name calling. These emotional scars are hidden scars, which can be more damaging to the child's self worth and identity than physical scars. The verbal abuse has an insidious impact on the child's sense of being as the child feels splintered, insecure, demeaned, and enraged, and may want to retaliate. Given how demanding, provocative, and unrewarding a dissociative child can be periodically, it is a most challenging task for the tired, frustrated, and angry parent to maintain a calm, low voice when the child is screaming or refusing to listen.

When a child is out of control, it may be best not to try to reason with the child, but to separate the child from the parent. The parent may send the child to his or her room with the instructions that when the child has calmed down, then he or she can come out of the room to discuss what had occurred. Sometimes it may be advisable for the parents to remove themselves from the provocative child who is attempting to incite the parent's anger. This approach would be appropriate if the parent was not worried about the child harming himself/herself or others or destroying property. The parents can go to their bedroom or to the bathroom for privacy until the provocative cycle is broken.

One parent of a DID child reported that his petite 8-year-old adoptive daughter's alter would scream in his face inches away when he was attempting to deal with her oppositional alter personality. If he yelled back, she would escalate, and the situation would quickly worsen. If he kept his voice low and calm, she was able to calm down sooner. Then, they were able to work out the conflict without a full-blown crisis.

It is very difficult for parents to separate out angry responses which their child has toward them and see their behavior as symptomatic of the abuse rather than a personal affront to them as parents. One adoptive mother, who was in a helping profession, reported to me that she could deal more effectively with her dissociative teenage daughter's angry outbursts by viewing her as a client rather than as her adoptive daughter who was resistant and fearful of attaching. Maintaining a psychological distance kept the mother from becoming entangled and embroiled with her angry, demanding, and unattached daughter. This "clinical" distance also provided some protection for the mother, who was psychologically hurt by her daughter's rejection.

3. When discussing with the dissociative child consequences, ask the child to have "all your parts (alters, fragments, ego states) watch and listen" so everyone is aware of the undesirable behavior and consequences.

The parent's goal is to encourage the child to develop co-consciousness by requesting that the child's alters, ego states, or fragments watch and listen when the parent is instructing the dissociative child.

Parents should not assume that the child and the alters, fragmented personalities, or ego states are aware of the discussion following an inappropriate behavior, even when the child has expressed co-consciousness, because the alters may be "sleeping" or preoccupied with some other activity internally. Several dissociative children whom the author has treated stated that a helpful alter (one who has a positive influence) was "sleeping," even when it was agreed that all alters were to be attentive.

Another common dilemma with parents is managing the dissociative child's aggressive behaviors, e.g., hitting, swearing, breaking objects, when the child reports that the alter who committed the offense quickly disappeared leaving the host personality "holding the bag." These alters may "go into hiding" to escape from listening to the reprimand. To avoid or minimize this from occurring, the parent needs to make reference to the child and alters, if known, or "to any and all parts" that were involved in the misbehavior to be aware of the consequences decided. For example, the father can say to his dissociative daughter, "I want you and your parts to watch and listen while we talk about what just happened, and decide how it should be handled. Everyone needs to listen so they know the consequences."

Due to dissociative features, these children need frequent reminders about the rewards and consequences of unacceptable behaviors. Parents should not assume that the child will remember and learn from one incident to another what is acceptable and unacceptable behaviors. Until the child is further along in treatment in which amnestic barriers have eroded, and there is coconsciousness and cooperation, he or she will require continuous discussion of expectations, rules, and consequences.

4. No matter who was out or internally influenced the child at the time of the inappropriate behavior (alter, fragmented personality, ego state), the child still has to be held responsible for his or her behavior.

It is my general position that the dissociative child needs to be accountable for his or her behavior. Understandably, this will present conflicts of responsibility and ownership of behavior in the initial phase of therapy in which the identification of the dissociative system is unknown and amnestic barriers are still present. Therapist and parents can use judgment and flexibility in determining the degree of the child's accountability for inappropriate behavior by weighing many factors.

One critical factor to weigh in determining consequences is this question: "Is this behavior linked to a traumatic incident which the child is remembering and therefore acting out?" For example a child's inappropriate sexual behavior with a peer or a much younger child may be rooted in his or her own unresolved trauma. It is important that the therapist explores with the child the underlying dynamics and the motives of the behavior. The therapist assists the child to deal with the traumatic memory of sexual abuse and stresses to the child the serious legal and social consequences of sexually inappropriate behavior. The therapist, then, helps the parent understand the motives of the child's behavior.

Nevertheless, the parent would need to set up necessary environmental precautions to prevent or greatly reduce the opportunity for the child to sexually engage with or abuse another child, such as playing only in supervised areas, prohibiting sleepovers, or allowing only structured activities with peers outside of the home. These restrictions give the child the message that the sexually inappropriate behavior is unacceptable, and the child will have to learn ways to control future sexual impulses in order to be allowed more freedom with peers.

5. When the child denies a witnessed, problematic behavior, the parent gives the firm message that the child needs to sort out with the alters what occurred as the parent provides an understanding atmosphere.

Even though dissociative children are encouraged by parents and therapist to engage in coconsciousness and cooperation, the child may not always have an awareness of a destructive behavior exhibited by an alter. Restrictions should be accompanied by the strong message that the patient needs to do an internal check to find out what role an alter may have played in the behavior. This encourages inner communication, the eroding of amnestic barriers, and cooperation. The child's task is to learn to work together with the alters to control any impulses.

When a parent is faced with a child's denial of a witnessed behavior, the parent should calmly instruct the child to go to his or her room and explore internally what may have occurred, and later they will discuss the behavior and consequences. One astute adoptive mother of an 8-year-old DID girl told her when conflicts occurred between her and her alters, "It's not up to me to fix it. You have go inside and fix it!" The adoptive mother understood her limits and encouraged her daughter to fix her conflict with her alters, and to arrive at an agreed solution. This approach worked well to minimize jealousy, competition, and resentment among the child's alters, and to encourage communication, cooperation, and conflict resolution with them.

Another factor in evaluating the child's denial and accountability for his or her actions is to consider if the child is manipulating to avoid responsibility for behavior by blaming an alter for the actions. The author knew one 10-year-old DID girl who would frequently try to fool the author and the child's parents by pretending to be her male alter in order to blame him for her misbehavior. When she learned that it did not matter if it was her or her male alter, but that there were clear consequences for the misbehavior, her attempts to deceive her parents and the author decreased. In addition, her male alter was instructed to come out and take control, if needed, to prevent the child from getting into trouble and being grounded. The child and her alters had to work out together a way to deal with projection of blame, internal conflicts, and accountability for the misbehavior.

6. The therapist, child, and parent confer and identify internal helpers who are requested to assume control if the child or an alter attempts to engage in destructive or abusive behavior.

The author has instructed alters to be "watchers" and to take over, if needed, to prevent the child from engaging in destructive or aggressive behavior. Parents need to be aware who the "watchers" are and encourage them to take executive control or warn the parent if the child is going to engage in destructive or abusive behavior.

7. The therapist, parent, and child confer and agree on modified treatment techniques to be employed at home for safe discharge of feelings. The child is rewarded with an agreed-upon privilege.

Traumatized children need safe and varied methods to express and discharge their feelings. Frequently they have rage, which may be expressed in violence toward their family members, peers, or property. Providing acceptable discharge of such rage can minimize these destructive episodes. Arranging in advance privileges for safe discharge of intense feelings will encourage the child to employ these techniques.

The following are some suggested bargains that the parent can negotiate with a dissociative child to help with expressing anger:

1. punching a pillow or punching bag to earn points toward a toy;
2. drawing a picture of their feelings and ripping it up to earn points toward renting a video;
3. making a snow sculpture symbolic of feelings and then smashing it to earn the privilege of a favorite bedtime snack;
4. making a sand sculpture symbolic of feelings and stepping on it to earn the privilege of inviting a friend over;
5. making a clay figure symbolic of feelings, and smashing it to earn points toward the privilege of ice skating, roller blading, or roller skating;
6. running down the driveway or around the block three times a week to discharge anger to earn the privilege of attending a favorite sports event;
7. using an exercise machine to expel anger in exchange for time playing a computer game;
8. shooting baskets to expel anger in exchange for watching a favorite television show that day;
9. journal or write poetry about feelings three times a week in exchange for going to a movie.
10. Most importantly, verbalizing to the parent the anger felt and requesting parent's help in processing thoughts and feelings in exchange for spending special time with the parent.

Each family needs to evaluate what opportunities are available and acceptable in their home environment to express rage. One family, who resided in a rural area, agreed on a creative solution for their adopted 10-year-old DID girl. She was permitted to go to the woodshed, which also contained garbage cans, and shake them, scream, and swear. She understood that this was the only place in which she was allowed to use vulgarities toward the abusers who had sworn at her profusely.

Another devoted adoptive mother who also resided in a rural area would make use of her quarter-mile driveway when her 8-year-old DID daughter would become rageful at bedtime. The mother would bundle up her daughter and march her up and down the driveway until her daughter was able to calm down and verbalize her anger, hurt, and fears. Then the mother would rock her daughter and put her to bed.

The therapist and parents need to review techniques which they find acceptable and agreeable and permit their child to voice what she is willing to do to safely discharge negative feelings. Children can suggest creative techniques that adults might have overlooked. Children need to decide with parents what rewards would be meaningful to them when they use appropriate expression of unpleasant feelings instead of destructive behaviors.

8. Therapist, parent, and child agree on code words or symbols to signify the presence of intense, and uncontrollable feelings, thoughts, and behaviors.

It is advisable for the therapist, parent, and dissociative child to select code words or symbols which can be verbalized by the child, parent, therapist, teacher, and other appropriate adults to signify that the child is in need of quick stabilization. Code words or symbols can be used for the following purposes:

a. The child may be experiencing intense and uncontrollable feelings, thoughts, and behaviors which could result in destructive behaviors.
b. The child may be experiencing a flashback of a traumatic memory and needs to be reoriented to the present.
c. The child may be dealing with conflicts with alters over executive control of the body or over a desire to hurt someone or oneself.
d. The child may be disoriented and switching personalities and needs to maintain coconsciousness and cooperation.

The expression of code words or symbols can be a quick way to halt the escalation of serious behaviors without exposing the child to humiliation in front of peers or other adults. This is an intervention tool to redirect the child to being appropriately oriented and under control.

The code words "get it together" have been used by parents, teachers, and therapists with DID and DDNOS children who appeared disoriented and had uncontrollable switching of alters or ego states influencing the child to act developmentally inappropriate, exhibit extreme mood switches, or experience difficulty in performing needed tasks, e.g., homework or chores. This word signified to the child and his or her parts the need to come together in co-consciousness and cooperation.

The symbolic word "spike" was used by a DID child to report to her parents when she was experiencing intense feelings or new memories. Sometimes her parents would use the word when they suspected that their daughter was having a new memory, saying, "Are you having a spike?" One child used the symbolic word "bubbles" to signify when he felt that he was "going to burst" with overwhelming emotions and might hurt himself or someone else.

For one child the symbol of the child's hero figure, Power Ranger, was employed to reorient the child to the present when the child was experiencing a flashback. The hero figure was seen as the child's protector who gave the child the emotional support to come back to the present environment because his hero was watching over him.

In order for code words or symbols to be effective, the child and alters should select the code words or symbols and agree to comply with the use of them. Sometimes children may become resistant or oppositional to using them. A frank discussion with the child about effective ways to help him to have control over himself to spare him any embarrassment or a long discussion may be required to regain the child's commitment to responding to the code words or symbols. Hypnotherapy (Kluft, 1985b) may be employed to instill code words to help stabilize the child, if the child is agreeable to this technique.

Summary

Therapeutic approaches involve assessment of the family's functioning, counteracting any abusive elements in the dissociative child's environment, and contracting with the parents to provide a safe and supportive setting for effective treatment. Making appropriate referrals and close collaboration with protective service agency are essential when there is a threat of abuse. A multidisciplinary team approach with schools, criminal justice system and others can provide the different interventions needed to treat chaotic families, while the therapist works with the parents on specific techniques to maintain the child at home. Treating the child in a safe and nurturing environment with caring and stable parents is necessary for the child to begin to remove dissociative barriers, uncover the personality system, reveal traumatic material, and reach a state of personality integration.

Parents of dissociative children face many obstacles in managing their children. By learning to accept and interact with the dissociative aspects of the child, learning how to manage difficult traumatic memories, and helping the child manage his extreme emotions, the parent serves as a therapeutic collaborator in the child's treatment. With adequate knowledge, support, and commitment, parents can play an integral role in facilitating their child's recovery. Therapeutic work with parents is an essential component in the full treatment plan. Parental perseverance will facilitate the dissociative child's attainment of trust and attachment and promote the child's development into a functioning adult.

References

Benjamin, L. R., & Bejamin, R. (1993). Interventions with children in dissociative families: A family treatment model. *Dissociation, 7*, 47–53.

Berenstain, S., & Berenstain, J. (1987). *The Berenstain Bears Series.* New York: Random House.

Braun, B. G. (1985). The transgenerational incidence of dissociation and multiple personality disorder: A preliminary report. In R. P. Kluft (Ed.), *Childhood antecedents of multiple personality* (pp 127–150). Washington, DC: American Psychiatric Press.

Bryant, D., Kessler, J., & Shirar, L. (1992). *The family inside: Working with the multiple.* New York: Norton.

Coons, P. M. (1985). Children of parents with multiple personality disorder. In R. P. Kluft (Ed.), *Childhood antecedents of multiple personality.* Washington, DC: American Psychiatric Press.

Dell, D. F., & Eisenhower, J. W. (1990). Adolescent multiple personality disorder: a preliminary study of eleven cases. *Journal of the American Academy of Child and Adolescent Psychiatry, 29*, 359–366.

Eth, S., & Pynoos, R. S. (1985). Developmental perspective on psychic trauma in childhood. In C. R. Figley (Ed.), *Trauma and its wake* (pp. 36–52). New York: Brunner/Mazel.

Fagan, J., & McMahon, P. P. (1984). Incipient multiple personality in children. *Journal of Nervous and Mental Disease, 172*, 26–36.

Hornstein, N. L., & Tyson, S. (1991). Inpatient treatment of children with multiple personality/dissociative disorders and their families. *Psychiatric Clinics of North America, 3*, 631–648.

Hornstein, N. L., & Waters, F. S. (1995). Developmental perspective on childhood trauma and dissociative disorders (Summary). Workshop. Department of Psychiatry. Institute of Juvenile Research. The University of Illinois at Chicago.

Kluft, R. P. (1985a). Childhood multiple personality disorder: Predictors, clinical findings, and treatment results. In R. P. Kluft (Ed.), *Childhood antecedents of multiple personality* (pp. 167–196). Washington, DC: American Psychiatric Press.

Kluft, R. P. (1985b). Hypnotherapy of childhood multiple personality disorder. *American Journal of Clinical Hypnosis, 27*, 201–210.

Kluft, R. P. (1986). Treating children who have multiple personality disorder. In B.G. Braun (Ed.), *Treatment of multiple personality disorder.* Washington, DC: American Psychiatric Press.

Krugman, S. (1987). Trauma in the family: Perspectives on the intergenerational transmission of violence. In B. A. van der Kolk (Ed.), *Psychological Trauma* (pp. 127–151). Washington, DC: American Psychiatric Press.

McMahon, P. P., & Fagan, J. (1993). Play therapy with children with multiple personality disorder. In R. P. Kluft & C. G. Fine (Eds.), *Clinical perspectives on multiple personality disorder* (pp. 253–276). Washington, DC: American Psychiatric Press.

Ritual Abuse Task Force. (1994). *Ritual abuse: definitions, glossary. The use of mind control.* Los Angeles: Los Angeles County Commission for Women.

Silberg, J., & Waters, F. S. (1995). *Advanced workshop in the diagnosis and treatment of childhood dissociation.* Presented at Eastern Regional Conference on Multiple Personality and Dissociative States, Alexandria, VA.

Waterbury, M., & Waters, F. W. (1992). Treatment of childhood dissociative disorders (Summary). Proceedings of the Ninth International Conference on Multiple Personality/Dissociative States, Chicago, IL.

Waters, F. W. (1990). Profile of nine cases of childhood multiple personality disorder (Summary). Paper presented at Seventh International Conference on Multiple Personality/Dissociative States, Chicago, IL.

fourteen

━━━━━━━━ The Pediatric Management
of the Dissociative Child

David B. Graham

Dissociative disorders are unfamiliar to most pediatricians, as these conditions are relegated to the mental health literature. Yet, unbeknownst to pediatricians, dissociative disorders may confuse the diagnostic picture and affect typical practice response to treatments. Review of the professional literature on dissociation revealed only one publication in a pediatric journal (Whitman & Munkel, 1991). This is not surprising, because it is only within the past decade that cases of childhood dissociative disorders have been published in mental health journals. Without information and awareness of these conditions, dissociative behaviors in children and adolescents are attributed commonly to other disorders.

Dissociation is a psychophysiological process that alters a person's thoughts, feelings, or actions, so that for a period of time certain information is not associated or integrated normally or logically with other information (West, 1967). Certain forms of dissociation, such as daydreaming, fantasizing, or relating to an imaginary playmate, are normal in children. Normative dissociative behavior tends to peak at 9–10 years, then decreases with age (Putnam, 1993). The pediatrician or family physician hears about the normal types of dissociation almost daily. How often we hear a parent say "He (or she) just won't listen to me; he tunes me out; he spaces out; he's in his own world; it's like he doesn't hear me!" While it may seem appropriate to relegate such comments to the realm of manipulation, in fact, dissociation may cause the behavior that triggers such comments.

It is generally agreed that pathologically dissociative behaviors are associated with early childhood traumatic experiences. The child uses dissociation as an adaptive coping mechanism to protect against the potentially overwhelming nature of the trauma. With repeated trauma, such as recurrent sexual or physical abuse, the child learns to dissociate as soon as a stressful situation threatens. When dissociation affects the continuity of memory or disturbs integration of self, a dissociative disorder results.

The Diagnostic and Statistical Manual of Mental Disorders (American Psychiatric Association, 1994) categorizes five types of dissociative disorders: dissociative identity disorder (DID, formerly called multiple personality disorder or MPD), dissociative disorder not otherwise specified (DDNOS), depersonalization disorder, psychogenic fugue, and psychogenic amnesia. DID and DDNOS are the disorders most commonly described in children. Patients with DID present with episodes of amnesia, and alternate states of identity (alters) that feel autonomous, and have unique characteristics. The diagnosis of DDNOS is used frequently with children who do not display rigid barriers between identity states but feel influenced by "voices" or "parts" (Hornstein & Putnam, 1992). Dissociative disorders in childhood (both DID and DDNOS) may present as puzzling, fluctuating behavior, impulse control problems, attention problems, sleep problems, and problems with depression.

It appears that the vast majority of adults with DID experienced recurrent trauma—usually from emotional, physical, and/or sexual abuse—as a young child. A National Institute of Mental Health (NIMH) survey of 100 DID cases found that 97% of all DID patients reported experiencing significant childhood trauma, with incest being the most commonly reported trauma (68%). Two thirds reported experiencing both sexual and physical abuse (Putnam, Guroff, Silberman, Barban, & Post, 1986). Furthermore, adults with DID may report sadistic abuses during childhood, often with bondage and insertions of various objects into mouth, anus, and vagina. In addition, these adults report burns and being physically tortured in various ways. They report emotional abuses such as being constantly demeaned and denigrated as children and adolescents. Awareness and understanding of dissociative disorders is of particular importance for pediatricians, as they may become the first professional to pick up signs of ongoing emotional, physical, or sexual trauma.

Dissociative disorders as a group may affect as much as 10% of the adult population (Ross, 1991). According to Kluft, only 3% of DID diagnoses are made in children less than 12 years old (Kluft, 1985b). Since there is strong consensus that severe dissociative disorders begin in childhood, it is potentially tragic that so few diagnoses are made in the early years. The pediatrician may be the first professional to be confronted with many of the symptoms of dissociative disorders. However, without a high index of suspicion for dissociative disorders, other diagnoses may seem more likely. Childhood dissociative disorders must be differentiated from attention-deficit/hyperactivity disorder, conduct disorder, oppositional defiant disorder, and separation anxiety disorder (Dean, Giem, Guerro, &

Leard, 1989). Dell and Eisenhower (1990) report in a series of 11 adolescents with DID that criteria were met for mood disorders (65%), disruptive behavior disorders (55%), and post-traumatic stress disorder (45%); thus co-morbidity with other disorders is high and the issues of differential diagnosis complex. Nonetheless, the perspicacious primary care physician can initiate an appropriate early referral and set the stage for appropriate intervention. Compared to adults, early intervention with children is more likely to be successful with shorter, less expensive therapy (Kluft, 1985a; Fagan & McMahon, 1984).

Many symptoms associated with a dissociative disorder will bring a child into a physician's office: headaches, abdominal pain, skin rashes that come and go unpredictably, various assortments of aches and pains without clear etiology, intermittent blurry vision, variable responses to the same allergen, significant physical trauma without evidence of pain, seizures (especially temporal-lobe type), symptoms of eating disorders, symptoms of attention deficit hyperactivity disorder, and almost any constellation of behaviors and emotions consistent with almost any childhood psychiatric diagnosis. The list becomes legion because DID and DDNOS are polysymptomatic disorders with frequent somatic complaints. Presently, most of the research has been done on adults with dissociative disorders. Perhaps in the future we will have an entire book on the physiologic properties of childhood dissociative disorders, but for now we can look briefly at some of the more common physical symptoms and symptom complexes that may bring a child into a primary care physician's office and how to differentiate them from dissociative disorders.

Differential Diagnosis

The physician needs to be alert to possible pathologic dissociative phenomena in a child during the parent and child interview as well as the physical examination. Since amnesia is usually a significant aspect of dissociative states, note should be made of the child who frequently forgets or denies behaviors or statements he/she has made. If the physician has a sense that the child is not purposely denying, then the possibility of dissociation should be entertained. A clue that a child's denial may be unconscious is frequent denial of actions witnessed by adults.

Dissociative children often act "spacey." Often I have seen them become distracted, forgetful, or dazed in the office, especially when being asked to comment on their own reported behaviors. Dissociative defenses may be used to avoid painful memories or physical pain during office procedures. The child may go into a trance just as they get an immunization or as a procedure (removing cerumen from the ear, lumbar punctures, EKGs, etc.) is performed. Other signs of dissociation I have seen in the office include: unexpected mood changes; moods that are inappropriate to the situation; sudden regressed behavior, especially in a latency aged child who begins acting quite infantile; striking changes in speech including pitch, rhythm, rate, tone, vocabulary, and grammar; numerous contradictory statements, sometimes back to back; and parent or teacher report of the child having conversations with himself or herself.

As a help in screening, several checklist and self report forms have been devised (Evers-Szostak & Sanders, 1992, Putnam, Helmers, & Trickett, 1993; Reagor, Kasten, & Morelli, 1992). The most widely used and most extensively validated is the Child Dissociative Checklist (CDC) (see Appendix A). This is a 20-item checklist completed by the parent or other observer who knows the child well. It has been normed on samples of normal children, sexually abused girls, and dissociative children (Putnam, Helmers, & Trickett, 1993). Scores of 16 or more suggest evidence of significant dissociation, and scores above 24 suggest DID (Putnam & Peterson, 1994). The authors point out that this is a screening instrument rather than a diagnostic test and that the diagnosis must include a clinical interview.

For pediatricians interested in behavior, the CDC is a useful tool, particularly when a psychogenic etiology is being considered for somatic complaints. A screening instrument called the Adolescent Dissociative Experience Scale (A-DES) is currently being tested (see Appendix A). Even without current norms available, it does provide useful clinical information that can suggest the need for further assessment.

These instruments may be a helpful addition in the clinical evaluation of pediatric patients who present with a variety of disorders that share common symptom presentations with dissociative disorders. Some of these disorders for which pediatricians are most likely to be consulted—ADHD, Eating Disorders, and Seizure Disorders/Conversion Disorders—will be discussed below.

Attention-Deficit / Hyperactivity Disorder (ADHD)

All of the symptoms occurring in ADHD can occur in children with dissociative disorders, especially with DID. It is not clear whether this is due to comorbidity or whether it is actually part of the dissociative disorder. Inattention and distractibility are two of the hallmarks of ADHD. Children and adolescents with DID are often inattentive and distracted because they hear internal voices speaking to them. The voices may command them to do certain things, some of which may be ego-alien. Resultant behaviors may appear impulsive, oppositional, or inappropriate. The voices may tell a child to call out in class, to push another child, or to call a parent a "name." The child may resist complying, but when the demand is repeated numerous times the child loses patience and may comply just to silence the voices.

The observer often interprets dissociation as inattention because the child's mind no longer attends to the present activity, conversation, or task. In school the teacher observes the child as daydreaming, staring, or tuning out. Peers and parents say the child is "spacey." When questioned about what he or she is thinking about when not paying attention to the teacher or class work, the child with DID often responds, "I wasn't thinking of anything," or "My mind was blank," or "I don't know." The child with ADHD responds similarly.

I have seen several children, initially diagnosed by me or others with ADHD, who I have subsequently discovered had a dissociative disorder. Now I look for symptoms during the initial evaluation that help to differentiate ADHD from dissociative disorders. A cluster of the following symptoms leads me to do further evaluation for a dissociative disorder.

By history
1. frequent daydreaming, dazed expressions or blank stares at home and school during which the child does *not* respond easily to prompts to regain their attention;
2. rapid, spontaneous mood changes without apparent precipitating events;
3. frequent age regression;
4. denying behaviors that are directly observed by parents or others;
5. frequently forgetting things that the child is interested in and has obviously been attentive to;
6. significant variability in skills requiring fine motor functioning (writing) or gross motor functioning (throwing, catching, batting, etc.);
7. frequent variability within subjects in which the child shows interest (in ADHD interest and motivation foster recall).

By observation
1. spontaneous trances;
2. amnesia;
3. frequent contradictory statements—often back to back;
4. numbness to pain or a variable response (e.g., from passive acceptance of immunizations or venipunctures to extreme resistance in the same child on successive occasions).

I often check for amnesia by asking the child toward the end of the session to tell me some of the things we discussed. If I notice any age regression, dazed expressions, or changes in voice quality or mannerisms, I will ask during that time for information discussed prior to those changes.

In the case of a child or adolescent with DID, the behavioral characteristics of alters differ so that it is possible to identify certain alters that meet the criteria for ADHD, whereas other alters may not meet or even come close to meeting the criteria. A 13-year-old girl was brought to me by her foster mother with complaints of fidgetiness, short attention span, impulsivity, distractibility, forgetfulness, lying, sleepwalking, talking to herself, and intermittent poor hygiene. In addition, she occasionally appeared dazed and was quite moody. There was a history of sexual abuse as a young child. Connor's abbreviated teacher questionnaires completed by five different teachers showed considerable variability ranging from scores of 1 to 19. She was initially diagnosed with ADHD and treated with Ritalin. Impulsivity and fidgetiness decreased but attention increased only slightly. After I saw her a few times it became clear that sometimes she would recall certain events from her past but other times could not recall the same events. A CDC completed by her foster mother scored 17, a fairly high score. Further interview with the child revealed that she occasionally heard voices talking to her in her head. I strongly suspected she had DID but could not make that diagnosis because I had not knowingly observed any alters. Referral to a child psychologist specializing in dissociative disorders confirmed that she did have DID. In fact she had five named alters in addition to the host personality. One of the alters was an hyperactive 5-year-old girl. Whenever she was "out" (i.e., assuming executive control) in the office, she became dramatically more fidgety, distractible, and inattentive. The other alters and host personality were much less fidgety. The diagnosis of ADHD would likely be made if someone frequently observed the hyperactive alter, but not if other alters were observed.

To date no studies are published on the use of stimulant medication in children with dissociative disorders. However, as in the above vignette, some physicians have noted that stimulant medication has effected a decrease in hyperactivity and impulsivity in children and adolescents with dissociative disorders, but dissociation or internal auditory hallucinations may still cause symptoms of inattention and distractibility.

In recent years physicians have recognized that high levels of comorbidity exist with ADHD. Available literature suggests frequent occurrence of ADHD with conduct, mood, and anxiety disorders, as well as learning disabilities in children, adolescents, and adults (Biederman, Neuroin, and Sprich, 1991). In a study of 106 adolescents with borderline personality disorder, Andrulonis (1982) found that 25% had a current or past history of ADHD. As borderline pathology is also heavily associated with physical and sexual abuse (Westen, Ludolph, & Misle, 1990) it would not be surprising if some of these adolescents also had undiagnosed dissociative disorders. Hornstein & Putnam (1992) found that 12.5% of dissociative patients had been diagnosed with ADHD.

Researchers usually define ADHD study populations based on criteria found in the most current edition of *DSM-IV*. Previous *DSM* editions have not included dissociative disorders as exclusionary criteria for defining ADHD. However, exclusionary criteria for ADHD in *DSM-IV* state that the symptoms "are not better accounted for by another mental disorder (e.g., Dissociative Disorder)." Most studies in ADHD have not included screening for dissociative disorders in the study populations. Thus, the results of some studies may be contaminated because ADHD research populations may contain dissociative disordered children and adolescents. Future researchers should use a screening device such as the CDC to exclude children with dissociative disorders.

The primary care physician should bear in mind that dissociative disorders may complicate the diagnosis and/or treatment of ADHD. All children who present with ADHD-type symptoms should be screened for possible dissociative disorders. Treatment resistant ADHD patients should be thoroughly reassessed for dissociative disorders before physicians resort to high levels of medication, changing medications, or adding additional medications to the treatment regimen.

Eating Disorders

Dissociative disorders appear quite frequently in adults with eating disorders. In one study of both inpatients and outpatients with eating disorders ranging in age from 19 to 35, 28% were found to have dissociative disorders and 10% had DID (McCallum, Lock, Kulla, Rorty, & Wetzel, 1992). Likewise both anorexia and bulimia are found in patients with dissociative disorders (Miller & McCluskey-Fawcett, 1993). In Dell & Eisenhower's (1990) sample, 18% of the DID adolescent patients presented with eating disorders. Thus, it would seem wise to rule out dissociative processes in adolescents presenting with eating disorder symptoms. Questions regarding feelings associated with self-induced vomiting or precursors to the onset of vomiting may help to bring dissociative phenomena to the forefront. Some patients have described self-induced vomiting as a trancelike dissociative experience. Questions about body image may help uncover information related to abuse. Screening for dissociative disorders in adolescents with eating disorders with the A-DES may be prudent and may provide a springboard for subsequent discussions of these issues. It should be kept in mind during interviewing that eating disorder symptoms may be confined to one alter personality.

Seizure Disorders / and Conversion Disorders

In reviewing single case reports, Putnam (1989) reported 21% of adult cases had seizures, primarily of a temporal lobe variety, or seizure-like behaviors. Although abnormal EEGs were found in 10% of DID patients (Putnam, 1989), many apparent seizure-like occurrences are best understood as dissociative or posttraumatic (Bowman & Markand, 1996). In a study of 45 patients with pseudo-seizures, Bowman & Markand found that 91% had dissociative disorders.

When pediatric patients are referred for evaluation of possible seizures, inclusion of dissociative disorders in the differential diagnosis is suggested. If the referral is based on observations of momentary attentional lapses, the possibility of brief dissociative episodes should be considered. Sometimes adolescent patients may present with repetitive seizure-like episodes for which no medical basis can be found. Goodwin, Simms, and Bergman (1979) and Gross (1979) described pseudo-seizures in adolescents that clearly related to incestual experiences. As Bowman and Markand determined in their sample of adults with pseudo-seizures, many cases of pseudo-seizure can be explained when the traumatic origins of the behaviors are understood.

A 16-year-old teenage girl was referred to me who suffered from strange "seizures" that only occurred between 11:00 p.m. and 1:00 a.m. There was apparent loss of consciousness with flailing of arms, followed by guttural noises, mumbling, and then occasional statements like, "Don't kill me!" or "Please don't!" She was being treated by a neurologist with tegretol, but the "seizures" continued. Neurologic examinations and EEGs were all normal, and a 3-day inpatient evaluation failed to reveal any organic pathology.

Three years later, this patient was diagnosed with DID. During outpatient therapy, one alter explained that preceding the onset of these seizure-like episodes, the young woman had been tied at gunpoint, threatened to be killed with a gun placed in her mouth, and made to breathe some unknown chemical on a cloth covering her face. This all occurred between 11:00 p.m. and 1:00 a.m. Her "seizures" were actually partial reenactments of these traumatic events by one of her alters.

Pseudo-seizures such as the one above are commonly seen as "conversion disorders," which involve unexplained symptoms or deficits affecting voluntary motor or sensory function. Somatization disorders and conversion disorders, both characterized by physical complaints without known organic etiology, are commonly found in dissociative patients (Putnam, 1989; Saxe et al., 1994). Putnam, Guroff, Silberman, Barban, and Post (1986) reported that about 55% of 100 reported cases of DID had conversion symptoms. Conversion disorders may appear in prepubescent children but usually begin in adolescence and, in fact, are more common in adolescents than in adults (Gold & Friedman, 1995). Conversion disorders in children and adolescents are associated with a history of sexual abuse and family pathology (Nemzer, 1991).

Often adolescents presenting with pain, motor dysfunctions, or sensory impairment without organic cause are diagnosed with a conversion disorder without considering a more encompassing diagnosis such as a dissociative disorder. If all medical causes for a symptom have been ruled out and a conversion disorder is being considered, a dissociative disorder must be included in the differential diagnosis. If the primary care physician is unable to screen for dissociative disorders, referral should be made to a mental health provider who can assess the child with an unexplained physical symptom to uncover the possible traumatic roots of the symptom and assess for a possible dissociative disorder.

Referral Guidelines

Treatment of children with dissociative disorders is a specialty. Unless the primary care physician has particular interest and training in this area, a child suspected of pathologic dissociation should be referred to someone with expertise in dissociative disorders. In most localities this is easier said than done, because there are few with such expertise. Child psychiatry, psychology, and social work training programs are just beginning to incorporate dissociative disorder training in some localities. The problem of the paucity of treatment providers is compounded by controversy within the mental health professional community: even though dissociative disorders are considered legitimate diagnoses with specific criteria for diagnosis in *DSM-IV,* some mental health professionals refuse to consider a diagnosis such as DID.

To identify appropriate referral resources, begin by contacting your usual referral sources for children with behavior problems. Find out what their experience and training has been with children with dissociative disorders. Many therapists have been trained to work with abused children but have not been trained to assess or treat dissociative disorders. If they are unable to provide the needed assessment and treatment, find out if they know any professionals trained in dissociative disorders. Other sources that can be contacted include the International Society for the Study of Dissociation; the American Academy of Child and Adolescent Psychiatry, the American Psychiatric Association, and your state chapters of the American Psychological Association and the National Association of Social Workers.

Treatment Challenges of the Dissociative Patient

Now that a dissociative patient has been diagnosed in the primary care physician's practice, many unique treatment issues arise. A newly diagnosed dissociative patient may have complicated legal issues related to a presumed history of abuse, sleep problems, a multitude of somatic complaints, confusing psychophysiological changes, and many issues related to conduct, school performance, and family relationships. The pediatrician must work conjointly with the therapist, social service worker, or lawyer when necessary to help coordinate the management of the patient.

The pediatrician may have information that each of these professionals might require and sharing information and observations can help keep the patient's treatment on course.

Exams for documentation of abuse

A pediatrician may be asked to do an exam to document physical injuries for legal purposes. The parent or caretaker should be interviewed separately from the child. A detailed history concerning the injury should be obtained and recorded from each of them. A note should be included about the child's mental status, especially noting any changes, during the interview and exam. This is particularly important, because the history from a dissociative child can change depending on the particular dissociative state the child may be in. If the physician suspects a change in dissociative states during the course of the interview, retaking the history or part of the history may be helpful to assess for supplementary information. During the physical examination of what might be a tender area, a dissociative child may overreact or underreact to pain, and this should be recorded as well.

Interviewing and examining the dissociative child or adolescent about sexual concerns must be done with great care. It is likely to precipitate dissociation, which can lead to unpredictable behavior. Total withdrawal, hostility, histrionics, seductive behaviors, and indifference are all possibilities. In addition, I have seen several instances of false accusations of sexual abuse by a dissociative child (though none were directed at a physician during an examination). False accusations by children with dissociative dissorders are often due to distorted perceptions related to previous sexual abuse. The child may superimpose part of an abuse memory onto a present event. Therefore, a few caveats are worth noting. It will be viewed as less threatening to interview the child with their clothes on, and have the child seated in a chair rather than on the examining table. It is advisable to sit a reasonable distance from the child, as sitting close may be perceived as threatening. Consider having a nurse present for the interview to help verify what was observed or to document conflicting information from patients in different dissociative states. Always have a chaperon present for a breast, anal, or genital examination. Be sure to explain to the child ahead of time what you will be doing, and be gentle and move slowly during the course of the exam. Follow the "Guidelines for the Evaluation of Sexual Abuse of Children" published by the American Academy of Pediatrics, Committee on Child Abuse and Neglect (1991). For further helpful pediatric information on this subject see "Child Sexual Abuse" (Berkowitz, 1992).

Sleep Problems

One of the most common pediatric concerns of parents regarding their dissociative children is sleep difficulty. Most of the children I have seen experience frequent nightmares, sleepwalking, or periods when they are hypervigilant at bedtime. These symptoms may be due to having been sexually abused repeatedly either at bedtime or during the night. One 5-year-old boy, whom I evaluated and who was later diagnosed with DID, presented with destructive behaviors in the middle of the night, when he would get out of bed, go downstairs, and damage his foster parents' things. He would cut upholstery with a kitchen knife, cut pictures with scissors, urinate on the carpet, etc. The problem was resolved when the foster parents purchased a battery-operated alarm device at a local electronics store and fastened it to the top of his bedroom door molding. As most of the sleep problems in children with dissociative disorders appear to be related to the abuse they experienced, treatment needs to be closely coordinated with the psychotherapy. There may be instances when medication such as diphenhydramine may help to ameliorate sleep symptoms. Further psychotropic medications may be prescribed under the direction of a child psychiatrist (see Chapter 12).

Another common problem associated with sleep is nighttime (or daytime) enuresis, a symptom common in sexually abused children in general (Frederich, 1990). The physiological reason for the association of enuresis to sexual abuse is unclear, but may relate to the dissociation of genital sensation that the child uses to cope with the abuse. This dissociation of sensation could then become generalized to bowel or bladder function as well. Peterson (1996) has described enuresis among dissociative children that may relate to a younger alter's enjoyment of the warm feeling associated with wetting. Pediatricians must maintain contact with the therapist to assess the role of the symptom within the dissociative system, while prescribing appropriate medical interventions. Some families have simply accommodated to a routine of changing sheets every morning while avoiding stigmatizing the child or emphasizing the symptom.

Fluctuating Physiological Phenomena

Adults with DID have exhibited psychophysiologic phenomena in which physiologic changes are induced by psychologic states. Although specific data concerning psychophysiologic phenomena in children and adolescents with DID are less available, those working with this population have seen similar phenomena. Physicians may feel less bewildered if they recognize the "atypical" physiologic responses that may occur in children with dissociative disorders.

There are a variety of psychophysiologic changes that have been reported in adults with DID. Braun (1983) cites cases involving allergic responses, dermatologic reactions, and reactions of the autonomic and central nervous systems, among others. Interestingly enough, many of the same phenomena can be produced by hypnosis, which has many parallels to dissociation.

Differential allergic reactions have been reported in adults with DID, depending upon which alter has executive control of the person. For example, one or more alters may be allergic to cats, resulting in allergic rhinitis or allergic conjunctivitis, while other alters can play with cats without problems (Braun, 1983). In my experience, one 15-year-old boy with DID discussed with me that one of his alters was very prone to develop severe reactions to poison ivy, whereas other alters with presumably similar contact developed either no rash or much milder cases. In fact, when the highly reactive alter with poison ivy switched to another alter for awhile, the patient reported that the pruritus and erythema decreased. When I see a differential pathologic response amongst alters, I recommend to the patient that the alter experiencing the problem take the medication, apply the cream, or perform the treatment. Although I can offer no scientific or physiologic rationale, clinically this approach seems to help. Perhaps over time the medical profession will come to understand these perplexing variabilities in physiologic functions, and information gleaned from researching this may enhance our ability to treat a variety of medical conditions or fortify immune response in patients.

Adults with DID sometimes have alters who have experienced physical trauma that caused contusions, burns, or other skin traumata (Braun, 1983). When these alters assume executive control over an individual, perhaps years later, similar lesions may develop on the same body location as the original lesion. Neither the host personality nor most of the alters have memory of the original traumatic event. This "body memory" often seems incomprehensible to the observer unless the traumatic history and the DID are appreciated. The primary care physician's role is to document the history obtained, examine, and record the physical findings as accurately as possible. If a child is known to be dissociative, then obtaining a history of the child's mood during the occurrence of a physical complaint such as abdominal or limb pain or headache is important. Occasionally one will find that certain physical complaints are associated with certain moods or unusual behaviors. Such information should be reported to the therapist.

Investigators have found that persons with DID have differential autonomic nervous system responses to the same stimulus depending upon which alter has executive control (Putnam, 1991). Heart rate, blood pressure, respirations, galvanic skin responses, cerebral blood flow, evoked potentials, EMG, and brain mapping can vary with different alters. However, the studies in these areas have small populations, so the results should be interpreted with caution (Brown, 1994). Headaches are the most common physical complaints (Putnam, 1989) of DID patients. Some headaches have migraine characteristics with auras, excessive sweating, and visual changes. There are other headaches that seem to relate to switching among alters. Patients report headaches when there is rapid switching as well as when there is conflict over which alter will obtain executive control. "Switching" headaches seem to be reported less often in children than in adults with DID. I have had an opportunity to observe several adults with DID, all of whom had "switching" headaches. These seem to be focal, unilateral, and often migratory headaches, i.e., they begin in one area such as right temporal and move to another, lasting seconds to minutes. In adults these headaches sometimes respond to clonazepam. Surprisingly, I have seen very few of these headaches in dissociative children or adolescents.

A variety of sensory changes can occur in people with DID. Visual acuity differences have been noted among different alters in the same individual (Miller, Blackburn, Scholes, White, & Mamalis, 1991). Thus, depending upon which alter is "out," vision screening may produce different results. In adults, "hysterical" diplopia and blindness have been reported (Bliss, 1980). Psychogenic deafness and parathesias have also been reported among some alters (Putnam, Guroff, Silberman, Barban, & Post, 1986; Bliss, 1980).

One of the most disconcerting psychophysiologic phenomena for physicians is state-dependent differential responses to medications by various alters within the same individual (Loewenstein, 1991). Acetaminophen may relieve pain in some alters but not in others. Some alters may report relief from antihistamine/decongestants, while others do not. Compliance with medications also can vary among alters. It is often helpful, especially with adolescents who may be responsible for taking their own medications, to work closely with the therapist to identify an alter who will be responsible to take medications. When speaking to an adolescent with DID about medications, it can be helpful to state that you want to speak to "that part of the person who will be responsible to take the medication" and that you want that part to "listen carefully." This may seem awkward or strange to the physician, but it will not seem so to the patient with DID. It is a simple way to increase compliance. Presumably this is unnecessary in the younger child, since the parent should be responsible to give medication.

Behavioral Problems

Pediatricians are frequently confronted with questions about disruptive behavior, and it is important not to respond with the typical behavior modification approach when the patient has a known trauma history.

Some disruptive behavior at home, school, or elsewhere may be a flash-back or reexperiencing of a past traumatic event. For example, a child may suddenly start yelling for help or flailing at someone as they reexperience a past perpetrator of abuse approaching them, even though no perpetrator is present. In some cases, a child is reminded of a traumatic event by something in their environment that triggers a sudden mood change unexplainable to the observer. For example, a 7-year-old girl was brought to see me by her parents because she had unexplained moodiness, irritability, and intermittent withdrawal from the family. Her parents were bewildered by her behaviors. This girl had been sexually abused by an adult babysitter at age 4, disclosed it about 1½ years later and to outward appearances had functioned well until recently. What the girl had not disclosed to her parents were the mixed feelings of guilt, shame, and anger that were triggered each time she saw a "sexualized" TV commercial, or when she noted persons embracing on video movie jackets. Treatment of this child required more than employment of behavior modification techniques to reduce irritability. The parents needed to understand how environmental triggers stimulated certain feelings, such as guilt, shame, and anger, and the child needed an opportunity to discuss these feelings. Helping parents learn to identify triggers to flash-backs, tantrum behaviors, or sudden mood shifts may provide a framework for better parent-child communication and a more supportive environment.

It is common for an adolescent with DID to have one or more alters that "act out" in various ways. An alter may use street drugs and/or overindulge in alcohol. However, the host personality is often amnestic for such behaviors, and a history from the host will prove negative for use of alcohol and drugs. There may be another alter who "comes out" during the next office visit and "tells on" the imbibing alter, or the imbibing alter may assume executive control and admit to the behaviors. The host personality may then return and deny the behaviors again. Unless the interviewer is aware of the diagnosis, he or she may feel confused or will wrongly assume the adolescent is willfully denying the behavior. If a primary care physician discovers substance or alcohol abuse in a person with DID, the therapist should be contacted immediately. The therapist, in turn, may need the physician's assistance both for patient and family education and laboratory monitoring of substance abuse.

Repeated sexual abuse of a child sometimes leads to sexual acting out and promiscuity. Masturbation, initiation of sexual activities with peers (both homosexual and heterosexual), sexual molesting of young children by adolescents, indiscriminant adolescent sexual behavior, and other sexual behaviors can all occur in dissociative children and adolescents. A well-developed 12-year-old child with a dissociative disorder took her blouse and brassiere off on the street in front of her house in the afternoon with numerous people around. She was escorted quickly into the house by her foster mother, who witnessed the behavior. A few minutes later, the girl had a significant change in mood and denied being able to recall what had just occurred. When I saw her later that week, she continued to maintain that she could not recall what had happened. The juxtaposition of unusual sexual behavior, sudden mood change and apparent amnesia should suggest the possibility of a dissociative disorder.

Communication with parents

Based on our current knowledge, children with dissociative disorders and especially DID have often been abused. It should not be assumed, however, that a parent is the perpetrator. Presumption of guilt may negatively affect communication between physician and parent, which in turn will adversely affect the child.

It is difficult to parent a dissociative child. Parents can easily feel confused, frustrated, and angry at the child. They often need opportunities to talk and ventilate. Hopefully they have opportunities do this with the child's therapist, but these feelings may spill out at a well-child or sick visit as well. The physician can help by providing a listening, understanding, empathic ear. Appointments with these children may require extra time, and office staff need to be aware of this in scheduling.

I find that parents of dissociative children often bring up behavioral problems, even during the course of a sick visit. I tell the parent that they are raising an important concern that needs discussion and I would suggest discussing it with the therapist. I may be tempted to give a quick behavioral recommendation, but this could result in mistaken recommendations if the full meaning of the behavior is not taken into account. In fact, I find that in responding to questions about behavior from these parents, I usually need to review information about dissociation and how it influences behavior, a time-consuming prospect. Frequently parents will bring up the problem of the dissociative child's lying. Responding to this concern of the parents requires reviewing amnesia and how to recognize it in the dissociative child. Unless the physician has the time, interest, and knowledge, responses to this type of concern are best left to the therapist.

Summary

Children and adolescents with dissociative disorders can present with a variety of somatic or behavioral complaints in a physician's office. These patients may respond poorly or only partially to standard therapies. Pediatricians who are aware of dissociative disorders may help facilitate early referrals for appropriate assessment and treatment. Use of the Child Dissociative Checklist in preadolescent children can be a helpful screening tool. The primary care physician may need to work in collaboration with the therapist and other treatment team members from time to time.

In treating patients with DID, physicians must be aware of the variability of physiologic responses depending on which alter has executive control of the individual. In adolescent patients who may be responsible for taking their own medication, compliance can be improved by asking that the responsible alter listen to the instructions. Physicians treating children with ADHD should be aware that children with dissociative disorders can have the same or similar symptoms. If medical treatment fails to significantly alleviate symptoms or if the child has dissociative behaviors, referral for further assessment is indicated.

Future research in ADHD, eating disorders, psychosomatic illnesses, and behavioral disorders should rule out dissociative disorders in the study populations to avoid spurious results. Improved clinical research on diagnosis of dissociative disorders and associated physiological correlates in children will facilitate the management of this difficult patient population.

References

American Academy of Pediatrics, Committee on Child Abuse and Neglect. (1991). Guidelines for the evaluation of sexual abuse of children. *Pediatrics, 87,* 254–260.

American Psychiatric Association. (1994). *Diagnostic and statistical manual of mental disorders* (4th ed.). Washington, DC: Author.

Andrulonis, P. A. (1982). Borderline personality subcategories. *The Journal of Nervous and Mental Diseases, 171,* 670–679.

Berkowitz, C. D. (1992). Child sexual abuse. *Pediatrics in Review, 13,* 443–452.

Biederman, J., Neuroin, J., & Sprich, S. (1991). Comorbidity of ADHD with conduct, depressive, anxiety, and other disorders. *American Journal of Psychiatry, 148,* 564.

Bliss, E. L. (1980). Multiple personalities: A report of 14 cases with implications for schizophrenia and hysteria. *Archives of General Psychiatry, 37,* 1388–1400.

Bowman, E. S., & Markand, O. R. (1996). Psychodynamics and psychiatric diagnosis of pseudoseizures. *The American Journal of Psychiatry, 153,* 57–63.

Braun, B. G. (1983). Psychophysiologic phenomena in multiple personality and hypnosis. *American Journal of Clinical Hypnosis, 26,* 124–136.

Brown, P. (1994). Toward a psychobiological model of dissociation and post-traumatic stress disorder. In S. J. Lynn & J. W. Rhue (Eds.), *Dissociation: Clinical and theoretical perspectives* (pp. 94–122). New York: Guilford Press.

Dean, G., Giem, D., Guerro, J., & Leard, R. A. (1989). Comparison of incipient MPD and MPD predictors to disorders commonly diagnosed in children and adolescents (Summary). *Proceedings of the sixth international conference on multiple personality/dissociative states, 177.*

Dell, P. F., & Eisenhower, J. W. (1990). Adolescent multiple personality disorder:

A preliminary study of eleven cases. *Journal of the American Academy of Child and Adolescent Psychiatry, 29,* 359–366.

Evers-Szostak, M., & Sanders, S. (1992). The children's perceptual alteration scale (CPAS): A measure of children's dissociation. *Dissociation, 5,* 91–97.

Fagan, J., & McMahon, P. P. (1984). Incipient multiple personality in children. *The Journal of Nervous and Mental Disease, 172.* 26–36.

Frederich, W. N. (1990). *Psychotherapy of sexually abused children and their families.* New York: W. W. Norton.

Gold, M. A., & Friedman, S. B. (1995). Conversion reactions in adolescents. *Pediatric annals, 24,* 296–306.

Goodwin, J., Simms, M., & Bergman, R. (1979), Hysterical seizures: A sequel to incest. *The American Journal of Orthopsychiatry, 49,* 698–703.

Gross, M. (1979) Incestuous rape: A cause for hysterical seizures in four adolescent girls. *The American Journal of Orthopsychiatry, 49,* 704–708.

Hornstein, N. L., & Putnam, F. W. (1992). Clinical phenomenology of child and adolescent dissociative disorders. *Journal of the American Academy of Child and Adolescent Psychiatry, 31,* 1077–1085.

Kluft, R. P. (1985a). Childhood multiple personality disorder: Predictors, clinical findings, and treatment results. In Kluft, R. P. (Ed.), *Childhood Antecedents of Multiple Personality* (pp. 167–196). Washington, DC: American Psychiatric Press.

Kluft, R. P. (1985b). The natural history of multiple personality disorder. In Kluft, R. P. (Ed.), *Childhood antecedents of multiple personality* (pp. 197–238). Washington, DC: American Psychiatric Press.

Loewenstein, R. J. (1991). Rational psychopharmacology in the treatment of multiple personality disorder. *The Psychiatric Clinics of North America, 14,* pp. 721–740.

McCallum, K. E., Lock, J., Kulla, M., Rorty, M., & Wetzel, R.D. (1992). Dissociative symptoms and disorders in patients with eating disorders. *Dissociation, 4,* 227–235.

Miller, D. A. F., & McCluskey-Fawcett, K. (1993). The relationship between childhood sexual abuse and subsequent onset of bulimia nervosa. *Child abuse & neglect, 17,* 305–314.

Miller, S., Blackburn, T., Scholes, G., White, G. L., & Mamalis, N. (1991). Optical differences in multiple personality disorder: A second look. *The Journal of Nervous and Mental Disease, 179,* 132–135.

Nemzer, E. D. (1991). Somatoform disorders. In M. Lewis (Ed.), *Child and adolescent psychiatry: A comprehensive textbook* (pp. 697–706.). Baltimore: Williams and Wilkins.

Peterson, G. (1996). Early onset. In J. L. Spira (Ed.), *Treating dissociative identity disorder* (pp.135–173). San Francisco: Jossey-Bass.

Putnam, F. W. (1989). *Diagnosis and treatment of multiple personality disorder.* New York: Guilford Press.

Putnam, F. W. (1991a). Recent research on multiple personality disorder. *Psychiatric Clinics of North America, 14,* 489–502.

Putnam. F. W. (1993). Dissociative disorders in children: Behavioral profiles and problems. *Child Abuse and Neglect, 17,* 39–45.

Putnam, F. W., Guroff, J. J., Silberman, E. K., Barban, K. L., & Post, R. M. (1986).

The clinical phenomenology of multiple personality disorder: Review of 100 recent cases. *Journal of Clinical Psychiatry, 47,* 285–293.

Putnam, F. W., Helmers, K., & Trickett, P. K. (1993). Development, reliability, and validity of a child dissociation scale. *Child Abuse and Neglect,* 17, 731–741.

Putnam, F. W., & Peterson, G. (1994). Further validation of the child dissociative checklist. *Dissociation, 7,* 204–211.

Reagor, P. A., Kasten, J. D., & Morelli, N. (1992). A checklist for screening dissociative disorders in children and adolescents. *Dissociation, 5,* 4–19.

Ross, C. A. (1991). Epidemiology of multiple personality disorder and dissociation. *Psychiatric Clinics of North America, 14,* 503–517.

Saxe, G. N., Chinman, G., Berkowitz, R., Hall, K., Lieberg, G., Schwartz, J., & van der Kolk, B. A. (1994). Somatization in patients with dissociative disorders. *American Journal of Psychiatry, 151,* 1329–34.

West, L. J. (1967). Dissociative reaction. In A. M. Freeman & H. I. Kaplan (Eds.), *Comprehensive textbook of psychiatry.* Baltimore: Williams and Wilkins.

Westen, D., Ludolph, P. , Misle, B. (1990). Physical and sexual abuse in adolescents with borderline personality disorder. *American Journal of Orthopsychiatry. 60,* 55–66.

Whitman, B. Y., & Munkel, W. (1991). Multiple personality disorder: a risk indicator, diagnostic marker and psychiatric outcome for severe child abuse. *Clinical pediatrics, 30,* 422–428.

f i f t e e n

School Interventions for Dissociative Children

Marcia Waterbury

In order to work effectively in the school system, a mental health clinician must be attuned to local and national educational objectives. Even within an educational locale, individual differences exist amongst schools. Three essential concepts will assist you in establishing an entry into the traumatized child's academic environment: School-Based Mental Health Services, Definition of Seriously Emotionally Disturbed, and Multiculturalism.

School-Based Mental Health Services

The recognition that the prevalence of emotional and behavioral disorders was increasing at an alarming rate led Educators in 1994 to institute a much stronger proactive plan to bring mental health services into the school. Much of the impetus was sparked by the need to service increasing numbers of offspring of drug abusing parents, teen mothers, single parents, and families of diverse cultural background. Public Law (PL) 94-142 in 1975 mandated schools to provide whatever services were necessary to educate handicapped children and introduced the category of

The author wishes to express appreciation for the contributions of Julie Gaynor, M.Ed., SED/LD Specialist, her assistant Francis Simmons, and Principal Sheila Graham for their commitment to helping traumatized children and to their students at Sandy Plains Elementary School, Baltimore, Maryland, who have reaped the benefits of their efforts.

the Seriously Emotionally Disturbed (SED). PL 99-457 extended those services to infants and toddlers.

Traditional mental health services required considerable involvement with the parent—often the entire family—and regular attendance at sites often distant from the school and home. A family's failure to keep regularly scheduled clinic visits resulted in prompt termination. Alternative therapeutic services that went directly into the home met obstacles of parental resistance related to their not wanting outsiders to invade the family's privacy. The time-limited nature of the home involvement many times forced the therapist to refer families in need of prolonged services back to the local mental health agency where the aforementioned drawbacks pertained. Through the efforts of many multidisciplinary coalitions, a major revision in the state and federal funding of health care permitted primary providers to be reimbursed for services given at school sites through third party billing (Maryland Governor's Office for Children, Youth and Families, 1995). Consequently health care organizations have been establishing an increasingly broad range of mental health services within individual schools. A host of problems, including transportation and intensive parental participation, have been obviated, as the students are a captive audience. The powerful legal sanction that the child must attend school or the parent be subject to criminal charges adds even greater clout. A variety of avenues for positive interventions to dysfunctional children are now accessible, independent of responsible parental participation. Such services set a model for cooperative interaction between mental health and educational disciplines.

Definition of the Seriously Emotionally Disturbed

Legislation regulating education for the handicapped was revolutionary in providing a mechanism for including mentally disordered children in its rubric under the designation *Serious Emotional Disturbance* (SED). Legislated health care policy provides legal definitions of what constitute mentally handicapping conditions (SEDs) and of the accompanying severity criteria required to establish the presence of marked functional limitations. For most of two decades behavioral maladjustment has been distinguished from emotional disorder. Educators have tended to view conspicuously misbehaving children as incorrigible, poorly parented, or not interested in learning—thus not meriting the expensive psychological services used to ameliorate genuine psychiatric dysfunction (Maryland Disability Law Center, 1994). Even where psychiatric disorder has been documented, very rigid proof is required to prove that the mental disorder directly caused the child to fall behind academically and that the requested specialized services are essential for the child's educational growth. Mainstreaming, keeping the child in his regular educational setting, is another major goal in special education because it lessens the potential for stigmatization. Interventions are viewed as "restrictive" if they draw attention to the child's difference from the typical, so-called "regular" student, thereby, increasing the potential for stigmatization. Levels of restrictiveness are ordered from lower to higher levels of intensity, each requiring smaller student to staff ratios and greater expertise of the educator in addressing the mental dysfunction as well as frequently coexisting learning dysfunction. Location and conditions of the educational environment are similarly rated for restrictiveness. At highest intensity the child is required to remain in a self-contained program at a facility not connected to the public school and often attached to a residential treatment program, psychiatric hospital, or day hospital. It is anticipated that the federal government will officially broaden the *SED* designation through legislation to include behavioral as well as emotional disorders. Many states are proactively modifying their terminology to allow aggressive, unsocialized children specialized services, whereas previously those children were viewed as "bad" and not amenable to therapeutic interventions. Mental health and educational specialists will be expected to address both emotional and behavioral features of mental illness.

Multiculturalism

Another national thrust in education involves attention to cultural differences within the school environment. A similar trend is occurring within the mental health field, as it has become increasingly apparent that traditional therapies based on Western notions of independence and personal responsibility have generally failed to meet the needs of most ethnic minority groups in the United States (Vargas & Koss-Chioino, 1992, chap. 1). Vargas and Koss-Chioino point out that terms such as *culturally sensitive* and *culturally responsive* have been coined to reflect the therapist's appreciation of the impact of culture in shaping multiple developmental trajectories, familial value systems, and societal expectations. They challenge the clinician or teacher to carefully evaluate personal prejudices and cultural biases when exploring the cultural patterning of the student's family life as well as the universal applicability of cherished professional beliefs.

The field of trauma shares a commonality with minority cultures. Society has strongly resisted accepting ideas of physical and sexual victimization of children as commonplace, preferring to see such phenomena as rare societal anomalies. As increasing numbers of cases have been reported, many political and civic leaders have insisted that the claims are falsely inflated and have resisted providing greater public support. The scientific community historically has given little attention to sexual and physical traumatization of children and other weaker members of society.

Without theory, established technique, or belief in the phenomenon of overwhelming traumatization of powerless segments of American society, academic institutions ignored and sometimes actively attacked professionals trying to understand and treat them. The minority disciplines devoted to the study of weaker members of society—traumatized children—were often segregated from mainstream collaboration, funding, and endorsement. They experienced stigmatization and discrediting by scientific politicalization rather than by results of careful research (Peterson, Prout, & Schwarz, 1991, pp. 133–139).

Professionals working with seriously traumatized children and their families should take advantage of society's current interest in the culturally different as they intervene in the school or related agencies. Many paradigm shifts are needed to successfully deal with abused and neglected children, just as Koss-Chioino and Vargas (1992) have observed for children of minority color and religion. In the current climate of increasing tolerance toward extreme deviations from traditional Western values, mental health professionals may find educators more flexible in learning about and accommodating more effective means to deal with the distortions and maladaptive coping responses of severely traumatized children.

Strategies for Initiating Collaboration with School

Observation and Assessment

Now armed with the above concepts, the therapist should assess the child's school regarding what school based mental health services are currently available. In addition to meeting with the teacher(s), principal, guidance counselor, school social worker, and school nurse if indicated, the therapist is urged to observe the child in the classroom. Traumatized children typically react to a myriad of seemingly neutral or insignificant stimuli with dramatic alterations in mood and behavior states. These minor stimuli symbolize some aspect of prior traumatic experiences. The therapist must be sensitive to this characteristic and take advantage of the opportunity to observe or learn about the child's patterns of behavior in the multiple settings of the school environment. Often the teacher and other staff can be enlisted to make numerous observations, once informed of the expectation that the child will show considerable deviations in functioning across settings. For example, the clinician may inquire if the child at times seems unusually childlike in speech pattern, facial expression, and posture, as well as in increased dependency and passivity. At other times the child might be extremely defiant, stubborn, hostile, even violent. At yet other times the child may behave in a pseudo-mature or precociously sexualized manner. Then at other times the child seems severely depressed, depleted, and withdrawn or ebullient, energetic, and full of enthusiasm. The child may seem to be an adequate student, then appear to have forgotten much of what had previously been learned. S/he may display distinctive fearful states or evidence somatization which requires frequent nonproductive visits to the nurse. Of course, school contact does require the consent of the caregiver and child, but generally consent is easy to obtain because the child's functioning has deteriorated to crisis levels which demand therapeutic intervention. Often the child has already been screened for special education services designed to address academic weaknesses and/or emotional/behavioral dysfunction. The therapist needs to determine precisely how the school views the problem, what is being provided, and what it is willing to do to ameliorate the problem. Whenever possible, it is in the child's best interest for the consultant to establish a positive collaboration with the school and work conjointly to improve interventions within the current program, while strategizing together regarding additional services or more restrictive placement in the future.

Working with School Staff

School staff are very aware that some of their students live in chaotic homes and have experienced horrific events. When describing how children have been severely traumatized, psychologically hurt (Donovan & McIntyre, 1990), and damaged, the therapist should expect to find a receptive audience. School staff in my experience are easily able to make their own personal connections when given the explanation that the human mind uses predictable mechanisms to survive life threatening events.

It is important to provide a number of familiar examples of such mechanisms to the staff, so that traumatic reactions can be normalized. In my experience it is better to avoid controversial terminology, such as *dissociation*. If asked directly about dissociation, I will generally ask for the staff's thoughts on what the term means and then describe the human brain's remarkable capacity to siphon off aspects of an overwhelmingly noxious experience by altering conscious awareness and by damping or otherwise modifying perceptual processing of the event (*DSM-IV,* pp. 477–491). Furthermore, I explain that animals other than humans do the same thing for similar survival purposes. After ascertaining that school staff are receptive, I frequently inquire about the child's changeability in various settings. Severely traumatized children habitually dissociate at school and are distinguished by their perplexing extremes of behavioral responses, often many times in a single day. Many observant teachers have already identified patterns such as difficulty with transitions, avoidance of restrooms, intolerance of competitive sports, refusal to do certain types of school work. Caregivers too may have seen shifting patterns in after school activities.

One strategy I may adopt is to describe common variations in a single child. For example, I might say that the severely traumatized child has usually experienced great harm in the preschool years and that a frequent result is the child escaping in his/her mind through walling off those memories. By such doing, the child has had to detach connections with her/his usual conscious experiencing of the ebb and flow of everyday events. Under certain stressful states the internal experience of being that small, vulnerable child may reappear and observers will see voice intonation, speech pattern, behaviors, interests, and expressions reproducing that of a toddler, even an infant. Then I might shift to a discussion of what strength of mind is required to withstand such abuse and betrayal. That capacity is often found in the child's refusal to give in, to be enslaved, in the holding on to some semblance of personhood through resistance, and in battling the adversary. The rage and overt violence such children display is reframed as a measure of their will to survive. Although the rage must be contained and certainly the safety of other children and staff must be secured, I challenge the staff to reassess attitudes that label these children as fundamentally bad, antisocial, and delinquent. I point out several things well recognized in the literature regarding destructive, dangerous behaviors of traumatized children, such as the need to display sympathy and respect for those attitudes by attaching values of strength and self-protection to their aggressive, threatening stances. Often such a strategy has the extraordinary effect of disarming the child. Many times, by granting a positive connotation of strength to his/her aggressive position, the combatant child can team up with the teacher to better monitor anger and avoid outbursts.

Generally I list a number of affective states to anticipate: sad, depressed, even suicidal states; giddy, silly, giggling attitudes; teasing, tricking, testing moods; mistrustful, suspicious mind-sets; confused, preoccupied mental sets. What distinguishes these states is their stereotypy. Staff typically will quickly recall regularly recurring clusters of patterned behaviors and generally can accept the construct that during such occurrences, one of those states described above has taken hold of the child's mind. For example, a child may develop a beet red face. With its appearance, the child will storm around the classroom, shout or growl in precisely the same way each time, and almost robotically refuse an activity that at other times is not a problem. Besides affective states, the child may display role-like behaviors. Examples might be model student, mother's helper, teenage delinquent, seductress, big sister, parent, or a popular character on television. Another vexing state for the integrity of the classroom involves the child adopting an animal role. He or she may be found barking and crawling on the floor, roaring like a lion, or with fingers and nails extended like a bear's claws. The child might be found contemplating jumping out of a window, with arms flapping while proclaiming he or she is a bird.

Interaction with Student

After those working with the child have caught on to the technique of identifying repetitive patterns of characteristic behavior, I suggest that they adopt as a vantage point a perspective that attempts to address the patterns collectively. Just as they routinely interact with specific students individually and in various combinations, they may speak to the child's many sides, interests, or attitudes. By labeling the child's familiar fragments of behavior, they enable the child to more consciously address these mood/behavioral configurations. A dialogue with a student displaying frantic, fearful, dependent behavior who at other times is exaggeratedly independent, bossy, and determined might sound like the following: "Susie, right now you are feeling very scared and it seems to you that you can't possibly do this math problem. I guess it seems that this is what only a very big person could do." (Susie decreases her sobbing and seems to be listening) . . . After playing up how enormous the task seems, the teacher might gently remind her, "I bet you've completely forgotten something. Do you remember when you were working in the arithmetic book on Tuesday?" (Expect that Sally will require a lot of prompting to finally retrieve that memory). "You rushed through that so fast, you were like a race car. You didn't need any help from anyone. You were sure you knew just exactly what to do and, you know, you got most of answers right." (Susie is showing in her facial expression that she is recalling some of the confidence she exuded then).

At this point the teacher should engage Susie in an activity that addresses two very different ways of being in the school environment. A useful technique is to get a peg board with a large supply of differently colored pegs (some colored peg sets are also stackable). Teacher may select a color for the "tiny, uncertain side" and another for the "big, confident thinking side." Depending upon the subtleties of the situation Teacher may inquire if the colors suited the child's "sides." Then Teacher can construct two pegboard scenes. One should reflect the situation when Susie is feeling strong and self-assured. Teacher should be sure to wonder where the tiny, uncertain side is, saying, "It surely must be there somewhere since both are parts of Sally. Do a similar pegboard for the fearful, tiny side. The teacher should make a lot out of just recalling how "the feeling of the confident side helped the scared side get weaker and that then the strong side could be strong for both."

Then Teacher may lead Sally into other activities such as inquiring if the strong side likes a particular heroine, super-hero, cartoon character, etc. (Mills & Crowley, 1986, chap. 2 & 8). Questions might include what that side enjoys eating and doing, or how old it feels and what interests, likes, and dislikes it has. The teacher can do the same for the tiny side. Then she should suggest an alliance on the inside between "the strength" (for coping) and "the tiny side" (for company and providing appreciation and admiration). Many variations are possible and should be selected on the basis of the unique features of the situation and child.

Continuing with the same child, suppose the teacher notices that Sally seems much more confused in her science class than when she is in social studies despite similar degree of difficulty for amount of required reading and content complexity. By observing her closely, the teacher may discover that Sally demonstrates strikingly different cognition and perceptual/motor behaviors as well as behavior patterns in the two classes. Further assessment may lead to other cognitive/behavioral clusters in other educational activities. After mapping these skill clusters or skill deficiencies, the teacher can pursue specific remedial interventions that augment strength or support weaknesses. My approach enlists the teacher's own capacities to participate in the diagnosing of variations of the child's sensory, neuro-representational capacities in the school's varied academic, recreational, and social settings. Once identified, I counsel her to strategize how to use that information to construct therapeutic interventions directly in the class. I remind her that the child's functional abilities may be available in some settings but not others.

The teacher may maximize the visual-motor strength of a particular mental state by providing opportunities for drawing or the use of other visual modes. Then the teacher could draw upon the linguistic skills of another mind-set by giving an assignment to the child to make up a story about a selected topic and dictate it into a tape recorder or to write it as a creative writing project. As these capacities are practiced, the child is gradually introduced to using them together in various combinations, thus enriching the imaginative processes and promoting more perceptual registry and greater cognitive processing through multiple sensory modalities. The principles I am applying are very familiar to special educators, as they have been using multisensory interventions for years to assist learning and communication impaired children (Rupley & Blair, 1983).

Expressive Arts Techniques

Many innovative techniques for dealing with trauma-specific issues have been developed in recent years by allied fields collectively referred to as the *expressive arts therapies* (art, dance, music, drama). As pointed out earlier, many profoundly traumatized children have disconnected aspects of their multisensory processing with resulting deficits in a number of areas of perceptual/motor functioning. Some of them have been cruelly admonished never to tell, never to speak of their victimization. Drawing and other forms of nonverbal artwork become a safe channel of expression. Having had their bodies repeatedly invaded and otherwise maltreated and disregarded, many children disconnect their inner experience of bodily sensations (Peterson, Prout, & Schwarz, 1991). They may cease to show spontaneous gestures or movement and become clumsy and uncoordinated. Through movement and dance, they may find a way to regain a relationship with their bodies.

Feelings, as described above, have similarly become distorted, unregulated, disconnected. Children may complain of having no feelings, only sad feelings, of never having known what a particular emotion such as joy or fear felt like. They may display states of such intensity that I refer to them as *purified states*, being 99.9% pure in raw emotional content. When such states are unleashed at school, teachers generally are highly alarmed, perceive the child to be in serious crisis, and expect the therapist to make some form of emergency intervention, perhaps even to hospitalize the child. As too often happens, the child begins to have affective storms of increasing frequency, intensity, and variability. Before long the school is holding an emergency screening for a more restrictive level of special education placement. Too often staff insist that the child be promptly removed from school, believing that they cannot maintain adequate safety for the child, other students, and often staff.

As the child is almost always doing poorly at home, an inpatient stay tends to be the initial outcome, followed by the child being placed on Home Teaching while the long term appropriate school placement is sought. It is not uncommon for the child to be cut off from the school's moderating effects for 6 months, often longer. While confined to the home environment s/he may be exposed to ongoing traumatization. Overwhelmed caregivers, frequently single and working to maintain a minimal standard of living, must provide supervision for an uncontrollable child, one an entire school felt powerless to manage. Caregivers may be forced to quit their jobs and even go on public assistance, as well as to be placed in greater proximity to their child where risk of further abuse is potentiated.

To avoid this unfortunate cycle, expressive arts therapies may provide a temporary holding environment for intense affects, so they do not accelerate in this way. I have found that educators are most receptive to techniques associated with expressive arts therapies. Almost every school curriculum includes instruction in art; also in music and physical development, where movement, exercise, and dance are often featured. The teaching of self-awareness and sensitivity to others is a major educational objective and is introduced in preschool programs. Through a creative integration of academic objectives, expressive arts techniques, and trauma-specific therapeutic strategies, the clinician may prevent the behavioral disintegration and eventual expulsion of the child. Regardless of the child's grade level, some portion of the child's course curriculum is dedicated to self-expression. In the early primary grades teachers can help their students learn the names of emotions, what they feel like, look like, sound like, and what they inspire in others.

Case example: Tory

I worked with a 2nd-grade teacher who sought help in dealing with a student named Tory, who screamed at full volume when asked to clean out his desk or put away items after completion of an activity. When Tory is teased by his classmates, the teacher describes how he may charge them, hurl nearby objects at them, or withdraw into an impenetrable shell. At other times he is described as silly and giggly, an irritating class clown. Then there are times when Tory is a tormenter, a trickster, bedeviling other students and the teacher with pranks, practical jokes, and sudden scares. Tory's history is well known to the school. His parents were cocaine addicts and dealers, the father killed in an attempted robbery and the mother imprisoned for 20 years after killing a boyfriend in a domestic dispute. Tory lives with a great-aunt who is single, harsh, and preoccupied with her own complicated family circumstances. Tory's three younger siblings had been placed for adoption. The great-aunt had informed the school that Tory had been severely neglected, had retained scars from repeated physical abuse, and had required treatment for gonorrhea when placed with her at the age of 5 years. She did not know any specific information, foster care never having volunteered it and she never having asked for it. Tory was sporadically seen at a nearby community mental health clinic. The great-aunt found it extremely inconvenient to bring him on a regular basis, disapproved of the use of medication to control his attentional and disruptive behaviors, and felt he had received no benefit from therapy.

With the great-aunt's permission, obtained by the guidance counselor, I interviewed Tory and watched him in the classroom. I observed the above mentioned mood/behavioral states. Indeed, the great-aunt was well aware of them herself. Fortunately the school had a self-contained special education class for severely emotionally disturbed children of his age range. It was, therefore, possible to make a rapid in-house transfer to that class.

His special education teacher was very receptive to my recommendation to work with Tory proactively on his feeling states. Through art work, he was encouraged to draw himself feeling *loud,* feeling *mean and angry,* feeling *silly and giggly,* feeling *tricky.* She kept his drawings, paintings, and finger paintings in a special folder that she entitled "Tory's Special Feelings Folder." Gradually his teacher had him develop stories that captured the essence of the identities represented by these mental sets. The teacher inquired about the color each might like, activities, interests, music, and so on. By use of the pegboard, he mapped out each morning upon arrival how much he felt of each state, thereby having a visual representation of what affective states were with him as he began his day. In addition the repetitive focusing of his attention on the collection of states that represented his inner experience was a constant reminder that he was one boy with a collection of many strongly felt self states.

Amongst our goals were the reduction in intensity of the above affective states; developing improved strategies of behaving in social settings that previously triggered his maladaptive actions; tension and frustration reduction; and improvement in his academic functioning. Most of his goals were, in fact, quite similar to those of other students in his classroom. A number of group activities were developed that had positive effects on his entire class. One activity involved the children painting angry, sinister, villainous faces on empty plastic throwaway containers. Children were free to create representatives of bad people, bad feelings, bad thoughts. When the containers were completed, the children each took turns with a plastic bowling ball "bowling for bad guys" (see Chapter 8). This activity was utilized frequently throughout the week, particularly if Tory or another child was struggling with a lot of anger.

A relaxation box containing a number of items for quiet fidgeting during periods of inactivity or during rest time enabled children to contain themselves during boring, nonstimulating circumstances. "Fidget-widgets" of many sorts were collected and tried out with the children. The teacher discovered she could keep the children well-behaved during assemblies or while waiting in line during a transition. The simple technique of providing her students with something to do with their hands enabled the children to participate in a number of activities heretofore inaccessible to them.

The teacher heavily emphasized social skills building, self-esteem training, and other cognitive/behaviors techniques such as a complex behavioral reward system. Such strategies and techniques are very helpful to traumatized children in that they provide structured, well-organized coursework using multisensory modalities, much individualized assistance, small group activities, a lot of audiovisual assistance, immediate feedback, and a system of rewards and consequences that provide considerable order and predictability to those whose inner life is often in chaos. Through the blending of the teacher's techniques and those of the expressive arts therapies, traumatized children can learn songs that build confidence, games that teach how to communicate with other children, lessons in morality, and stories that teach moral lessons, offer inspiration, and build character.

Storytelling is worth some additional comment. Children are particularly receptive to influence when told stories that captivate and enthrall them. In fact, it is well-known in the field of clinical hypnosis that children are highly suggestible and readily enter therapeutic trance when their attention is focused on a story (Olness & Gardner, 1988). Many books, educational tapes, and manuals have been developed to effect therapeutic change through the introduction of a story. Some particularly useful publications describe how to create stories or provide a series of stories that are effective for a number of traumatic circumstances (Davis, 1988). One delightful story, *Ignatius Finds Help* (Galvin, 1988), was provided to the teacher; she read it to Tory and it had a powerful impact on Tory's belligerent, challenging tendencies. During that time period the teacher was also doing a section in multicultural awareness. She was teaching the children about Japan and their customs of outward equanimity, politeness, and suppression of affective displays. She also told stories of the Samurai warriors and their complex traditions. Tory was fascinated by their control and tolerance of frustration. His teacher used his interest to develop a number of projects requiring additional study of the legendary Samurai to broaden Tory's capacities for anger management. His great aunt also made arrangements for him to participate in a karate class after school. He was similarly impressed with stories of the stoical American Indian and the quiet courage and patience of the African Pygmy.

Periodically Tory would revive his annoying penchant for pranks. After exploring with him a suitable label for this part, "Trickster," the teacher made a therapeutic connection by highlighting Trickster's sense of humor. She found a book of silly jokes and began telling them to him as a reward for abstaining from practical jokes during the school day. He decided to write the jokes in his own notebook, entitled "Trickster's Book of Jokes." Throughout the year he and the teacher added to it and he got much pleasure from entertaining the other children with a newly obtained ridiculous joke.

The first major crisis occurred when Tory was introduced to subtraction involving three number sets. Whenever he came to a problem that was too hard, he would begin to yell and scream, much as he had in his previous class. The teacher's assistant, also very active in his educational program, worked with him to clarify through drawings and story telling what he was experiencing. He drew a little boy who was three years old and named "Tweee" (Tory was too hard to pronounce) who had been screamed at and beaten repeatedly for not putting his toys away and particularly for not tying his shoes. No matter how hard he tried, he could not learn the skill. He recalled his mother's counting. Sometimes she got to 10; sometimes she kept counting for a long, long time. Eventually she would spank him brutally. His assistant teacher introduced a calculator to help him with subtraction and he soon got beyond his terror of numbers.

At another time a new area of social skills building was introduced to help the children address the many losses that were a natural part of living their lives. The school librarian had become interested in the subject of bereavement during the protracted illness of her husband as he succumbed to cancer. She purchased for the library a number of instructional resources including a curriculum for teaching children of various developmental ages how to deal with loss, including the death of a loved one (O'Toole, 1989). Over time Tory was able to develop better ways to handle disappointments and, in time, through individual work with the assistant teacher, to address the loss of his father and siblings.

The end of the academic year posed another set of concerns. Tory had been maintained at school through the interventions of his teachers with my provision of periodic consultation. Throughout the summer he would be without educational support, and his great-aunt was even more adamant that she did not want to reapply to the community mental health clinic. Fortunately another mental health program had been introduced that spring, providing school and home interventions. The services in the home were short-term in scope and lasted approximately 12 weeks. He was seen at home during the summer and his counselor was fully apprised of the many helpful therapeutic techniques used at school that would be carried on over the summer. The counselor was able to develop a strong tie to Tory and it was possible to enlist her help during the next academic year as she came to the school itself to provide therapeutic services. She focused on the coordination of Tory's various mental states into a team effort within himself. Since Tory was in a potentially explosive home situation, given the great-aunt's age, limited resources, and own family problems, his counselor did not delve into his traumatic history. Rather, she used many metaphors around teamwork, units within a larger organization, or parts of a machine working together, to illustrate the necessity of Tory's many sides to work in harmony. Although she did not achieve anything approaching a treatment cure, she was able in close collaboration with his teachers and me to assist Tory in much better academic and social functioning as well as to make an acceptable adjustment to his great-aunt's household. His achievement scores were almost at age level by the end of the following school year.

The techniques and strategies described above are imminently applicable to other age groups and clinical settings with appropriate developmental adjustments. Certainly the treatment interventions discussed here are suboptimal, since direct work with traumatic memories is avoided. Pathological dissociation has not been interrupted, although it does appear that Tory resorted to it less often as he learned to develop many adaptive resources within the educational environment. We also anticipate that serious problems will crop up in the future. He will have to be switched to another SED program for older aged primary school children when he reaches 9 or 10. Special educators of older children may be less comfortable with some of the techniques that draw on the play activities of young children. However, story writing and telling, drawing, and use of computer-based methods are adaptable for any age student. Given Tory's history of sexual abuse, we also speculate that sexual acting out or some problem associated with sexual dysfunction will manifest itself. Prior to Tory's actually developing overt symptoms, it would be wise for his teachers and counselors to institute a carefully thought-out plan for sex education, in the hope that therapeutic work can abort one of the most worrisome consequences, namely, sexual perpetration and involvement with the juvenile justice system. Tory is also at great risk for drug addiction and criminal behavior (Peterson, Prout, & Schwarz, 1991). Here also coordinated work amongst educators and mental health counselors might diminish, perhaps even interrupt, such tendencies.

Summary

The school is an under-used resource in treatment planning for traumatized children. Given the national and state objectives to assist school aged mentally disturbed children, as well as to provide climates for greater acceptance of diversity and alternative approaches to lifestyle and family perspectives, therapists should actively establish themselves as consultants and providers of treatment and crisis intervention directly within the schools. I have offered a conceptual framework and a number of treatment interventions, techniques, and game plans that can be adapted to the child's most consistent setting during his or her development, the school. Regardless of whether the class is in a public or private school, inpatient unit or residential treatment center, innovative interventions can be applied directly within the school environment, even when ongoing abuse is suspected and when outside therapeutic resources are not available.

Reference List

American Psychiatric Association. (1994). *Diagnostic and statistical manual of mental disorders* (4th ed.). Washington, DC: Author.

Davis, N. *Once upon a time . . . Therapeutic stories* (rev. ed.). (1988). Oxon Hill, MD: Psychological Associates.

Donovan, D., & McIntyre, D. (1990). *Healing the hurt child: A developmental-contextual approach.* New York: Norton.

Galvin, M. (1988). *Ignatius finds help, a story about psychotherapy for children.* New York: Imagination Press.

Koss-Chioino, J. D., & Vargas, L. A. (1992). Through the cultural looking glass: A model for understanding culturally responsive psychotherapies. In L. A. Vargas & J. D. Koss-Chioino (Eds.), *Working with culture, psychotherapeutic interventions with ethnic minority children and adolescents.* San Francisco: Jossey-Bass.

Maryland Disability Law Center. (1994). *Special education rights . . . and wrongs, an MDLC handbook* (3rd ed.). Baltimore: Maryland Disability Law Center.

Maryland Governor's Office for Children, Youth and Families. (1995, February). *Comprehensive school health readiness initiative (CSHRI) concept paper.* Baltimore: Author.

Mills, J. C., & Crowley, R. J. (1986). *Therapeutic metaphors for children and the child within.* New York: Brunner/Mazel.

Olness, K., & Gardner, G. G. (1988). *Hypnosis and hypnotherapy with children* (2nd ed.). Philadelphia: Grune and Stratton.

O'Toole, D. (1989). *Growing through grief, a kindergarten-12 curriculum to help young people through all kinds of loss.* Burnsville, NC: Rainbow Connection.

Peterson, K. C., Prout, M. F., & Schwarz, R. A. (1991). *Post-traumatic stress disorder, a clinician's guide.* New York: Plenum Press.

Rupley, W. H., & Blair, T. R. (1983). *Reading diagnosis and remediation: Classroom and clinic.* Boston: Houghton-Mifflin.

Vargas, L. A., & Koss-Chioino, J. E. (Eds.). (1992). *Working with culture, psychotherapeutic interventions with ethnic minority children and adolescents.* San Francisco: Jossey-Bass.

Appendix A:
Assessment Instruments

The Dissociative Features Profile
by Joyanna L. Silberg, Ph.D.

This measure was developed to help uncover dissociative pathology in children and adolescents. Research is continuing but initial results suggest that this measure can select 93% of a dissociative target group.

This measure was developed to be used with a typical psychologcial testing battery which might include the Rorschach, the TAT, Drawings, Sentence Completion, and a Wechsler IQ Test. The DFP may be used if at least two measures were administered.

The DFP consists of two parts—Part I (Behaviors) and Part II (Markers). The Behaviors section picks up unusual behaviors or presentations of the patient during the testing. Part II (Markers) describes actual test responses.

To order a set of 5 preliminary DFP forms and the scoring manual, send $10.00 to:

> The Sidran Foundation
> 2328 West Joppa Road
> Suite 15
> Lutherville, Maryland 21093
> Phone: 410-825-8888
> Fax: 410-337-0747

The Imaginary Friends Questionnaire

The Imaginary Friends Questionnaire can be used to help make the differentiation between normal imaginary friend phenomena and more pathological dissociative projections. Preliminary research suggests that item numbers 1, 3, 4, 5, 7, and 10 are more characteristic of children with DDNOS (dissociative disorder not otherwise specified) and DID (dissociative identity disorder). The remaining items are commonly acknowledged as "true" by normal children with imaginary friends. Research that further assesses the differences between normal and pathological imaginary friends is being conducted by Jenny Frost and Dr. Jeanie McIntee in England and by Dr. Joyanna L. Silberg.

The Adolescent Dissociative Experiences Scale

This instrument is in a preliminary stage of validation. Initial results show that a score of 4.8 is the mean for dissociative adolescents with a standard deviation of 1.1. The authors suggest a score above 3.7 would warrant further evaluation for a dissociative disorder diagnosis.

Child Dissociative Checklist

This instrument is designed to be used as a clinical screening tool for the identification of potential dissociative pathology in children. In the initial validation sample, DDNOS youngsters had a mean score of 16.8 with a SD of 4.7 and MPD (DID) youngsters had a mean score of 24.5 with a SD of 5.2. The mean score of the normal controls was 2.3 (SD of 2.7). Ninety-six percent of the dissociative sample scored 12 or higher, and this score may be considered a cut-off above which a dissociative disorder should be suspected.

Putnam, F. W., Helmers, K., & Trickett, P. K. (1993) Development, reliability, and validity of a child dissociation scale. *Child Abuse & Neglect, 17,* 731–741.

IMAGINARY FRIENDS QUESTIONNAIRE

1. My imaginary friend(s) is more than just a pretend friend.
   T   F

2. My imaginary friend(s) gives good advice.
   T   F

3. I have more than one imaginary friend and they disagree.
   T   F

4. My imaginary friend bugs me and I wish it would go away.
   T   F

5. My imaginary friend(s) takes over and makes me do things I don't want to do.
   T   F

6. My imaginary friend(s) tells me to keep secrets.
   T   F

7. My imaginary friend(s) tries to boss me.
   T   F

8. My imaginary friend(s) has knowledge about my life that I don't have.
   T   F

9. My imaginary friend(s) has skills or abilities that I don't have.
   T   F

10. My imaginary friend(s) does not like others to know about him/her.
    T   F

11. My imaginary friend plays with me when I am lonely.
    T   F

12. I wish everyone could see my imaginary friend(s) like I do.
    T   F

13. My imaginary friend helps me when I am afraid.
    T   F

Joyanna L. Silberg, Ph.D.
Sheppard and Enoch Pratt Health System

A-DES (version 1.0)
Judith Armstrong, Ph.D.; Frank Putnam, M.D.; Eve Carlson, Ph.D.

Directions
These questions ask about different kinds of experiences that happen to people. For each question, circle the number that tells how much that experience happens to you. Circle a "0" if it never happens to you, circle a "10" if it is always happening to you. If it happens sometimes but not all of the time, circle a number between 1 and 9 that best describes how often it happens to you. When you answer, only tell how much these things happen when you *HAVE NOT* had any alcohol or drugs.

EXAMPLE:

0	1	2	3	4	5	6	7	8	9	10
(never)										(always)

ID _____ Age _____ Grade _____ Sex _____ Date _____

1. I get so wrapped up in watching TV, reading, or playing video games that I don't have any idea what's going on around me.

0	1	2	3	4	5	6	7	8	9	10
(never)										(always)

2. I get back tests or homework that I don't remember doing.

0	1	2	3	4	5	6	7	8	9	10
(never)										(always)

3. I have strong feelings that don't seem like they are mine.

0	1	2	3	4	5	6	7	8	9	10
(never)										(always)

4. I can do something really well one time and then I can't do it at all another time.

0	1	2	3	4	5	6	7	8	9	10
(never)										(always)

5. People tell me I do or say things that I don't remember doing or saying.

0	1	2	3	4	5	6	7	8	9	10
(never)										(always)

6. I feel like I'm in a fog or spaced out and things around me seem unreal.

| 0 | 1 | 2 | 3 | 4 | 5 | 6 | 7 | 8 | 9 | 10 |

(never)   (always)

7. I get confused about whether I have done something or only thought about doing it.

| 0 | 1 | 2 | 3 | 4 | 5 | 6 | 7 | 8 | 9 | 10 |

(never) (always)

8. I look at the clock and realize that time has gone by and I can't remember what has happened.

| 0 | 1 | 2 | 3 | 4 | 5 | 6 | 7 | 8 | 9 | 10 |

(never) (always)

9. I hear voices in my head that are not mine.

| 0 | 1 | 2 | 3 | 4 | 5 | 6 | 7 | 8 | 9 | 10 |

(never) (always)

10. When I am somewhere that I don't want to be, I can go away in my mind.

| 0 | 1 | 2 | 3 | 4 | 5 | 6 | 7 | 8 | 9 | 10 |

(never) (always)

11. I am so good at lying and acting that I believe it myself.

| 0 | 1 | 2 | 3 | 4 | 5 | 6 | 7 | 8 | 9 | 10 |

(never) (always)

12. I catch myself "waking up" in the middle of doing something.

| 0 | 1 | 2 | 3 | 4 | 5 | 6 | 7 | 8 | 9 | 10 |

(never) (always)

13. I don't recognize myself in the mirror.

| 0 | 1 | 2 | 3 | 4 | 5 | 6 | 7 | 8 | 9 | 10 |

(never) (always)

14. I find myself going somewhere or doing something and I don't know why.

| 0 | 1 | 2 | 3 | 4 | 5 | 6 | 7 | 8 | 9 | 10 |

(never) (always)

15. I find myself someplace and don't remember how I got there.

0	1	2	3	4	5	6	7	8	9	10
(never)										(always)

16. I have thoughts that don't really seem to belong to me.

0	1	2	3	4	5	6	7	8	9	10
(never)										(always)

17. I find that I can make physical pain go away.

0	1	2	3	4	5	6	7	8	9	10
(never)										(always)

18. I can't figure out if things really happened or if I only dreamed or thought about them.

0	1	2	3	4	5	6	7	8	9	10
(never)										(always)

19. I find myself doing something that I know is wrong, even when I really don't want to do it.

0	1	2	3	4	5	6	7	8	9	10
(never)										(always)

20. People tell me that I sometimes act so differently that I seem like a different person.

0	1	2	3	4	5	6	7	8	9	10
(never)										(always)

21. It feels like there are walls inside of my mind.

0	1	2	3	4	5	6	7	8	9	10
(never)										(always)

22. I find writings, drawings or letters that I must have done but I can't remember doing.

0	1	2	3	4	5	6	7	8	9	10
(never)										(always)

23. Something inside of me seems to make me do things that I don't want to do.

0	1	2	3	4	5	6	7	8	9	10
(never)										(always)

24. I find that I can't tell whether I am just remembering something or if it is actually happening to me.

   0   1   2   3   4   5   6   7   8   9   10
(never)   (always)

25. I find myself standing outside of my body, watching myself as if I were another person.

   0   1   2   3   4   5   6   7   8   9   10
(never)   (always)

26. My relationships with my family and friends change suddenly and I don't know why.

   0   1   2   3   4   5   6   7   8   9   10
(never)   (always)

27. I feel like my past is a puzzle and some of the pieces are missing.

   0   1   2   3   4   5   6   7   8   9   10
(never)   (always)

28. I get so wrapped up in my toys or stuffed animals that they seem alive.

   0   1   2   3   4   5   6   7   8   9   10
(never)   (always)

29. I feel like there are different people inside of me.

   0   1   2   3   4   5   6   7   8   9   10
(never)   (always)

30. My body feels as if it doesn't belong to me.

   0   1   2   3   4   5   6   7   8   9   10
(never)   (always)

Child Dissociative Checklist (V 3.0—2/90)
Frank Putnam, M.D.
Unit on Dissociative Disorders, LDP, NIMH

Date _____ Age ____ Sex M F Identification _____

Below is a list of behaviors that describe children. For each item that describes your child NOW or WITHIN THE PAST 12 MONTHS, please circle 2 if the item is VERY TRUE of your child. Circle 1 if the item is
SOMEWHAT or SOMETIMES TRUE of your child. If the item is NOT
TRUE of your child, circle 0.

0 1 2   1. Child does not remember or denies traumatic or painful experiences that are known to have occured.

0 1 2   2. Child goes into a daze or trance-like state at times or often
appears "spaced-out." Teachers may report that he or she 'day-
dreams' frequently in school.

0 1 2   3. Child shows rapid changes in personality. He or she may go
from being shy to being outgoing, from feminine to masculine,
from timid to aggressive.

0 1 2   4. Child is unusually forgetful or confused about things that
he or she should know, e.g. may forget the names of friends,
teachers or other important people, loses possessions or gets
lost easily.

0 1 2   5. Child has a very poor sense of time. He or she loses track of
time, may think that it is morning when it is actually afternoon, gets confuses about what day it is, or becomes confused
about when something happened.

0 1 2   6. Child shows marked day-to-day or even hour-to-hour variations in his or her skills, knowledge, food preferences, athletic
abilities, e.g. changes in handwriting, memory for previously
learned information such as multiplication tables, spelling, use
of tools or artistic ability.

0 1 2   7. Child shows rapid regressions in age-level of behavior, e.g.
a twelve-year-old starts to use baby-talk, sucks thumb or
draws like a four year-old.

0 1 2   8. Child has a difficult time learning from experience, e.g. explanations, normal discipline or punishment do not change his or her behavior.

0 1 2   9. Child continues to lie or deny misbehavior even when the evidence is obvious.

0 1 2   10. Child refers to him or herself in the third person (e.g. as she or her) when talking about self, or at times insists on being called by a different name. He or she may also claim that things that he or she did actually happened to another person.

0 1 2   11. Child has rapidly changing physical complaints such as headache or upset stomach. For example, he or she may complain of a headache one minute and seem to forget all about it the next.

0 1 2   12. Child is unusually sexually precocious and may attempt age-inappropriate sexual behavior with other children or adults.

0 1 2   13. Child suffers from unexplained injuries or may even deliberately injure self at times.

0 1 2   14. Child reports hearing voices that talk to him or her. The voices may be friendly or angry and may come from 'imaginary companions' or sound like the voices of parents, friends or teachers.

0 1 2   15. Child has a vivid imaginary companion or companions. Child may insist that the imaginary companion(s) is responsible for things that he or she has done.

0 1 2   16. Child has intense outbursts of anger, often without apparent cause and may display unusual physical strength during these episodes.

0 1 2   17. Child sleepwalks frequently.

0 1 2   18. Child has unusual nighttime experiences, e.g. may report seeing "ghosts" or that things happen at night that he or she can't account for (e.g. broken toys, unexplained injuries).

0 1 2   19. Child frequently talks to him or herself, may use a different voice or argue with self at times.

0 1 2   20. Child has two or more distinct and separate personalities that take control over the child's behavior.

Appendix B:
Reading Lists

Books about Abuse and Disclosure for Parents

Adams, C., & Fay, J. (1992). *Helping your child recover from sexual abuse.* Seattle: University of Washington Press.

Hagans, K. B., & Case, J. *When your child has been molested.* (1988). New York: Lexington.

Hillman, D., & Solek-Tefft, J. (1988). Spiders and flies: Help for parents and teachers of sexually abused children. New York: Lexington Books.

Matsakis, A. (1991). When the bough breaks: A helping guide for parents of sexually abused children. Oakland, CA: New Harbinger.

Monahon, C. (1992). *Children and trauma.* New York: Lexington.

Books about Abuse and Disclosure for Teens

Alexander, D. W. (1992). *Something bad happened.* (Series of 6 books.) Huntington, NY: Bureau for At-Risk Youth.

Aliki, (1984). *Feelings.* New York: Mulberry.

Gil, E., & Bodmer-Turner, J. (1994). *Someone in my family has molested children.* Rockville, MD: Launch Press.

Jessie. (1991). *Please tell!* Center City, MN: Hazelden Foundation.

Johnsen, K. (1986) *The trouble with secrets.* Seattle, WA: Parenting Press, Inc.

Porett, J. (1994). *When I was little like you.* Washington, DC: Child Welfare League of America.

Books about Abuse and Disclosure for Parents to Read with Children

Alexander, D. W. (1992). *The way I feel* (Set of 6 books.) Huntington, NY: Bureau for At-Risk Youth.

Bean, B., & Bennett, S. (1993). *The me nobody knows.* New York: Lexington.

Boat, Barbara W., & Peterson, Gary. (1991). *MPD explained for kids.* Lutherville, MD: Sidran Press.

Polese, C. (1985). *Promise not to tell.* New York: Beech Tree.

Gil, E. (1983). *Outgrowing the pain: A book for and about adults abused as children.* Rockville, MD: Launch Press.

Gil, E. (1990). *United we stand.* Walnut Creek, CA: Launch Press.

Sessions, Deborah. (1994). *My mom is different.* Lutherville, MD: Sidran Press.

Seuss, Dr. (1982). *Hunches in bunches.* New York: Random House.

Fairy Tales

The following fairy tales may be used with traumatized children:

Hansel and Gretel, to illustrate anger and lying as a response to fear and abuse.
Rapunzel, to illustrate intergenerational aspects of abuse.
Beauty and the Beast (the story, not the movie) with the Beast as an alter.

Books about Abuse and Disclosure for Therapists

Amatea, E. S. (1989). *Brief strategic intervention for school behavior problems.* San Francisco: Jossey-Bass.

Briere, J. N. (1992). *Child abuse trauma, theory and treatment of the lasting effects.* Newbury, CA: Sage.

Cohen, J. J., & Fish, M. C. (1993). *Handbook of school-based interventions, resolving student problems and promoting healthy educational environments.* San Francisco: Jossey-Bass.

Ehly, S., & Dustin, R. (1989). *Individual and group counseling in schools.* San Francisco: Jossey-Bass, 1989.

Elias, M. J., & clabby, J. F. (1992). *Building social problem-solving skills, guidelines from a school-based program.* San Francisco: Josesy-Bass.

Forman, S. G. (1993). *Coping skills interventions for children and adolescents.* san Francisco: Jossey-Bass.

Furrer, P. J. (1982). *Art therapy activities and lesson plans for individuals and groups, a practical guide for teachers, therapists, parents and those interested in promoting personal growth in themselves and others.* Springfield, IL: Charles C. Thomas.

Gil, E. (1996). *Treating abused adolescents.* New York: Guilford.

Gil, E., & Cavanagh Johnson, T. (1993). *Sexualized children: Assessment and treatment of sexualized children and children who molest.* Rockville, MD: Launch Press.

James, B. (1989). *Treating traumatized children: New insights and creative innovations.* Lexington, MA: Lexington Books.

Kluft, R. P. (Ed.) (1985). *Childhood antecedents of multiple personality.* Washington, DC: American Psychiatric Press.

Kluft, R. P., & Fine, C. F. (Eds.). (1993). *Clinical perspectives on multiple personality disorder.* Washington, DC: American Psychiatric Press.

O'Callaghan, J. B. (1993). *School-based collaboration with families, constructing family-school-agency partnerships that work.* San Francisco: Jossey-Bass.

Putnam, F. W. (1989). *Diagnosis and treatment of multiple personality disorder.* New York: Guilford Press.

Sue, D. W., & Sue, D. (1990). Counseling the culturally different, theory and practice (2nd ed.). New York: John Wiley.

Wiglesworth, M. F. (1990). *Willie and his friends, a manual for creating stories to build a child's self-esteem.* Cynthiana, KY: Potentials.

Young, S. B., & Keplinger, L. (1988). *Movement is fun, a preschool movement program.* Torrance, CA: Sensory Integration International.

Zins, J. E., Curtis, M. F., Graden, J. S., & Ponti, C. R. (1993). *Helping children succeed in the regular classroom.* San Francisco: Jossey-Bass (1993).

Zins, J. E., Kratochwill, T. R., & Elliott, S. N. (Eds.). (1993). *Handbook of consultation services for children, applications in educational and clinical settings.* San Francisco: Jossey-Bass.